P9-CFA-930

CRITICAL ISSUES
IN CONTEMPORARY
HEALTH CARE

CONTRIBUTORS TO THIS VOLUME

Joseph Boyle, Ph.D.
Professor of Philosophy
St. Michael's College
University of Toronto
Toronto, Ontario, Canada

The Reverend Philip J. Boyle, O.P.
Associate Director, Center for Health
Care Ethics
St. Louis University Medical Center
St. Louis, Missouri

The Reverend David E. Brinkmoeller, M.A.
Executive Director of the Secretariat
for Priestly Life and Ministry
N.C.C.B.
Washington, DC

The Reverend Monsignor James P. Cassidy, Ph.D.
Chancellor, New York Medical
College
Valhalla, New York

Christopher M. DeGiorgio, M.D.
Assistant Professor of Neurology
USC School of Medicine
Los Angeles, California

The Reverend Joseph P. Gillespie, O.P., D.Min.
Visiting Professor of Pastoral Care
and Counseling
Eden Theological Seminary/Aquinas
Institute of Theology
St. Louis, Missouri

The Reverend Benedict J. Groeschel, C.F.R., Ph.D.
Trinity Retreat House
Larchmont, New York

Sister Margaret John Kelly, D.C.
Provincial Superior,
Northeast Province of the Daughters
of Charity of St. Vincent DePaul
Depaul Provincial House
Albany, New York

Mrs. Rita Marker
The Human Life Center
University of Steubenville
Steubenville, Ohio

The Reverend Gerald R. Niklas, M.Div.
Director of Pastoral Care
Good Samaritan Hospital
Cincinnati, OH 45220

The Reverend Kevin O'Rourke, O.P., Ph.D., S.T.M.
Director, Center of Health Care
Ethics
St. Louis University School of
Medicine
St. Louis, Missouri

Fred Plum, M.D.
Anne Parrish Titzell Professor of
Neurology
Cornell University Medical
Center
Neurologist-in-Chief
The New York Hospital

D. Alan Shewmon, M.D.
Assistant Professor of Pediatrics
and Neurology
UCLA Medical Center
Los Angeles, California

John R. Silber, Ph.D.
President
Boston University
Boston, Massachusetts

Janet E. Smith, Ph.D.
Assistant Professor, Liberal Arts
University of Notre Dame
South Bend, Indiana

CRITICAL ISSUES IN CONTEMPORARY HEALTH CARE

Proceedings of
The Eighth Bishops' Workshop
Dallas, Texas

Russell E. Smith
Editor

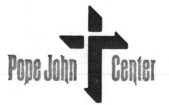

Pope John Center

Nihil Obstat: Reverend James A. O'Donohoe, J.C.D.

Imprimatur: Bernard Cardinal Law   Date: October 19, 1989

The Nihil Obstat and Imprimatur are a declaration that a book or pamphlet is considered to be free from doctrinal or moral error. It is not implied that those who have granted the Nihil Obstat and Imprimatur agree with the contents, opinions or statements expressed.

Copyright 1989
by
The Pope John XXIII Medical-Moral
Research and Education Center
Braintree, Massachusetts 02184

Library of Congress Cataloging-in-Publication Data

Workshop for Bishops of the United States and Canada (8th : 1989 : Dallas, Tex.)
    Critical issues in contemporary health care : proceedings of the Eighth Bishops' Workshop, Dallas, Texas / Russell E. Smith, editor.
        p. 356   cm.
    Proceedings of the Bishops' Workshop, January 30–February 3, 1989, Dallas, Texas.
    Includes bibliographical references.
    ISBN 0–935372–27–X : $17.95
    1. Health—Religious aspects—Catholic Church—Congresses. 2. Medical care—North America—Congresses. 3. Public health—North American—Congresses. 4. Medical ethics—Congresses. 5. Christian ethics—Catholic authors—Congresses. 6. Catholic Church—Doctrines—Congresses. I. Smith, Russell E. (Russell Edward) II. Title.
BX1795.H4W67   1989
241'.642—dc20   89–22935
                                                          CIP

Printed in the United States of America. All rights reserved. This book, or any part thereof, may not be reproduced without the written permission of the publisher.

W
50
W926c
1989

Contents

3 0001 00206 5003

2031993 9

The Pope John Center presented its eighth workshop in Dallas, Texas from January 30 to February 3, 1989. In attendance were bishops from the Caribbean, Canada, Central America, the United States, Mexico and the Philippines. This week of study, prayer and reflection for the bishops was made possible once again by a generous grant from the Knights of Columbus.

During each of the Bishops' Workshops, the Center has attempted to provide information, analysis and theological reflection upon timely issues in bioethics and moral theology. The papers delivered at each of these gatherings have been collected and published as a volume of Proceedings. Several of these workshops have focussed on human sexuality and personhood: *Human Sexuality and Personhood* (1981), *Technological Powers and the Person* (1983) and *Reproductive Technologies, Marriage and the Church*

(1988). This latter symposium was a detailed examination of the then recently published *Instruction on Respect for Human Life in its Origin and on the Dignity of Procreation (Donum vitæ)* from the Congregation for the Doctrine of the Faith.

Other Workshops dealt with specific topics of pastoral concern in the field of moral theology: *New Technologies of Birth and Death* (1980), *Moral Theology Today: Certitudes and Doubts* (1984), *The Family Today and Tomorrow: The Church Addresses Her Future* (1985) and *Scarce Medical Resources and Justice* (1987). The content of the workshops has been both theoretical and pastorally applicable. The faculties for these gatherings have been composed of scholars renowned in their respective fields.

The general theme of this eighth workshop was *Critical Issues in Contemporary Health Care.* Into this one thematic pavilion were gathered several diverse topics treated by over a dozen highly articulate scholars who comprised the faculty. A personal message to the bishops from our Holy Father opens this volume, with greetings from the Knights of Columbus, the opening homily on health care and the keynote address. The first part of workshop dealt with the medical, moral, political and pastoral aspects of the artificial provision of nutrition and hydration. The second part dealt with the interrelationship between health care facilities, their institutional ethics committees and the local bishop; the question of the constitutive elements of Catholic identity in health care delivery, especially in light of corporate merger with non-Catholic institutions; and the role of pastoral care personnel in Catholic health facilities.

The third part of the workshop dealt with the recently much publicized interest in fetal research, the desirability of fetal tissue and its medical promise, the medical anomaly of anencephaly, and the encumbent moral issues. The health of the clergy comprised the fourth segment of the presentations, dealing with such issues as health and well-being in general and the psychological, moral and legal problems involved in psychic disorders. The finale of the workshop was a panel discussion presented by three bishops who had previously taught in seminaries. Together they examined the issue of a consistent presentation of the moral doctrine of the Church in light of the pluralistic backgrounds of their clergy. *Tolle, lege ... fruere!*

* * *

The late Cardinal-designate Hans Urs von Balthasar wrote a book entitled, *The Truth is Symphonic*. The wisdom of this title applies not just to the divine genius expressed in the Creed, but also to something as mundane as the orchestration of an international gathering such as the Dallas Workshop. Scores of individuals are responsible for the planning, content and hospitable ambience of this event. Specific recognition of any individual or group entails the risk of omission and oversight of others. However, with sincere apologies to anyone who finds himself in this latter group, we believe that gratitude and indebtedness necessitate an attempt to publicly acknowledge a few.

We are once again very grateful to the Supreme Knight, Mr. Virgil C. Dechant, and to the Knights of Columbus for their generous sponsorship of this workshop. Also, heartfelt thanks go to the members of our faculty for their time, concern and cooperation.

Sincere thanks go to the Most Reverend Thomas Tschoepe, Bishop of Dallas, for his gracious hospitality. Thanks also to Father Thomas Cloherty for the liturgical arrangements and to the staff and seminarians of Holy Trinity Seminary, University of Dallas, for their assistance. Thanks also to the local councils of the Knights of Columbus and the Catholic Women's Guilds of the Diocese of Dallas, as well as to Father Rudy Vela and his Spanish language translators from San Antonio and Fort Worth for their generous service, and to Laurie Ungarsohn from New York City for the taping and transcription of the conference. Also, we are grateful to the staff of the Doubletree Hotel at Lincoln Centre for their graciousness and service. A very special word of thanks goes to the Nuns of the Poor Clare Federation of Mary Immaculate who prayed for the success and for the participants of the conference. Last, but certainly not least, a word of profound thanks to Mrs. Jeanne Burke and Mr. Donald Powers for their indefatigable assistance from the conception of this project to its birth.

The Reverend Russell E. Smith, S.T.D.
Editor

Feast of the Portiuncula, 1989
Boston, Massachusetts

GREETINGS

INTRODUCTIONS

KEYNOTE

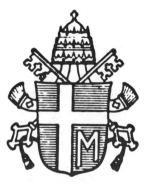

To My Brother Bishops
from North and Central America
The Caribbean and The Philippines

I greet you with great joy in Christ Jesus our Lord as you gather together for study and prayer. You come from dioceses in Canada, the Caribbean, Central America, Mexico, the Philippines and the United States, and thus your ministry as Shepherds and Teachers of the Christian faithful encompasses diverse and widely scattered lands and peoples. This Workshop, organized by the Pope John XXIII Medical-Moral Research and Education Center, will once again offer you the opportunity to reflect on the implications for suffering humanity of the Lord's Paschal Mystery. I wish to thank the Knights of Columbus for their generosity which has made it possible for you to come together in a visible manifestation of your communion with one another and with the Successor of Peter.

The general theme of your Workshop, "Critical Issues in Contemporary Health Care", suggests that the meeting is devoted in part to issues which result from the continual progress being made in the medical arts and from the ever expanding horizon of scientific capability. These issues include an examination of the technological ability and the moral requirements for sustaining life by artificially providing nutrition and hydration, as well as the ethical implications of euthanasia and the so-called "right to die" movement. Other questions which arise from advances in medical technology include the transplantation of organs and tissues from unborn and severely handicapped new-born infants.

Beyond questions of scientific skill lies the deeper aspect of human activity, namely, its moral dimension. No adequate consideration of human endeavor can neglect this essential truth. As indicated in the *Instruction on Respect for Human Life in its Origin and on the Dignity of Procreation,* published by the Congregation for the Doctrine of Faith, "one cannot derive criteria for (moral) guidance from mere technical efficiency... Thus science and technology require, for their own intrinsic meaning, an unconditional respect for the fundamental criteria of the moral law: that is to say, they must be at the service of the human person, of his inalienable rights and his true and integral good according to the design and will of God" (February 22, 1987, No. 2).

The moral character of all human activity is more clearly identified in the light of our Christian faith, which must permeate and animate the corporate identity of all Catholic institutions. This is particularly true of the Catholic hospital. Your study of the Bishop's role with regard to Catholic health facilities and institutional ethics committees will no doubt seek to ensure a more effective corporate witness to the Church's teaching. This witness, essential to Catholic identity, must be safeguarded in any cooperative undertaking between Catholic hospitals and non-Catholic health facilities.

Your study and reflection will also focus on those who provide pastoral care for patients and their families. These pastoral workers are in a unique position to perform both the corporal and spiritual works of mercy, as they bear witness to Christ the healer, who showed compassion for the sick wherever he went (cf. Mk 6:56), and to Christ the sufferer, who by his Passion and Death brings his followers to glory (cf. Heb 2:10).

A particularly significant concern is the health of priests. This Workshop will provide you with an opportunity to reflect on the many dimensions of health as it applies to the physical, psychological and spiritual dimensions of God's ministers. For the priest, as for every Christian, health that is all-embracing is rooted in surrender to God through conversion and prayerful discipleship. Sacramental nourishment—particularly through the Sacraments of Penance and the Eucharist—is also an essential element for spiritual well-being and for holiness, as I pointed out in my *Letter to Priests* for Holy Thursday of 1986.

Finally, you will also consider the importance of the Church's moral teaching in a rapidly changing cultural environment and at a time of intellectual ferment. Fidelity to this teaching in the face of indifference or even hostility constitutes a great service to a world in search of meaning and love. By following Christ along the path of truth, you, as pastors, and all those associated in Catholic health care, bear witness to the grace of God at work in our world.

May the Holy Spirit guide you, dear brothers, in the way of understanding during these days of study, helping you to explain the truths of faith and apply them with prudence and compassion. And may the intercession of the Blessed Virgin Mary, Seat of Wisdom and Comfort of the Sick, assist you in your service to her Divine Son, the Incarnate Word of God. With fraternal affection I gladly impart my Apostolic Blessing.

From the Vatican, January 6, 1989

Joannes Paulus PP. II

GREETING FROM THE KNIGHTS OF COLUMBUS

The Most Reverend Thomas V. Daily
Supreme Chaplain

May it please Your Eminences, Your Excellency the Apostolic Pro-Nuncio, Archbishop Laghi, Your Excellencies, my brother priests, distinguished guests, members of the Knights of Columbus Supreme Council and Staff, members of the Board of Directors and Administration of the Pope John Center, distinguished speakers and presenters, and friends all:

As the Supreme Chaplain of the Knights of Columbus, I feel singularly privileged to be at the podium this evening in order to speak in behalf of the Supreme Knight of the Knights of Columbus, Virgil C. Dechant. Regretfully, the Supreme Knight is unable to be present because of the duties of his office that require him to fulfill a long-standing commitment to Knights of Columbus insurance agents at their annual incentive meeting.

This is the eighth workshop presented by the Pope John Center and enabled through a grant from the Supreme Council of the Knights of Columbus. The topics for presentation and discussion at this Eighth Bishops' Workshop have evoked no little interest.

My brother bishops: One of the best pronouncements, or perhaps better, instructions, given by the Holy Father to the Church in the United States was presented by Pope John Paul II to the bishops of the New York Province on October the 15th, 1988. And while his instructions and his words pertain particularly to Catholic colleges and universities, it seems to me that his words can well be applied to this workshop and, indeed, to the atmosphere and context in which the presentations and discussions are to take place. Let me quote the Holy Father: "Today we are gathered together as pastors, conscious of the words of Jesus to His apostles: 'Go, therefore, and make disciples of all nations ... teaching them to observe

7

all that I have commanded you.' (Mt. 28:19–20). These words must find a constant echo in our minds and hearts. As successors of the twelve, we have as our preeminent duty the proclamation of the Gospel to all people (cf. *Christus Dominus*, No. 12). This is a task that is always necessary, but it is even more urgent wherever there is ignorance, error or indifference to the truth." The Holy Father goes in his instructions to say: "After commanding us to teach, Jesus assures us of His presence and support: 'Behold I am with you always, to the end of the age.'" (Mt. 28:20). May this be the context in which presentations and discussions take place during this Eighth Workshop.

Finally, the position of the Knights of Columbus has been, is now and always will be in total and complete conformity with the teachings of the Church as taught by the Magisterium. Especially where life is concerned, from conception to natural demise, there is no compromise, for while encouraging the debate or even providing the means for the debate, the Knights of Columbus is a Catholic Fraternal Order dedicated to truth and united to the Holy Father and the bishops with the Holy Father, uncompromisingly.

I look forward to an enlightening and productive week. Thank you very much.

CATHOLIC HEALTH CARE:
THE TOUCH OF THE MASTER
Reflections on the Gospel Text,
"Talitha, koum" (Mk 5, 41)

Homily at the Opening Mass
The Most Reverend Diosdado A. Talamayan, Ph.D., S.T.D.
Metropolitan Archbishop of Tuguegarao
Chairman, Episcopal Commission on Health Care
Catholic Episcopal Conference of the Philippines

Your Excellencies, Brothers and Sisters:

"Taking the child's hand he said to her: 'Talitha, koum' which means, 'Little girl, get up.' The girl, a child of twelve, stood up immediately and began to walk around."

It was certainly something that inspired a sense of awe and wonder for Jesus to have raised a little girl who appeared to all to be dead. But there is something in the story of the raising of Jairus' daughter that strikes me even more: it is the distinctiveness of the Master's touch; the compassion and love with which he takes the child's hand and addresses her, but also the authority over sickness and weakness and death with which he raises her up.

There may have been miracle-workers in Jesus' day and there may have been occurrences as wonderful as the raising of Jairus' daughter. These possibilities, however, would in no way diminish the mystery, the distinctiveness and singularity of the episode today's Gospel narrates. It is an elemental theological principle that who Jesus is and what his mission was are what give meaning to his acts, and therefore, there will always be something special, something irreplaceable and wonderful about Jesus' touch, because it is the touch of the Master. It is the touch of the Creator who surveys the work his hands have wrought, and finds it good! It is the touch of God that raised humanity to glory through the incarnation of the

Son! It is the touch of Life Eternal that breaks through the gloom of death and shatters the fetters of the tomb.

We have met to discuss the issue of health care from within the context of the pastoral ministry. These concerns we have then put us in direct contact with man in his frailty and weakness, and it was in its vulnerability that the Son of God took upon himself our nature. At the same time we have to do with the excellence of the human mind and the genius of his spirit, for we address ourselves at the same time to the medical and nursing professions.

The specific charism of a commission on health care can be formulated in many ways, but I suggest, in the light of today's Gospel that we consider its main task that of transforming health care in its varied forms into the touch of the Master. This means such basic things as seeing in the sick, not numbers in a hospital ward, but persons who suffer and who need the soothing hand of the compassionate Lord. This means enhancing a Christian conscience throughout the whole of the medical and nursing professions so that they consider their expertise and skill gifts God has given them to be shared with those who suffer.

But Jesus' voice had authority, the dominion of the Creator over the weakness and frailty of man, over sickness and death, over the despondency of his spirit and the chaotic forces of his life. To transform health care then into the touch of the Master is to make the ministering hands and hearts of surgeons, physicians, nurses, and health-care workers resonate with Jesus' own authority. This means that from lives steeped in the values of the Gospel, in the charity that is at the heart of Christianity, surgeons, physicians, nurses and health-care workers reach out with skill and expertise, yes, but also with tenderness, mercy, compassion and faith. Then they will not only strengthen nerve and tissue; they will raise crushed and bruised spirits and make the world feel that God has indeed touched our world and has made it beautiful beyond belief.

Today, St. John Bosco is remembered by the Universal Church. He understood fully well what the Master's touch is. In one of his letters, we find a passage that bears testimony to the sanctity and nobility of his soul:

"I have always labored lovingly for our foster children and carried out my priestly duties with zeal ... Yes, indeed, it is more fitting to be persistent in punishing our own impatience and pride than to correct the boys. We must be firm but kind, and be patient with them ... Let us regard those boys over whom we have some authority as our sons. Let us place ourselves in their service."

Authorities, but servants, firm but kind, expertise and compassion born of faith—this is the example of St. John Bosco, this is the wonder of the Jairus story, this is what the Master's touch is, this is what health care ought to be.

ETHICS IN THE PRACTICE OF MEDICINE

John R. Silber, Ph.D.

Your eminences and excellencies, members of the Knights of Columbus, and other distinguished guests, I am grateful to the Bishops' Workshop and to Cardinal Law. I deliver this keynote address with some misgivings because I realize the limitations of the perspective that I bring to issues about which each of you has thought deeply and long, and about which there is a great body of Catholic doctrine. I speak not as a Roman Catholic but as a philosopher, and must leave it to you to extend and apply my philosophical reflections by means of your knowledge of Catholic dogma and Catholic experience.

Despite our wealth and power, we live in a society and in a world of severely limited resources. When we decide to invest our resources for one purpose, we decide simultaneously to withhold them from other purposes. When we exhaust our energies in one or more causes, we deny them to other causes. Limits of time, energy, and wealth freight our choices with important ethical implications. And in no area of life are choices more critical than in the area of medical practice.

As I indicated a moment ago, I address the complex issues of medical practice not as a Roman Catholic but only as a philosopher concerned to bring as much light as reason can to this discussion. I believe there is natural law, descriptive in those areas of life subject to scientific understanding, and normative in others. To the extent that reason can guide, I will attempt, in the time available, to delineate that law. Your program director has, by restricting my time, guaranteed the presence of error—not that error wouldn't have been there anyway—since I have time for little more than a sketch of key issues. I shall devote about half of my time to the nature and methods of ethics so that my conclusions, whether sound or in error, are not arbitrary but follow from the methods that I have set forth.

Although making use of the light of reason is not alien to or offensive to Catholic tradition, the Church has other means to arrive at its dogmas and doctrines—means that transcend the limits of reason. Some of my arguments and conclusions diverge from centrally held doctrines and practices of the Church, while others are clearly orthodox. Whatever the merits of my position, I trust that by considering it you may find ways, in some cases, to make the Catholic position more convincing to non-Catholics and even to Catholics. In other cases, I hope can help you understand why there is opposition to the Catholic position even from those who, like myself, hold the Church in the highest esteem and diverge from its teachings only with great reluctance and concern.

The Nature of Ethics

The first and the most important thing we can say about medical ethics—or any so-called "professional ethics"—is that there is no such thing. To speak of the ethics of the medical profession is as misleading as to talk of the physics of civil engineering or the physics of electronics. Most people recognize that there is only one physics, which has different applications in different fields.

Ethics and physics are fundamental disciplines. Seen at the most basic level, they are the application of logic, one logic, to different human purposes. All human effort to think clearly is dependent upon logic, for logic is the science of sound thinking. There is not one logic for scientists, a second for bookmakers, a third for physicians, a fourth for artists, and a fifth for politicians. Those who want to think clearly and rigorously must subordinate themselves to the laws of thought, those canons of rigorous thinking whereby one moves from true assumptions by valid reasoning to true conclusions. All ethical and scientific thinking makes use of and exemplifies logic which applies in all areas in which mankind strives to think clearly.

Ethics is that branch of philosophy devoted to the examination of universal principles of conduct. It is a normative science dealing with the principles and procedures in accordance with which individuals and society should act, just as logic describes the principles and procedures according to which individuals should think. Neither attempts to describe the ways in which individuals and groups actually think or act.

Correctly understood, there is one ethics, one set of principles for the guidance of human conduct. And it is wholly consistent with the objectivity and universality of ethical principles that they are applied differently in a variety of fields. The moral obligations of doctors, soldiers, scientists and other professionals may differ from the moral obligations of farmers, bankers, bureaucrats, bus drivers, chimney sweeps and homemakers, but the ethical principles by which their conduct is guided and judged in these various contexts are the same.

This distinction may be made more clearly in the context of physics. What a faddist might call the physics of field artillery is, correctly understood, no more than the correct application of Newtonian physics to short-range trajectories. The application of Newtonian physics is made easy for artillerymen by the provision of range tables that indicate the proper elevation of the artillery piece for the myriad possible ranges, projectile weights and propellant charges. This situation is not altered by the introduction of computerized weapons. Newton and his laws are alive and well inside the computer. The equations on which the range tables are based are all derived from the law of gravity and the laws of motion, which Newton was the first to formulate accurately. None of these need be modified because they are used by soldiers rather than bridge builders, clergymen, organ grinders, or small boys throwing stones. If you ask a child of ten to throw a one-half pound stone twenty feet and then ask him to throw the same stone forty feet he will, without knowing anything about Newton or physics, put greater force behind his second throw. And if one could accurately measure the force of each of his throws, one could develop a range table for rock-throwing small boys.

What holds for physics holds also for ethics. The currently popular courses and books in "business ethics," "medical ethics," "legal ethics," and the like, are frequently grounded on a fundamental mistake—namely, that there are different ethical principles for doctors, businessmen, ministers, or soldiers. There is one ethical or categorical imperative which must be applied in all walks of life—the responsibility to act according to principle.

It is interesting to note that when we speak at the level of principles we can use "ethics" and "morals" interchangeably, although ethics is the study of principles whereas morals may also refer to practices normative in a given community or group. It may also be of interest to note that there are communities in which it is said that there are neither ethics nor morals. It is frequently said, for example, that Bostonians have no morals, only manners. (Indeed, some say that Bostonians have no manners, only customs.) But if we move beyond the world of professional philosophy, we find that there is general confusion between ethics on the one hand and morals on the other. Non-philosophers tend to use the terms interchangeably. More precisely, however, the term "morals" describes generally the normative practices of communities: what is done and what is not done. Cannibalism, thus considered, can be moral or immoral, depending on the community in which it is practiced. Any student of comparative anthropology or the history of normative practices in his own culture will find apparent relativity in morals. But this does not prove a relativity in principles or, for example, that cannibalism is ethically justified. If cannibalism can ever be ethically justified, its justification must depend upon a very unusual set of circumstances, and on a practice whereby ethical issues are taken carefully into account.

16

Some of the apparent relativity in moral practices comes simply as a reflection of sound applications of objective and universal ethical principles in a variety of different contexts. There is no reason for doing exactly the same thing in two different contexts from a moral standpoint any more than from the standpoint of applied physics. Other instances of apparent relativity may reflect a genuine relativity deriving from ignorance or error in the determination of the relevant ethical maxim, that is, an error in the application of the ethical principle in a specific context. Such relativity as this likewise occurs in science, in engineering, in artillery practice. Additional instances of relativity may reflect nothing more than deliberate failure on the part of some individuals and communities to live up to what they recognize as their moral, that is, ethical obligation. (In this context, "ethics" and "morals" are used interchangeably by both non-philosophers and philosophers.)

No one has formulated the principles of ethics or morality more rigorously than Immanuel Kant. This does not mean that Kant invented ethics or morality—any more than Newton invented gravity. Rather, Kant described ethical principles in formulations that met strict philosophical standards. He recognized that Confucius' statement, "Do not do unto others as you would not have them do unto you," and Jesus' statement, "Do unto others as you would have them do unto you," were first steps toward the formulation of the fundamental principle of morality. These partially expressed a sound ethical point of view, but unfortunately they were inadequate as formulations of the principle of ethics. George Bernard Shaw observed in *Man and Superman,* "Do not do unto others as you would that they should do unto you. Their tastes may not be the same." In his humorous comment Shaw identified a problem that Kant had corrected a century before. The principle "your moral obligation is to do unto others as you would have them do unto you" can be faithfully carried out by two heroin addicts. One is pleased to give the other a heroin injection, provided that his good deed, so-called, is reciprocated. As each of the addicts gives and receives a shot, each does unto the other as each would be done by.

This is obviously a grotesque misapplication of the intent of the Golden Rule; nevertheless, it is a perfectly consistent and reasonable application based on the literal but inadequate formulation of the Rule. Kant recognized that the true nature of the moral principle was disfigured in the formulation of the Golden Rule and in Confucius' principle, and he tried to formulate that principle without distortion.

He began by examining the nature of the person, to discern those characteristics as entity must possess if the personal pronoun is to apply. No one, Kant showed, is a person unless capable of acting in accordance with his own idea of law. If one's only ability as an individual is to act according to the stimuli that impose themselves on him, then he lives the life of a thermostat. He is nothing more than a mechanical device responding to an influence such as heat. Such a life would not justify using personal pronouns or names. (We do not name our thermostats—"This is Paul, who works in the living room; John here works in the bathroom.") We apply personal pronouns and names to beings who can act independently of forces impinging upon them. To express himself as a person in genuine action, as initiator of a sequence of events for which he is responsible, a genuine person must have the capacity to transcend those influences.

The human capacity to conceive of acting and to act independently of forces, whether external or internal to the individual, is what Kant meant when he said that the will is free. This freedom can be expressed negatively as the person's immunity from determination by all such influences. But freedom in this negative sense is incomplete, because the person would still lack the capacity for individual, personal action. To be genuinely or fully free, the individual must also be free in a positive sense. That is, he must have the positive capacity to act, while preserving his personal transcendence of influences upon him. The only way an individual can achieve this transcendence is by acting according to a principle which—because it is universal—transcends any and all particular motivations, stimuli or influences affecting him.

This, in very short form, is the analysis and argument behind Kant's derivation of the categorical imperative. "So act that the maxim [that is, the applied principle] of your act can be a universal law." Or, "so act that the maxim of your act can, through your will, become a universal law of nature." Or, "so act that you treat other persons never as means merely but always as ends in themselves." Or, "so act that you become a law-giver in a kingdom of ends·of which you are also a member." Kant provided these various formulations of the single categorical imperative simply in order to clarify its meaning and thus to offer guidance in applying this abstract principle concretely in daily life.

To explain the meaning of that single imperative, Kant offered a variety of formulations. The formulations were not different imperatives, but simply alternative ways of expressing the meaning of that single imperative. Kant's alternative formulations parallel his formulation of his three basic procedures of sound thinking: first, to think for oneself, second, to put oneself in thought in the place and point of view of others, and third, always to think consistently or coherently. These three logical formulations were, Kant held, the guides to sound thinking. The various formulations of the categorical imperative are similarly guides to sound volition.

The rule to think for oneself requires the universalization of the principles of thought, just as the categorical imperative requires the universalization of the maxim of action. The rule of thinking oneself into the viewpoint of others describes the procedure by which one comes to know what he must do in order to treat others as ends in themselves. The rule to think consistently requires that the ruler in the kingdom of ends assess his laws from the perspective of one who must also obey them.

In order to think and act soundly, one must think and act for oneself. But in addition, nothing is more important than the ability, by means of imagination, to put oneself in the place or point of view of others. By this means one comes closest to achieving that universality which is the hallmark of moral action.

By placing oneself in the point of view of others, one comes to know the nature and consequence of his acts from their point of view. This enlargement of understanding is of fundamental importance in all aspects of life, including the ethical fulfillment of one's professional responsibilities.

Disciplining oneself to think and examine one's professional activities by this procedure is of obvious importance to doctors. A doctor must examine the situation from his patient's perspective as well as his own, and from the point of view of the patient's family and of the community in general. The patient's point of view must be taken into account when developing a plan of treatment. In addition, the plan of treatment must be well-conceived in terms of the knowledge and art of medicine available to the doctor.

I have not here turned from applied ethics to merely professional considerations. When speaking about the application of ethics to a profession, it is a common mistake to suppose that what an individual does professionally is separate and distinct from his ethical responsibility. On the contrary, the professional's paramount ethical obligation is to be professionally competent. The moral assessment of an active professional must be based on the quality of his professional performance.

The ethical surgeon is not the one who does not overcharge, or who is unfailingly polite. He is the one who performs his operations effectively, thereby restoring the patient's health. The ethical internist is not the one with the irresistible bedside manner, but the one whose diagnosis is correct.

If we assume that a correct diagnosis can be made and proper surgical conditions are available, an internist who misdiagnoses and a surgeon who butchers his patient are not merely incompetent. They are moral failures.

There is, however, no way in which the individual himself can provide all the knowledge on which sound application of the categorical imperative finally depends. Even if one applied the categorical imperative conscientiously and in accordance with the most enlightened views of his time, his act might be wrong. But it would not be wrong from the point of view of his moral assessment, since his actual moral responsibility can never exceed the limits of enlightenment accessible to him. If his ignorance is not due to his negligence, it cannot be held to his moral account. Perhaps at a later time, from a perspective of greater enlightenment, one might find that the decision of a morally good person was nevertheless wrong. This subsequent assessment would in no way diminish the moral worth of the individual who acted at a time when additional insight was not available. Kant, and everyone else who has thought seriously about the subject, has recognized that every individual is the creature of his time, limited to a significant degree by the scientific, artistic, and social milieu of his day.

There are ideas we know to be ridiculous that were not known to be so at some earlier time. Cotton Mather, for example, was perhaps the best educated and most thoughtful American intellectual of his day, and recognized as such in England by his election to the Royal Society. Mather could, nevertheless, quite seriously and con scientiously put himself in the place and point of view of the villagers of Salem convicted of witchcraft. And he could, after a most conscientious and intense examination of the ends and the issues involved, hang the witches. From all the evidence and knowledge available to him, Mather believed them possessed by devils; as a Christian of his day he believed that the possibility of saving their souls was more important than saving their bodies, and he tried to achieve that greater end by hanging those bodies. In his *Preface to St. Joan,* George Bernard Shaw detailed the conscientious procedures followed by officers of the Inquisition in determining the guilt of those accused of heresy, and demonstrated that these clerics were not insensitive men who cared nothing for justice or truth. They had acted in accordance with the best knowledge available to them at their time, from a profound concern for the eternal well-being of those who became victims of their judgment. It is sobering, humiliating, and tragic to realize that we all suffer in all we do the limitations of the knowledge of our time. Our posterity, no doubt, will have their favorite examples of our profound ignorance.

All of us are trapped by the limited enlightenment of our time, and we are thus limited in our ability to apply without error the universal ethical principles. We can only try to transcend our times by thoughtful, considerate, and scientific examination of what we are about. But despite our best and most honest efforts we can be influenced and misled by those general ideas of our time that are so pervasive that we are unaware of them and therefore fail to examine them.

The Issue of Abortion

Of the issues of our time that call for careful examination, abortion is among the most important. Abortion is a public issue recognized to have a moral component, but the quality of debate on this moral issue is too often appalling. Many who advocate abortion speak of it in terms of a woman's right to do as she sees fit with her own body. But one must ask "What does this have to do with the issue of abortion?" No woman gives birth to herself; she gives birth to a child that is a body and personality distinct from herself. Consequently, even if we agree that every woman has a right to do with her own body as she sees fit, we cannot conclude that she therefore has the right to take the life of her child.

Another argument is based on hedonism. Why, it is asked, should a pregnant woman be compelled to suffer the ordeal of childbirth or the burden of unwanted children? If a woman can justify the termination of a pregnancy following voluntary coition, the same line of reasoning can be used by healthy and able-bodied men to justify abandoning wife and children and refusing to pay child support. In either case, personal convenience and comfort replace moral responsibility.

The Supreme Court holds that the government may not prohibit abortion before the third trimester on the ground that for the first six months the fetus is not viable outside the womb. This is a peculiar use of the term "viable." It ignores the fact that nearly all fetuses which survive until the second trimester would be viable if left in the womb until birth. Moreover, the fetus is not really viable early in the third trimester. If it is born then, doctors must work furiously to save its life, for it is a dangerously premature infant.

In fact, of course, no baby is in any realistic sense viable at birth. It is anything but easy or simple to nurture a newborn child. A human being is not really viable until age four or five, that is, until it has learned enough to cope on its own. If viability is the criterion, infanticide at any age up to four could be justified.

In any event, if potentiality is to be considered, how can an abortion after conception be justified? Who would undertake the burden of caring for a newborn infant if one knew that it would always remain a neonatal creature? A newborn baby, incontinent, speechless, instinctively demanding and gyrating though totally unaware of self or others, would be a creature of abhorrence and terror were it not for the vision of the adult potential in the infant. Imagine that the baby would always be a baby: such a creature, substantially less satisfactory as a companion than a dog or cat, would be lucky to attract the legal protections now bestowed upon animals.

Without considering potentiality we could in fact justify terminating life at almost any stage. If we recognize the importance of potentiality to the love and appreciation of the newborn infant, why should we deny the importance of potentiality in the assessment of the fetus, whether in the first, second, or third trimester—

or at the moment of conception? The ovum unfertilized is not potentially human. The sperm in isolation is not potentially human. The normal fertilized egg is potentially human. It is on its way.

This analysis does not by itself provide a sufficient moral basis for resolving all the legal complications of abortion law. But it does indicate the superficiality of the moral reasoning that has dominated the public debate on this complex question.

My own position on abortion is that the fertilized egg is human, that therefore the fetus is human, and that consequently abortion is homicide. Some homicides are, of course, justifiable. For example, if the continued development of the fetus poses a clear and credible threat to the life of the mother, it is my opinion that the doctrine of self-defense can justify its removal. Just as clearly, the mere convenience or preference of the mother, or the father, or anyone else, could never justify killing the fetus. On such a rationale abortion is ethically indistinguishable from first-degree murder of a particularly callous sort.

But I do not advocate embodying this view in the statute books. Absent a consensus that abortion is in most cases tantamount to murder, any law maintaining that position will be unenforceable. Consequently, prior to its passage, we should try to secure a consensus of opinion on the subject. In the absence of that consensus, it would lead to widespread contempt for the law without improving the moral climate. On the other hand, given the fact that a substantial proportion of the people in this country regard abortion as murder, it does seem wrong to pay for abortions with tax money. And indeed, the "pro-choice" advocates, by arguing that an abortion is a purely private matter, cannot consistently demand that public funds should be used to carry it out. Our most urgent priority in this area should be developing an understanding of the morally degrading nature of the argument that abortion is simply a case of what women do with their bodies, or that abortion can be justified as a matter of convenience.

Contraception and Abortion

As you can see, I am in considerable agreement with the Catholic Church on the issue of abortion. But on another closely related matter, I would like, respectfully, to raise some questions. I think it unlikely that the Catholic Church will win the intellectual and moral consent of thoughtful, spiritually sensitive people if the Church argues both in opposition to abortion and in opposition to contraception.

To oppose contraception on the grounds of natural law raises questions which I do not believe can be easily answered. The female human being has thousands of ova that can never be fertilized. The loss of ova, the loss of spermatozoa do not in either case represent loss of a human life. Neither the ovum nor the spermatozoan is in isolation a human being. Each is merely one-half of what is naturally or biologically speaking, essential to the creation of a human life.

Can we explain God's purpose in creating so many millions of superfluous spermatozoa in every man, and so many thousands of superfluous ova in every woman, on the assumption that it was the will of God that each and every one of them be joined in a union giving birth to human beings? Such a notion evokes, in imagination at least, the vision of human beings all over the earth to a depth of 17 or 18 feet. Suppose there were 25 billion persons, weighing an average of 150 pounds each. Their combined weight would be some 37.5 trillion pounds which, if distributed unevenly, might send the earth out of its orbit, spiralling into the sun. Of course, it is inconceivable that we could find food to produce 25 billion reasonably healthy individuals. The nightmare of this thought-experiment dissolves when we recall the doctrine that matter can neither be created nor destroyed—except by God.

I am, of course, using a geometrically expansive *reductio ad absurdum* here, merely to suggest that the Church might do both itself and mankind the greatest service by reexamining their conclusion that the natural law sustains the Catholic view on contraception.

The issue, as I know you are aware, is a vital one, in the most literal sense of the word "vital." If there can be no control of population on the basis of contraception, and if we are not to encourage the wanton destruction of human life through starvation or a widespread disease such as AIDS, there is only one other historically demonstrated form of population control—war. It is, for many of us, all too plausible that the Four Horsemen of the Apocalypse will appear, not as God's vengeance but as the consequence of our inadvertence. Our humane concern to put an end to abortion, combined with our dogmatic concern to proscribe contraception, may release Disease, Famine, War, and Death.

Sexual promiscuity, it is important to note, is an entirely different issue from that of contraception. Continuing to discourage the use of contraception by unmarried men and women, is, it seems to me, an area in which the Catholic Church can and should continue to speak with great authority and persuasiveness. No one has the right to create human life, or to engage in that activity by which human life is normally created, without having made a commitment to his or her partner, and having together made a commitment to the support and nurture of the child should it come. The Catholic Church would be historically, ethically, and socially true to its mission in opposing contraception for unmarried persons while recognizing the legitimacy of contraception within the limitations of a consecrated marriage. The Church's prohibition of contraception for devout, responsible married couples who seek parenthood to the fullest extent of their capacity to support and nurture their children, compels such parents to blind obedience or to sin. Blind obedience may be required, but would it not be wise to ask: why, if the Church's position is sound, a better justification than blind obedience cannot be offered?

Transsexual Operations

Among other ethical issues arising from medical practice is the question of transsexual operations. The main point to be observed here is that, strictly speaking, such operations are impossible. The castration of a man does not produce a woman; it produces an ox. Renée Richards, despite the claims of Billie Jean King, was a castrated male tennis player. It is an insult to womanhood to suppose that a woman is nothing more than a mutilated man. It leads to the absurd conclusion that, after the intervention of Heloise's uncle, she and Abelard had a lesbian relationship. The Church cannot approve the misuse of hundreds of thousands of dollars in medical services for the debased purpose of engaging in what is nothing more than a patent fraud.

Transplants of Fetal Tissue

Transplanting of tissue from preborn and anacephalic infants is a difficult moral issue. In examining this question, one must surely ask whether the fetal material is available as a consequence of an induced abortion. In this case, the Church might properly object that to permit the use of such tissue is to invite and encourage abortion. Consistent with its opposition to abortion, the Church may argue that one cannot make a moral use of such materials if they are acquired through an immoral practice.

If the fetal tissue is available through natural causes, however, as a consequence of miscarriage, accident, or the premature death of the mother, there is nothing immoral about its acquisition. If it is available through death of the infant, caused by profound malformation, as in the case of anencephalics, its acquisition may again be without moral blame. In these situations, the central question, I believe, is this: should we deny medically helpful materials to human beings in serious physical and mental need when that material becomes available without any wrongdoing on the part of any human being?

To deny the use of such material, I think, would be as difficult to justify as the refusal to use the blood from a matching donor. Suppose, for instance, that an otherwise healthy donor was, because of a severe brain injury, in a profound coma and incapable of giving consent. Would there be any sound moral reason for refusing to use blood of that donor—assuming that the taking of a pint of his blood would do no physical harm to him while saving the life of another patient?

Although morally justified, a physician might refuse to make the transfusion because of legal obstacles. But if the moral argument is correct, we should then advocate reforms in the legal code to permit such life-saving interventions.

My thought-experiment of the blood transfusion reveals the same moral structure, I believe, as the use of tissue available through natural miscarriages and the birth of fatally deformed infants. In neither case is the being who is the source of the needed material capable of exercising judgment. Placing ourselves through imagination in their point of view, however, must we not conclude that they would favor, if they were morally sound, using what was of no benefit to them for the benefit of others?

The use of material from fatally deformed infants would require parental consent, as the taking of blood from a comatose person would involve the consent of the legal guardian, or, in his absence, the attending physician. But how would parents in the former case, or guardians in the latter, justify their refusal to make use of such material in saving human life?

Animal Rights

On the issue of animal rights, it seems to me the Catholic Church needs to be heard, because such individuals as the Australian philosopher Peter Singer, who have argued against speciesism on the grounds that all species are of equal value, fly in the face of all Christian, Moslem, and Jewish theology. Yet twelve states, including Massachusetts, have passed laws prohibiting the use of pound animals for medical research. And medical research is suffering as a consequence.

Views such as Singer's may be quickly reduced to an absurdity. The fallacy of the position that opposes all forms of speciesism is seen in the fact that those who oppose the use of animals in research have availed themselves of medical procedures and medicines that are the products of animal research. Consequently, they are parasitic on the use of animals for medical research even as they denounce and oppose it. There is something wrong with a person who is alive today because of the polio vaccine or because of the vaccine against smallpox going out and proclaiming the moral wrong of those who have used animals to produce those vaccines. Those who welcome the protection of doctors, policemen, and soldiers who, at the risk of their lives, protect members of our society, must explain how they can accept these sacrifices while refusing to permit rats, cats, dogs, or monkeys to risk their lives in the service of society.

If one seriously holds that all species are equal in their claims upon our moral consideration, we have lost the moral basis for denying the pit bull its pleasure in destroying a young child. How dare we, all species being equal, presume to do such a thing? This is the way of pit bulls. This is what they enjoy. How dare we intervene on behalf of children?

If we reject any hierarchical arrangement of the species, we must look with equanimity over Alexander the Great and Theatetus. One can imagine bands of E. coli gathering together in the colon of a great man to say, "Today, the colon! Tomorrow, the world!"

What could possibly be moral about denying scientists the opportunity to advance medical research through the use of animals abandoned in pounds when, in the absence of adoption, those animals are exterminated without benefitting anyone? In the spirit of speciesism, let us place ourselves in the place and point of view of the abandoned dog or cat. Are we to believe that the animal in question prefers to end its life in a meaningless death? Would it not prefer to give its life for the benefit of other animals and possibly of human beings? If the anti-speciesist objects to my supposition that a dog or cat might prefer to share the nobility we prize in human existence, is he not acknowledging by his objection their inferiority?

This is not to deny the need for guidelines to prohibit the abuse of experimental animals, and the imposition of needless suffering. But I know of no responsible doctor or scientist who does not hold this position.

It is unfortunate that Catholics who have been strong in the pro-life movement have seriously avoided taking a stand with regard to the right to use animals in medical research. It is an oversight that I hope will soon be corrected.

The Wanton Prolongation of Human Life

Can doctors justify the expenditure of scarce medical resources in the prolongation of human life after the last vestige of rational capacity has vanished when, by so doing, they deny lifesaving services to infants and to others who might be saved? How can a church that proclaims, on the basis of natural law, the right of the fetus to be born, deny the right of the physician or the family to cease medical intervention in the prolongation of suffering in an elderly patient for whom recovery is impossible? Why is the doctor or the family under any obligation to defeat the natural law? Have they no obligation to conserve limited medical resources for the benefit of those patients for whom recovery is possible?

We live in a world of finite resources. Highly expensive medical resources are in particularly short supply. How then can one justify squandering these resources on those who have lost self-awareness and the terminally ill? I am not arguing for euthanasia. I am arguing against deliberately and unnaturally prolonging the suffering of those terminally ill, or wastefully and unnaturally prolonging the existence of those lacking self-awareness and even consciousness, and who cannot recover these. The use of expensive resources for these unnatural purposes denies those resources to infants and children who are in greater need and for whom a compelling case for medical care can be given.

Closing Remarks

The limits of time have ensured the superficiality of my views. But I hope I may have been of help, because the importance of the Church to the future of mankind has never been greater than today.

When I was a young Protestant seminarian, I was critical of the Catholic Church for having set standards of belief and conduct that then seemed to me far too low. I then believed that we could and should expect individuals to reach higher standards of faith and conduct strictly on their own.

But, in light of the experience of 40 years of virtually unrestrained pursuit of individualism, I realize how naive and wrong-headed I was. We have witnessed the degeneration of our people in orgies of sex, drugs, and immediate gratification, and in the disfigurement of faith through a "Bakker's dozen" of TV evangelists and others who have reminded us of the historic role of authority in restraining the wayward nature of sinful man, and, with rare exception, the beauty, the nobility, the goodness, and truth of that authority as exercised by the Catholic Church. It seems to me that the need for that authority was never greater than it is today.

Bishop: Thank you very much, Dr. Silber. You were introduced as a philosopher and thinker and, from your remarks you did provoke a lot of stimulating thoughts in our minds and some of your insights were truly—what do I say?—penetrating.

We are grateful for your presentation. I must say, however, that the reasonable people do differ and I, being a reasonable person, a man of faith, would like to ask a question. We live in a culture and in a society that is, as you indicated, very individualistic. I think the methodology by which our culture proceeds is inductive.

That is, we study the situation and from that, we try to come up with the imperative. And it seems to me that in your lecture you started with a conscience imperative and then proceeded to a methodology which became deductive proceeding from this conscience imperative.

In the Church, we are people of faith and our methodology is deductive in its approach to life and problems. And in that methodology, we feel that our reason is enlightened by faith. And therefore we can come to very different conclusions—given that that first principle, that faith, be very, very reasonable and offer to our people and to society, indeed, a very reasonable way in which to live, and hopefully one which has been given by God.

Having given that little speech, the question simply is: have you not done, by creating the Kantian imperative and coming to some conclusions with which we would agree, and some with which we would disagree, haven't you usurped the prerogative of the Church that says that these are our imperatives and this is our faith and this is the way we rationally live it out?

Dr. Silber: Well, first of all, I think the Catholic Church is a very complex institution. It has struggled over the years to accommodate views that at certain periods of time were thought to be heterodox. The Church has assimilated at least some of these once heterodox views into the general body of the faith. The Church has engaged in a good deal of rethinking.

Now, the extent to which I made use of Immanuel Kant was not in any way to set him up as an authority for the Catholic Church. I recognize the rather ludicrous implications of that idea. It was rather to say that, as I have read St. Thomas and other Catholic theologians, many of them seem to agree with the notion that a sound ethical principle has a universality in its application. I think St. Augustine and St. Thomas would certainly agree to a very large extent with Kant in his delineation of what is required if a moral principle is to be sound. In developing a sound principle one can't just pick and choose, but must strive for something with some universality about it. Now, that being the case, I apply that test of universality to doctrines of the Church.

However, I think that the Church is quite privileged from the standpoint of faith to say, "Despite the fact that we run into a problem of universality, we are going to make an exception because faith requires it." I would not presume for one moment to suggest the contrary. I think that faith no less than argument is a very important aspect of life, and the *credo ut intelligam*—where one believes in order to understand—is an important move within the tradition of the Church.

But, likewise, a fundamental part of the tradition of the Church has been a concern to understand so that one could defend and support the faith. The Church, particularly within Catholic theology, recognizes that being able to argue the case for something is no less important than to have the original insight, whatever its source may be.

It does appear to me that the Catholic Church has, at times, gotten it wrong, so that at times, when it had reached a false conclusion, it has recognized the need to correct itself. For that reason I call some of these issues to your attention.

With regard to animal rights, I don't think that anything I have said is potentially different from any position of the Church—I say "potentially" because the Catholic Church has, traditionally, bypassed that issue, perhaps for political reasons, saying, "Well, we don't want to take on too much." But it is consistent, I would say, with the sacredness of human life, to refuse to become sentimental about the lives of dogs, cats, rats, and E. coli. The Catholic Church could deliver a devastating counterargument against the anti-speciesist movement before it begins to be taken as a serious philosophical position.

The point that I was making with regard to contraception within the context of a serious and devout Catholic marriage is one of which every member of the faith is undoubtedly acutely aware, because it concerns a crisis within Catholicism. I sit there on the outside—although I have seven children and my father once remarked that, there I was, a Protestant living like a Roman Catholic—and I see the problem. It bothers me when I see young Catholics who simply acknowledge that they engage in sin, having several children, and wanting several children. I sit there looking at Catholic doctrine and asking, "What is it that brings this situation into coherence?" I am not at all sure that further enlightenment on this subject is not required. But you know this.

As a final remark, let me say that I think it is far better for the Catholic Church, even from my point of view, to remain in what I would consider to be a mistake on one small matter or another, than for it to engage in a series of accommodations in order to become more popular. The extraordinary popularity of the Pope all over the United States—among Catholics, non-Catholics, Christians and non-Christians, among people who are indifferent or even antagonistic to religion—is, I believe, because in him we ran across a person over 40 years of age who is not going through an identity crisis. It is remarkably reassuring, it is contagious to find a group of individuals united in a matter of opinion who are not trying to accommodate their views to the multitude in order to become more acceptable, but instead stand for something. By standing for something they can become a beacon and a source of guidance to the multitude, hoping that the multitude will eventually guide itself by the greater enlightenment of the Church.

So, if I had to choose between one or the other, I would clearly choose the position that the Church has in fact followed. Nevertheless, I believe that there are certain areas in which the Church is not fundamentally committed. And I say that with all humility as an outsider. I know perfectly well that any one of you should know better than I whether that is so or not. But I also have read enough, and read closely enough, in Catholic publications to know that there are persons who adhere to the faith, participate in the Mass, and who yet share many of the doubts that I raised with you.

Bishop: Dr. Silber, I understand very well that I'm not going to change your mind, particularly in some of these areas and with reference to your argument of the limited use of contraceptives in the proper form.

I am trying to follow the logic. The question is very simple, I suppose. If contraception, in your view, is acceptable for use by the married in the sexual act, why can't it be used by the unmarried, since it's not hurting anybody, assuming they are adults?

Dr. Silber: Okay, sure, that's a fair comment. Let us make the argument even a little more difficult by assuming that there are methods of contraception available which are 100% effective so that we are not arguing the prudential matter—we are not saying that the reason why we are opposed to non-marital sex is because something might go wrong and you have got to be protected against the accident. Let's suppose that accidents were impossible,

33

and consequently anyone could engage in premarital or extramarital sex without any chance of producing a human life. There still seem to me to be other issues involved.

Extramarital sexual relationships involve the betrayal of trust between two individuals. The lack of mutuality that follows from that seems to me so thoroughly to undermine the relationship of marriage, so thoroughly inimical to the proper nurture of the married couple's children, as to provide a substantial argument in opposition to extramarital sexual relationships. In an extramarital relationship you either are committed to secrecy, in which case great dishonesty and the corrosion of the individual's relationship to his or her family is an inevitable consequence, or you take the bolder step of informing your spouse of the infidelity. In the latter case you avoid secrecy and the corrosion of the perpetrator's own moral conduct, but you have undermined the relationship from many points of view.

With regard to a premarital sexual relationship: that seems to me to be more difficult to argue about. I would think that the difficulty in arguing for it derives from the low level of sensitivity that can be retained when one trivializes something as fundamentally important as sex. Only a low level of sensitivity can make sex seem a matter of relative unimportance.

It is the possibility of conception that gives the sex act its sacramental dimensions, its sacred dimensions. When that is removed, it seems to me, one has so trivialized a relationship that a certain aspect of human fulfillment and human realization is removed for the individual who has decided to go that route.

Speaking philosophically, marriage is not always and only a religious act. Marriage as a religious act is very important in expressing what is sacred about a committed relationship between a man and a woman, about their sexual relationship. But it seems to me that the importance can also be stated to some extent even in terms of a civil marriage. But to suggest that two human beings can share a sexual relationship as a matter of convenience to be initiated or terminated without regard to its very special nature—to suggest this is to comply in the demeaning of the human experience itself. It is to so trivilialize this wonderful and central opportunity for human joy and expression as to involve a reduction in human experience that to me seems deeply unfortunate.

I am not saying that these observations are going to pick up a lot of converts, but it doesn't seem to me that the argument against promiscuity is gone simply because one says, "Well, you don't have to worry about having a baby."

Bishop: I think we disagree about the issue of contraception from a religious point of view. But I would like to bring up the issue of situating the issue of contraception in terms of all that has gone on this century of trying to make a better society. I think I am hearing you say that we could improve the quality of life if there were a better balance in our doctrines concerning contraception and abortion. And my concern is, the eugenics movement, all this century, has continually employed birth control, contraception, and several other means, in the belief by social planners that the quality of life could be thereby improved. And it has always been one of those things that has been pushed by scientists as well as social planners to improve the quality of life—improve it by reducing the number of persons. They probably are considered to be poor and marginal because most of our social problems are considered to put the greatest drain on our social resources.

The Catholic position has been that contraception and abortion and all the other positions really do nothing more than to marginate even further those who are poor or marginal—working, in other words, a further injustice.

In point of fact, the use of contraception without any real serious addressing of the injustices that exist in this society concerning the distribution of wealth and possession of the means of production seems to be nothing more than what the old eugenicists would think and the newer eugenicists are doing today: they basically try to preserve the power and the money in one area by using contraception as a means of keeping the balance.

So, I am wondering whether or not your perhaps clear and well-intentioned position does not play into the hand of the eugenicists that have been really unjust, I think, in this century.

Dr. Silber: Well, I don't think so. American Catholic families might be able, let's say, to support a family of four children, whereas they simply might reach the point where they could no longer educate or even adequately care for and nurture the seven, eight, or ten children they might have without contraception. I think it is pretty hard to move from a concern for that situation to saying that the purpose of contraception is to try to limit the number of poor people—let's say, blacks or Hispanics or something like that—who might get themselves born.

I agree with you if what you are saying is that, in so-called third world countries, straightening out some of the social problems is a first stage toward trying to make any kind of improvement in the quality of the lives of the poor. But it is interesting to note that in every society in which the quality of life has been improved, you have seen a reduction in the number of children per family. I don't believe you can find a single society in which there is an exception. With a substantial improvement in the standard of living, you get a substantial decrease in the number of children born to each woman, which means that with the substantial improvement in the economic way of life, somehow they have learned to engage in contraception. They have not reduced the number of children by the rhythm method; that too can be verified in society after society.

Instead of seeing acceptance of contraception come about as a result of a callous disregard of faith and a growing materialism, I would rather see it come as a part of disciplined spiritual life, recognizing the responsibilities of parents to children—not simply out of a materialism that says, "This is the way in which the mother and father can become more selfish and give less to other people," but out of concern for children. But I am not going to worry about the eugenics point of view because I am not trying to pick any specific group and say that they should not be allowed to reproduce. I think I would have to go that next step in the advocacy of contraception—to say that it should be applied selectively—before any eugenics argument could be made.

Bishop: I would just like to comment and perhaps you would like to comment in return, but it's really not a question. When you were speaking about contraception I got the impression that you thought the Catholic teaching was based on a recognition that an ova and a sperm, because of their inherent "partial personhood" should be united. All I would like to comment is that the Catholic teaching abstracts completely from the nature of the ova and sperm and that it is founded more upon the meaning of the action and, as you mentioned before, the sacramental meaning of that action. I got the impression—and perhaps you would like to change that—that we're working on some misguided scientific apprehension of what ova and sperm are of themselves.

Dr. Silber: No, I recognize the complete validity of what you are saying there, and I can also understand how you might very well have supposed I was making an incorrect statement about Catholic doctrine in the comment I made. I was not saying, in that comment about the sperm and the ovum, that this was the Catholic position, but rather saying that one must be quite clear that it would be impossible to offer any such argument consistent with Catholic theology because that argument just won't wash at all. The number of spermatozoa and ova is so great for every individual that it would be a *reductio ad absurdum* to argue that there was anything about natural law that would suggest the union of each and every one of these in the creation of a human being. I was not suggesting that was in fact the Catholic position. The presence of the *reductio ad absurdum* ensures that it never will be a part of the Catholic position, because that argument just wouldn't wash at all.

Bishop: Even with that qualification, as you characterized the Catholic position, it did not convince at least this hearer that whatever you ultimately do about agreeing or disagreeing, that you understood the Catholic position. And I would simply state that, over the past twenty years, there has been a rich development of the Catholic teaching regarding the sacredness of the sexual union. Pope John Paul II has contributed to that in a very rich way. I believe that the answer that would give credence philosophically to our position is to be found more in the direction of the response that you made about how you could justify denying the possibility of extramarital sexual relations. It's more a consideration of the relationship and the meaning of that relationship, the intrinsic meaning of the act and not separating it out by simply a biological consideration. Furthermore, I also think that the great deal of investment has gone into natural family planning which takes us far afield from Vatican roulette. So I believe that while you may ultimately disagree with our position, the position itself has undergone tremendous development. One of the tragedies of the past 20 years, both within and outside the Church, is dissent within the Church.

We have been unable to articulate the beauty of this teaching in a way that could counter some of what I would consider the dismal consequences in contemporary society of the contraceptive mentality. And that contraceptive mentality is certainly in place.

Bishop: I have a question and I really want to make a comment about something quite different. I think that our problem in making the Catholic teaching in regard to contraception intelligible is that we fail to go to what's basically the philosophic core: the inherent union between the procreative aspect and the intimacy that is inherent to the marriage act, which derives its meaning from the marriage relationship itself.

You fail to admire the sanctity of the marriage relationship and the positive contribution the marriage act brings to that relationship. Then, we have not been forceful, although at certain times, the Church has probably been far more forceful than previous theologians.

Another thing that you failed to bring into the discussion is the legitimate need for a restraining factor in sexual activity. The world in which we live, having undergone the sexual revolution, labors against any kind of restraint, either self-restraint or imposed restraint. Actually, there is no imposed restraint and so the really last part of the battle is a breakdown of all imposed restraints or any kind of self-restraint. In our position, we must admire the concurrent unity between intimacy and appropriation in and outside of the marriage act and the need for some self restraint.

The natural method of family planning differs greatly from what you characterize as rhythm or what someone referred to as Vatican roulette. And it is in the pursuit of the perfection of these methods that we begin to see both the realization of the unity between appropriation and intimacy at the personal level and the acceptance of and certification for self-restraint. Now, that being said, still it has not been well packaged in a way which we can present to young people and have it assimilated and made part of married life.

Bishop: Dr. Silber, in a sense, you sounded like somebody in Catholic family in 1968. When the Encyclical came out, I know many thoughtful people who were unhappy with the Encyclical because they wanted the use of contraceptions within a family where they had good reason to not want any more children. And this restriction didn't seem to make much sense. But what happened concretely between 1968 and the present among our own is that once people said that they could decide for themselves on whether or not procreation was desirable in having marital relations, in a sense, they had turned the marital act into an act that was instrumental to secure their own purposes. The next thing that cropped up was people saying that for people who were not married because they couldn't afford housing or something but loved each other very much, it was all right for that group to have sexual relations. The next thing that came up was that every human being had a right to sexual expression and, if you were a homosexual, it was all right and maybe even desirable for them to go into some type of stable relationship rather than be promiscuous. The next step after that was to say that if two people really cared for each other, it was all right to have sexual relations. At the same time, in the sexual revolution that took place in the last 20 years whereby people felt much freer to go ahead and have sexual relations, contraception, at least theoretically, removed any kind of self-control.

So I find it hard to believe, not that your position is your position, but that it really carries much weight in society, that kind of an isolation for contraception within marriage apart from sexual promiscuity.

Dr. Silber: Well, I think that when you were arguing the slippery slope, and the way in which one argument about self-indulgence led to another, and you noted that if contraception is introduced then the marriage act itself becomes instrumental to purposes other than procreation—I think all of that is true. But it also seems to me that, to the extent that Catholics talk about family planning and about family practices that can avoid conception, they have already gone that route themselves, and they ought to face up to the implications of having done so.

Whether you use the currently accepted methods of Catholic family planning or whether you use some other form of contraception, this, it seems to me, is an instrumental and mechanical distinction. You have already made the decision that it is consistent with Catholic doctrine to decide to limit the size of a family and not simply allow it to burgeon beyond the capacity of the parents to handle it.

The fact that the point of view that I have been advocating is not widely influential in society—that I will stipulate right along with you. I think that you and I and everybody in this room hold in common the notion that there is something very special about the sexual relationship, something that is lost in the context of promiscuity, and that there is something grotesque about the substitution of the homosexual relationship for the heterosexual relationship, since the latter can lead to the fulfillment of birth, which is a fundamental part of the meaning of the sexual act.

I think we are in agreement on that. Consequently, I am not in any way averse to your notion that one can, once he starts talking about the accommodation of the sexual act for the purpose of gratification, very quickly reduce the meaning of that act, thereby providing a justification for instant gratification, the instant marriage, divorce, and remarriage, and, in short, that emptying of sex of all its importance which is characteristic of the present time. When sex is reduced to just one other form of instant gratification it becomes, unlikely as it may seem, uninteresting. The enthusiasm of young people in college today for—not one-night stands but for one- or two-minute stands, perhaps more than once per night with any number of partners—what these young people have lost in the loss of the romantic quest for a mate and so forth is terribly great. I quite agree with you that the movement toward promiscuity empties the meaning from a centrally important aspect of life.

So I don't see that, on that subject, the Catholic Church is in a very significantly different position from the one I am in. I think that it takes the subtlety of the learned doctors to differentiate the position that you are advocating with family planning in the Catholic Church and the one that I am advocating by saying that, within the context of the devout Catholic family, some form of contraception might be accepted as consistent with the sacredness of the sexual act and the sacredness of marriage. But I certainly would bow to you and to the other people here as being in a far better position than I am to assess the merits of the argument.

Bishop: As a young priest growing up a long time ago, there was no question about contraception. We were, to a certain extent, being too biological. And the whole concentration was on the biology of the sexual act. There are other values that are being lost and that's a valid criticism. So we realized that and appreciate it and addressed these other values of the sexuality and the act of sex. But I would just respectfully suggest that some have fallen into the same trap and have had only emphasized those values and have forgotten the integral biological fact that somehow you have to explain why this communication of persons with reference to biology or the human sexual act can't be separated from that.

So we have to integrate these values with the biological factors. That's why, as you pointed out, you have a question on how our promotion of certain forms of family planning are different from contraception. That has to be explained, of course.

But the very fact that we had to find something else, that we saw that the artificial act had a real problem and we went to something else—now, logistically, we say: well, how is that different? We think that it is, but how?

Dr. Silber: I think that is a very good point, and I think that is a point that needs a good deal of elaboration if it is to be understood, because there are a lot of things about Catholic doctrine that are rather well understood by people who are not Catholic or who are just interested laymen. To get a better insight into the significance of that difference in approach to what is, in many ways, a similar objective, one does need to emphasize the difference.

Another issue that I didn't mention because it is not, strictly speaking, medical—though it is, I think, very closely related to the family—is what the Catholic Church is going to do or try to do with the women's movement. And there I am not even interested in the religious vocation of women within the Catholic Church. I am seriously concerned about the responsibility of Catholic mothers for the nurture of their children at home. I raise this out of the experience of my own daughter who happens to have married a Catholic and who is herself now a Catholic and just is recently the mother of a child. She had a very good job, and she is now the beneficiary of a fine maternity leave. Her maternity leave will cover her for about 90 days, provided that she returns to work at the end of the 90 days, and works for a certain number of months thereafter—only under these conditions will the maternity leave be valid. These maternity leaves, which seem to be very benign and wonderful things, become a very serious temptation to young mothers to abandon their children shortly after birth and leave them in the hands of various babysitters or day-care centers whose adequacy is far removed from the adequacy of just the average mother in her relationship to her own child.

I would like my daughter to say, "Well, forget that maternity leave. We don't need it. We can live without it. I won't go back to work in order to pick it up. Just let it go and recognize this new vocation as a mother and stick to that at least until the youngest child is in the first grade at school." But this point of view is becoming a very abnormal, eccentric one. Increasingly it's being taken for granted that the mother does her job when she has the child, nurtures it for two or three months, and then abandons it for eight hours of the day while continuing in a career. It seems to me that this is an area in which the Catholic Church really needs to take an important stand. It is my opinion that the women's movement, taken as a whole, is going to result in enormous misery, in enormous human suffering, and the neglect of the nurture of children to the point that civilization becomes virtually impossible.

PART ONE

ARTIFICIAL NUTRITION AND HYDRATION

Chapter 2

MEDICALLY ALTERED STATES
OF CONSCIOUSNESS

Fred Plum, M.D.

It is a privilege to speak at this distinguished conference on medically altered states of consciousness. Few thoughtful persons, whether headed for science, medicine, philosophy or whatever, have grown up without asking the critical question about consciousness: *how* do we know *that* we know *what* we know? These introspective probings have intensified during the past forty years as scientific knowledge about the brain has remarkably increased. Discoveries about how we visualize objects, how and with what brain structures we recall memories and what awakens the thinking brain have offered unexpected and thrilling explanations of how the brain perceives, remembers, reacts, anticipates and directs the body to carry out its motor acts. Such discoveries must stimulate in all of us a sense of astonishment and humility that our vulnerable bodies can be guided by so delicate, sensitive and complicated an instrument. They cannot avoid influencing our view of what constitutes the essence of our humanity, how we construct our ethics or how we conduct the practice of medicine.

My goal today is to address from a medical biologist's perspective three questions: 1) What is the indispensible physiologic-psychologic core of human consciousness? 2) If permanent loss of consciousness, so defined, can affect a living human body, when can permanence of that state be concluded with reasonable certainty? 3) Does a living body that has lost permanently all capacity for consciousness retain its human individualistic identity, or is it acceptable to allow the remaining body to depart the temporal world peacefully since it can no longer know itself, think, love, feel, give or suffer?

Aside from its importance in defining the presence of a severe brain injury or illness, the subject of prolonged altered states of consciousness has attracted medical and social attention as an outgrowth of contemporary problems associated with an increasingly long-living population and, especially, the effectiveness of emergency resuscitative devices that have demonstrated repeatedly that the critical feature in judging the outcome of serious illness is what happens to the survivor's brain. Thus, while humankind has recognized forever that heart action is indispensable to the body's survival, it has been the discovery of our generation that so also is the vitality of the brain. This principle is now widely accepted without serious argument by church and state as well as medicine so that nearly all Western countries have without serious challenge passed laws defining brain death as equal to cessation of heartbeat in indicating the demise of the body. The much more difficult issue for physicians and religious leaders to resolve has become how to regard bodies which have forever lost their capacity for conscious awareness, i.e., that have entered the vegetative state. Before discussing this further it may be helpful to provide some definitions and describe the anatomy and pathology of consciousness from a medical standpoint.

Definitions

We define *Consciousness* as a state of wakefulness plus evidence of either self awareness or a capacity to express learned, purposeful behavior. Loss of consciousness indicates the loss of both these qualities. Books have been written expressing various views on the ramifications of consciousness, often with sharply contradicting opinions. Ours is a medical working description and implies that consciousness has two dimensions: arousal and the learned content of the aroused state. Patients in coma, defined below, have no capacity to express whatever psychological properties their aroused brains might retain. They are unconscious in our definition as are patients who are vegetative, i.e., are awake but have lost all evidence of a capacity to experience self-awareness and to make any kind of learned (rather than reflex) responses. Of this, more later. By contrast, some patients with severe but restricted left hemisphere damage may lose their capacity to express themselves verbally or even to recall events, but most of them retain the ability to respond purposefully rather than merely show a reflex reaction to exogenous stimuli, be those stimuli pleasant or unpleasant. We consider such patients to have retained consciousness, albeit in a limited way.

Brain Death is a state in which the tissues responsible for maintaining the vital functions of the brain have become irreversibly damaged or destroyed to a degree that no functional recovery is possible (1). As such, the term is absolute, not probabilistic, since it states that no evidence exists of any central nervous system functional activity which takes its origin within the skull nor, because of the nature of the causative injury, can such activity ever reappear. In such cases, body temperature regulation is lost, internal and external eye movements disappear and spontaneous swallowing, breathing or cranial nerve responses to stimuli applied anywhere to the body are entirely absent. To avoid tragic error, the diagnosis requires that no ingested or administered sedatives or toxins can be present in amounts that could cause an anesthetic state. Most medical and legal authorities require a twelve hour wait period to confirm the initial diagnosis of brain death, but this can be shortened in transplant donors if an appropriate laboratory test shows no cerebral blood flow or EEG activity. No reports anywhere in the world indicate that a body declared brain dead by experienced persons has recovered despite continuous subsequent efforts at resuscitation lasting days or weeks.

Coma describes a state of unarousable unresponsiveness unaccompanied by purposeful motor responses to external stimuli and lasting for at least several hours (2). In coma, the eyes are actively closed (i.e., not shut because of eyelid paralysis), and no evidence can be obtained of learned responses to even vigorous stimuli. Depending on the nature of its cause, the loss of arousal may last for hours, days or weeks, but true coma never becomes permanent unless exogenous agents such as sedatives are given concurrently.

The Vegetative State describes a condition in which cyclic arousal, i.e., waking and sleeping, remains (or returns after injury or acute disease), but no evidence of self-awareness or purposeful behavior can be elicited (3). Most patients in a vegetative state can breathe, swallow and often chew spontaneously, and they usually maintain a normal body temperature. Some will grimace, smile or make non-verbal phonations spontaneously. Others will startle to loud sounds or turn the head or eyes briefly toward a moving object. None, however, show consistent or sustained purposeful responses to vigorous stimuli or commands, and none speak. Many patients transiently go through a temporary vegetative state lasting a few hours or days on their way to recovery following an event causing acute coma. A few, however, for weeks or months fail to regain any evidence that they are aware of themselves or their specific surroundings or that they can learn even the most simple acts. This, we call a *persistent* or *chronic vegetative state.* Some have called this condition "cognitive death," and its tragedy is that it can last unchanged for many months or years until the rest of the body finally dies of some independent cause.

Three other conditions can be mentioned that represent less severe medical alterations of consciousness. *Delirium* is an acute state of confusion that can accompany a variety of toxic or structural illnesses affecting the cerebrum. Seriously delirious patients are usually disoriented, sometimes agitated, often hallucinatory, and occasionally amnesic even for close relatives or, occasionally, for the self. Most recover or at least improve. *Dementia* describes an incapacitating, chronic loss of intellectual powers characteristically affecting psychological integrating functions such as attention, judgment, memory for persons and events and the ability to learn new tasks. Severe or total dementia blends into the vegetative state.

Psychiatric pseudocoma can somewhat resemble unconsciousness to the untutored observer, but is readily distinguished by simple tests (2). Catatonic withdrawal in schizophrenia or severe depression can superficially resemble coma or an advanced dementia but usually can be distinguished by differences in the patient's thought content and the absence of any sign of organic abnormality of brain function. Hysterical pseudocoma is not uncommon but seldom lasts more than a few hours. It also can be identified by the absence of any abnormality on either the physical examination or any laboratory test. The *locked-in state* describes a condition in which the limbs and speech mechanisms become so severely paralyzed that the person cannot express thoughts or feelings except in some cases by coded eye movements (2). The condition can result from diseases that affect either the peripheral nerves or the descending motor pathways of the brainstem. The damage cuts the wires that normally carry the messages for voluntary movements from the normally working cerebrum to the muscles; and the condition is usually permanent except when caused by a reversible disease of peripheral nerves rather than damage to central pathways of the brain. Clinical diagnosis in experienced hands readily distinguishes the locked-in state from the vegetative state. Laboratory studies can confirm or rule out the diagnosis if any doubt persists.

The Anatomy of Consciousness and Unconsciousness

One cannot understand the special capacity of the human body for experiencing consciousness without at least a limited knowledge about those parts of the brain that control thought, arousal and the body's vegetative functions.

The brain can be anatomically divided conveniently into several large substructures. The *cerebrum* includes the two large cerebral hemispheres, covered on their cortical surfaces by grey matter containing nerve cells (Fig 1). Under the cortical surface lies subcortical white matter, composed of the nerve fibers leaving and entering the cortex, and two large groups of closely related subcortical nuclei termed the basal ganglia and the thalamus. The basal ganglia serve largely a motor function while the thalamus links the cerebrum to lower parts of the brain called the brainstem and to the body's sensory receptors from which we receive all signals about the outside world.

The cerebrum in human beings differs in appearance from that of all other species. It has more surface convolutions than in any other mammal, and its frontal lobes and visual areas are larger than even those of the higher apes. The corrugated external appearance results from a considerable infolding of the cerebral surface, nature's trick to accomodate an enormously evolved increase in the number of nerve cells without unnecessarily enlarging the head. The large frontal lobes function mainly to regulate behavior that relates to planning for the future and to generate the qualities that underlie abstract anticipation and discovery. Similar enlargements compared to other species mark parts of the temporal lobes devoted to language function.

The cerebral cortex and its deep lying nuclei contain the ultimate mechanisms by which humans convert complex visual, auditory or tactile sensations into perception. The hemispheres regulate language, memory and learned motor behavior. Normal human consciousness requires a relatively intact cerebral cortex for its experience and expression, and any severe loss of cortical activity almost always is accompanied by a decline in cognitive capacities. Extensive bilateral cortical damage even without serious injury to the deep nuclei or to other brain parts can lead to a severe or sometimes complete and permanent loss of consciousness.

Extending downwards beneath the cerebral cortex and its immediately interacting deep nuclei lies the deep central thalamus which contains the upper portion of the autonomic nervous system, described below, and also serves to relay forward messages coming from lower lying, more primitive regions of the brain called the mesencephalon, pons and medulla. Together, the last three make up the brainstem. Immediately on top of the brainstem, lies the cerebellum, a structure which coordinates the body's movements.

50

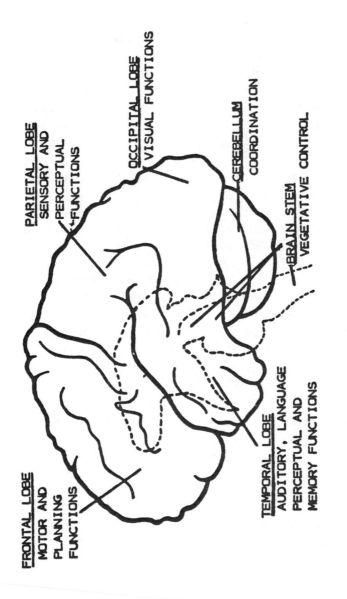

FRONTAL LOBE
MOTOR AND
PLANNING
FUNCTIONS

PARIETAL LOBE
SENSORY AND
PERCEPTUAL
FUNCTIONS

OCCIPITAL LOBE
VISUAL FUNCTIONS

CEREBELLUM
COORDINATION

BRAIN STEM
VEGETATIVE CONTROL

TEMPORAL LOBE
AUDITORY, LANGUAGE
PERCEPTUAL AND
MEMORY FUNCTIONS

Fig. 1. The lateral surface of the left side of the human brain. The cerebral and cerebellar hemispheres have been greatly simplified in this drawing.

The area where the lower thalamus and the mesencephalon join represents the crossroads between primitive, ascending brain influences that both arouse the cerebrum and integrate its psychological capacities and the descending cerebral and autonomic pathways (Fig 2). The latter automatically regulate many of the body's internal needs. The head ganglion of the autonomic nervous system is the hypothalamus, a tiny group of centrally placed cells that lie at the base of the thalamus and tie the cerebrum to the endocrine system through the pituitary gland. The hypothalamus also interconnects the cerebrum with the primitive emotional brain and through its downwards connection to the autonomic nervous system regulates systems which adjust life-maintaining functions such as breathing, heart rate, and temperature control during variations in behavior.

Both the cerebrum and the hypothalamus-brainstem (containing the autonomic nervous system) are indispensable to independent survival but in different ways. The autonomic nervous system, sometimes called the vegetative nervous system regulates the body's internal stability. It maintains body temperature, links the brain to the endocrine system, and even if separated from the cerebrum, it independently can maintain normal function in temperature regulation, the digestive tract, breathing, the cardiovascular system and even, to a degree, the body's immune system (Table).

Table

Autonomic (Vegetative) Functions of the Lower Brain

Endocrine balance

Stable body temperature

Sweating and shivering

Chewing, swallowing, digesting

Clearing waste by bladder and bowel

Automatic emotional expressions

Reflex limb-body movements

Circulation control

Breathing control

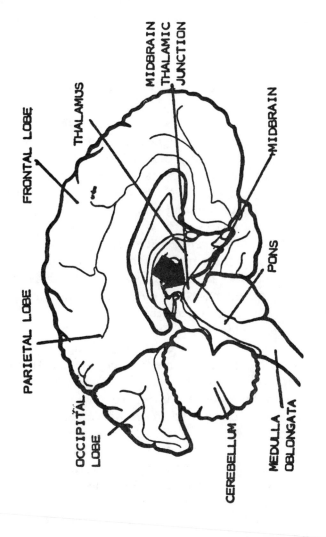

Fig. 2. A mid sagittal view of the human brain, simplified. The heavy black arrow marks the thalamic-mesencephalic junction, a region wherein lie structures critical for maintaining consciousness.

53

The vegetative nervous system is the body's automatic pilot; as long as caregivers supply food, water, cleansing and shelter, the vegetative nervous system can preserve the body's vitality indefinitely even if the cerebral cortex is totally and irreversibly damaged. By contrast, because respiratory, circulatory and digestive control would be lost, the cerebrum cannot long survive irreversible destruction of the brainstem even with the help of resuscitative machinery. Death of the brainstem is tantamount to brain death.

Brain Lesions and Altered Consciousness

Brief, reversible loss of arousal such as occurs with concussion or accompanies general anesthesia is not the concern of this discussion. What is our concern are prolonged losses of arousal, i.e., coma, that can last for days or weeks following severe injury or disease affecting any of several levels of the brain. Examples of coma-causing diseases include among others diffuse bilateral damage to the cerebral hemispheres such as occurs with examples of severe oxygen lack following cardiac arrest, head injury, certain strokes or tumors or, less often, brain infections such as acute encephalitis or meningitis. Prolonged coma is even more likely to follow damage to the general area where the deep midline structures of the thalamus join the upper brainstem.

The most frequent illnesses or injuries that cause prolonged coma or sustained unconsciousness do so by injuring the cerebral hemispheres and their immediately related deep nuclei. This part of the brain is much larger than the deep thalamus and brainstem, and it occupies a more exposed position to trauma, stroke and even infection, in part because it has more nerve cells and larger blood vessels. Furthermore, most patients in coma from severe damage to the brainstem die within a matter of days to weeks of their illness because of associated injury to the vegetative-autonomic nervous system. By contrast, most patients with injury to the cerebrum, if they survive the initial accident or specific disease, go on for long periods or indefinitely, no matter how severe their neurological disability may be. This principle applies even to those with extensive damage causing profound impairments of consciousness. Some cases in a persistent vegetative state have survived for more than 35 years!

It has already been mentioned that unarousable eyes-closed coma is never a permanent condition. It always gives way within days or a few weeks to at least some measure of cyclic wakefulness which then lasts as long as the patient survives. At this juncture, the psychological capacities of the reawakened brain become the critical elements in determining whether or not self-awareness and the capacity to make learned responses returns. Put another way, from the neurological point of view, mere wakefulness is not consciousness. Rather, it is the intellectual content of the awake state which represents the crucial dimension, for that determines the individual's personhood.

Prognosis in the Vegetative State

For some patients, the vegetative state consists of no more than a brief pause of improvement on the way to greater recovery, whereas in others it can remain unchanged indefinitely. The endpoint of the progressive, severe dementias is a vegetative state from which medicine knows that no turning back ever occurs. More difficult is the task of predicting the eventual outcome of patients who awaken but express no conscious behavior after an episode of acute coma caused, for example, by cardiac arrest or head trauma. The central question in these instances for doctor and family alike focuses on whether or not there is any way to predict whether or when meaningful improvement eventually will occur.

Several population studies have tested methods to estimate prognosis in patients in acute coma. The largest analyses come from two international working groups, one headed by neurosurgeons in Glasgow, Scotland, the other by our team in New York (4, 5, 6). These surveys found that within a few days after the onset of acute coma caused by head injury or medical illness such as cardiac arrest, one could identify some patients in whom it was possible to predict with a high degree of accuracy whether they would make an intellectually and physically independent recovery or would remain permanently disabled or die. Prognosis was especially poor in patients with signs of severe lower brainstem damage. In comatose patients who retained relatively normal brainstem function, however, it proved difficult to determine whether they would survive with only a moderate degree of neurological disability or would become indefinitely vegetative. In those situations, only the duration of unconsciousness served as a highly probable, i.e., better than 100 to 1 guide to the future, and this meant delivering maximum treatment while one waited out the early recovery period.

Most chronic vegetative patients survive because their brainstems and autonomic nervous systems are almost completely spared. For this reason, some may look comparatively well within the first few days after the onset of coma only to remain in their original vegetative condition indefinitely. Others initially look to be so badly injured that one cannot predict reliably whether they will survive or die. In the latter instances, a few recover but many of the others improve only to the point where brainstem function becomes relatively intact but they go no further. Either way, the longer the vegetative state lasts, the worse becomes the prognosis. Initially, in a relatively small group of 25 vegetative patients, unconscious principally after cardiac arrest, Dr. David Levy and I found that among those who were still unresponsive at the end of one month, only two regained even a fragment of verbal consciousness between the first and sixth months; neither retained those verbal capacities for more than a day or so after which they re-entered a state of permanent unconsciousness (7).

Long term studies on recovery from the vegetative state involving larger numbers of patients than the above confirm that it is uncommon to recover self-recognition after a vegetative period lasting three months and extremely rare to recover consciousness after six months (8, 9). Anecdotal reports of exceptions with later recovery of consciousness exist (10–14). Some of these patients may have entered an unrecognized locked-in state shortly after awakening from coma, but in at least a few instances continued unconsciousness was closely observed and well documented. Their late recoveries even though very limited in degree stand as puzzling exceptions to the overwhelmingly more frequent course of the chronic vegetative state.

How is one to act medically in the face of this knowledge? Progress in clinical and laboratory evaluations should eliminate errors in misdiagnosing locked-in patients. Furthermore, it must be recognized that regaining consciousness after 6 months in a vegetative state probably occurs less than once in a hundred cases and beyond 12 months, almost never. Sasbon (15), for example, whose hospital cares for every patient in Israel in sustained coma, noted that among 176 vegetative patients only 3 recovered consciousness between 6 and 12 months and none thereafter. Those who did recover were younger than 45 years and all were head trauma victims. Furthermore, all whose condition was described suffered from severe, incapacitating permanent neurologic disabilities. Such experiences combined with our own contacts with well over 100 patients have led us to counsel the families of all but the very young that by 6 months of the vegetative state, the chance of making an independent recovery is considerably less than one percent, and after a year it becomes practically nil. Even so, some of those who have been injured by head trauma or cardiac arrest may survive in the vegetative state for many years.

To summarize this section on prognosis and the vegetative state: International experience indicates that few such patients recover independent self-awareness after a six months' period of unconsciousness. Nevertheless, the remote possibility of improvement between 6–12 months, especially in persons under the age of twenty-five years means that prediction of a permanent vegetative state is necessarily probabilistic within this time frame. In advising families and others, the physician takes into account not only the patient's age and degree of neurological disability, but especially the patient's wishes and his own knowledge of what degree of neurological recovery the individual's damaged brain is likely to allow under even the best of circumstances. The experience of awakening from the vegetative state to face a permanent locked-in condition has been so intolerable for some patients that they have repeatedly pleaded to be allowed to die rather than suffer such overwhelming imprisonment. To observe such suffering can be a deeply troubling experience for caregivers.

What are the feelings of patients in a vegetative state? The evidence is that since such cases have lost all evidence of self awareness, they cannot perceive, think or suffer. Two major facts support this inference. The first is anatomic. In every postmortem study so far conducted on patients dying following a sustained vegetative state, the brain has shown extensive bilateral damage to the cerebrum and to its deep activating structures or both. In all of these brains the centers that regulate self-aware feeling states have been destroyed. The second is biochemical. Levy and I, together with our Cornell associates used a positron emission tomographic (PET) camera to study glucose fuel consumption of the brain in a group of patients in the vegetative state; we compared the results with similar examinations performed on normals and locked-in patients (16). The normal brain, even in its resting state, consumes enormous amounts of glucose amounting to one fifth of that of the entire body in order to carry out its continuous sensory and mental activities and maintain the vitality of its supporting cells. Our studies on awake vegetative patients showed in every instance that cerebral glucose consumption had fallen to only about forty percent of normal. The level was so low, in fact, that it resembled what one finds in normals only under conditions of deep surgical anesthesia. Cerebral glucose uptake in locked-in patients, each of whom had structural damage to somewhat different parts of the brain, lay at an intermediate level between that of the normals and the vegetative patients.

The matter of suffering, of course, is of much greater concern for locked-in patients. Patients whose working consciousness is locked-in by paralysis rather than destroyed by extensive cerebral disease have characteristic clinical and laboratory findings which should lead the examiner to an accurate diagnosis. Furthermore, most of them develop coding systems, e.g., by blinking, grunting, etc. that clearly distinguish their ability to understand from the absence of any such learned responses in patients who are vegetative.

The prevalence of persons in a chronic or persistent vegetative state is large and growing, emphasizing the condition's social, economic and ethical importance. Epidemiological studies in Japan carried out more than a decade ago estimated the number of vegetative patients to be approximately 3,000 in Japan's population of 100 million (9). For the U.S.A., the number is almost certainly considerably larger because lengthening life expectancy and an absolute enlargement of our old age population greatly increases the risk of developing a disease-produced chronic vegetative state. Additionally, we have adopted intense medical and legal pressures to resuscitate essentially all hospitalized patients irrespective of the nature of underlying disease, their pre-existing brain capacity or our careful and well substantiated predictions of whether or not their brains ever can recover. These considerations mean that the problem of the chronic vegetative state will almost certainly grow in numbers and create increasing problems in the future. How to meet the medical, spiritual and social implications of this issue is a challenge that no thoughtful person can ignore.

References

1. President's Commission for the Study of Medicine and Biomedical and Behavioral Research. (1981) Defining Death. U.S. Government Printing Office, Washington, D.C.

2. Plum F, Posner JB. 1982, *The Diagnosis of Stupor and Coma*; FA Davis Co., Philadelphia, 3d Ed, revised.

3. Jennett B, Plum F. 1972, The persistent vegetative state: A syndrome in search of a name. *Lancet* 1:734–737.

4. Jennett B, Teasdale G, Braakman R et al. 1979, Neurosurg. 4:283–289.

5. Levy DE, Bates D, Caronna JJ, et al. 1981, Prognosis in non traumatic coma. Ann Int Med. 94:293–30.

6. Levy DE, Caronna JJ, Singer BH, et al. 1985, Predicting outcome from hypoxic-ischemic coma. *JAMA* 253:1420–1426.

7. Levy DE, Knill-Jones RP, Plum F. 1978, The vegetative state and its prognosis following non traumatic coma. *Ann NY Acad Sci* 315:293–306.

8. Sato S, Ueki K, Arai H, et al. 1978, Epidemiological survey of vegetative state patients in Tohoku District in Japan. *Neurolog Med-Chir* 18:141–145.

9. Higashi K, Sakata K, Hatano M, et al. 1977, Epidemiological studies on patients with a persistent vegetative state. *J Neurol Neurosurg Psychiat* 40:876–885.

10. Berrol S. 1986, Evolution of the vegetative state. *J Head Trauma Rehabilitation* 1:7–16.

11. Rosenberg GA, Johnson SF, Brenner RP. 1977, Recovery of cognition after prolonged vegetative state. *Ann Neurol* 2:167–168.

12. Higashiki D, Hatano M, Abiko S, et al. 1981, Five-year follow up of patients with persistent vegetative state. *J Neurol Neurosurg Psychiat* 44:552–554.

13. Snyder BD, Cranford RE, Rubens AB, et al. 1983, Delayed recovery from post anoxic persistent vegetative state. *Ann Neurol* 14:152.

14. Arts WFM, Van Dongen HR, Hof-Van Duin, Lammens E. 1985, Unexpected improvement after prolonged posttraumatic vegetative state. *J Neurol Neurosurg Psychiat* 48:1300–03.

15. Sazbon L. 1985, Prolonged coma. *Prog Clin Neurosci* 2:65–81.

16. Levy DE, Sidtis JJ, Rottenberg DA, et al. 1987, Differences in cerebral blood flow and glucose utilization in vegetative state versus locked-in patients. *Ann Neurol* 22:673–682.

Chapter 3

DOES THE BENEFIT OUTWEIGH THE BURDEN IN THE ARTIFICIAL PROVISION OF NUTRITION AND HYDRATION? TWO ANSWERS

I. An Affirmative Answer

Joseph Boyle, Ph.D.

I. Introduction: The Moral Context.

Within the framework of Catholic teaching about ordinary and extraordinary treatments, the question posed in your program is the central moral question to be answered concerning the artificial feeding and hydration of the comatose. For according to this teaching a treatment may morally be withheld or withdrawn only if it involves a grave or disproportionate burden; and a treatment will involve such a burden only if these burdens outweigh the benefits of treatment. Thus, an affirmative answer to our question implies that it is *not* permissible to withhold artificially provided nutrition and hydration from the severely and permanently comatose.

The teaching on ordinary and extraordinary treatments suggests the steps needed to answer our question: one must first identify the burdens of treatment. Then one must identify the benefits of treatment. And finally one must determine whether the benefits outweigh the burdens.

For brevity's sake, I will use the expression "withhold food" as shorthand for "withhold or withdraw artificially provided nutrition and hydration."

II. Outer Limits Which Frame the Analysis.

It is possible to withhold life sustaining treatment from a patient not in order to avoid the burdens of the treatment but in order to end the patient's life. This, no doubt, is why the identification of the burdens of treatment is so central to Catholic teaching on this matter: if one is not choosing to avoid the burdens of treatment, then presumptively one is withholding treatment in order to bring about death.[1] Clearly, this possibility arises in cases of withholding food from the comatose.

There are well known cases of withholding food for the sake of ending life, for example, the highly publicized cases of refusal of food to handicapped newborns. And there appear to be examples of such decisions concerning comatose patients.[2] In these cases considerations about the burdens of feeding and their proportion or disproportion to the benefits are not relevant to the decision. The focus instead is on the patient's debilitated condition, which, taken by itself, is considered sufficient reason for withholding food. The withholding of food can be relevant in these cases only because it ends a life judged better off over. That is intentional killing, even though by omission, by choosing not to do something.

Our question does not concern these cases, but they should be noted because the public discussion of withholding food surely includes them, and Catholic teaching on this issue should not approve them. Furthermore, these cases define one end of the spectrum of cases we must consider, namely, those clearly wrong because they involve intending the patient's death.

Some moralists think that withholding food necessarily is killing, that is, always is killing by starvation. This position is often based on the special role food has in sustaining life, and sometimes on the conviction that providing food is not medical treatment but normal human caring, and so in a category to which the teaching about extraordinary treatments does not properly apply.[3]

This position is too stringent. This can be seen in cases in which the patient is not comatose, and in which the mechanisms for feeding are very annoying or painful, or prevent a person's carrying out important final activities before dying. In such cases withholding food clearly can be done to avoid burdens, and these can be grave or disproportionate. Analogous situations can arise for the comatose. Imagine a comatose person who is dying and who will die very shortly with or without feeding; or a comatose patient who can be fed only by a very expensive procedure such as hyperalimentation, of for whom all the ways of providing food are medically unfeasible or who is no longer able to assimilate food.

So, not all cases of withholding food from the comatose are killing by starvation. And some of these surely are treatments involving disproportionate burdens, even if the treatments are not *medical* in the strictest sense.[4] So, there is a spectrum of cases here, from those that clearly are immoral to those in which the withholding of food is permissible.

III. The Burdens.

Burdens of treatment are undesirable aspects of treatment which can provide reason for foregoing it—factors like cost, pain, psychological repugnance, and interference with a person's liberty or inner life.[5] The burdens in the cases just mentioned are easy to see, as is their disproportion to the benefits of feeding. But they arise because of special factors of specific cases. The question before us, however, is whether there is *always* a disproportionate burden involved in providing food to the comatose. In other words, if all we are considering about a proposed action is that it is withholding food from a severely and permanently comatose patient, does *that* provide enough moral information to allow us to judge that there is a grave burden involved? This admittedly abstract way of characterizing the action in question is not artificially abstract since it focuses precisely on the moral question to be resolved. Withholding food from the permanently unconscious is what is being considered in our society, not withholding food from the unconscious only within more specifically defined circumstances.

What, then, are the burdens involved in feeding the comatose? First, it seems that there are no *experienced* burdens to the patient. For such things as pain, discomfort and psychological repugnance are not experienced by one who is in deep coma. If they are to be considered, then we must wonder how deep a coma must be for it to be considered profound, and why, if there are experienced burdens of feeding, there are not also experienced burdens of dying without food.

Burdens to a person are not limited to those the person can experience. So, perhaps there are burdens to comatose patients beyond those they experience. But it is difficult to say what they might be. Let us consider one such burden: the indignity of treatment. Surely, unconscious persons can suffer indignities, and, more generally, can be treated wrongfully. But it is difficult to see how medical and nursing care involving artificial feeding in themselves constitute indignities or other wrongful actions, or how such activities are any more likely to be indignities or wrongs than foregoing them would be. In short, burdens which the comatose suffer but do not experience remain somewhat speculative, and so should not factor in our analysis.

It remains that the chief burden in these cases must be the costs, broadly construed, of the efforts to provide food. There are the obvious dollar costs of the procedures for providing the food, of the food itself, and the time and effort of those who provide it. There is also the cost in time and effort of others involved, and more generally the use of resources for which there could be other good uses.

The costs of feeding are morally relevant; considering them need not be a low form of utilitarianism but rather a realistic recognition of the relation of costs to the whole set of obligations people have.

IV. The Benefits.

The primary benefit of feeding the comatose is that it keeps them alive. Many deny that this is in fact a benefit when there is no prospect of recovery or return to a sapient condition. However, keeping a person alive is generally a benefit, and one can block the application of the generality to the comatose only by making the dubious value judgment that these human lives are not worth sustaining. We cannot say, if we are to hold to the Church's antidualistic anthropology, that the life of a comatose person lacks value and dignity. For the biological life of a human person is not something apart from the person; the organic life of a human being is not something which has value only insofar as it makes possible other good things, but has inherent value as part of the human person.[6] So, we may not intentionally kill the comatose. But if this judgment is true, how are we to ground a judgment that sustaining that same life is not good?

I conclude that there is a benefit just in keeping someone alive. This conclusion establishes nothing about how great the benefit is, or how significant the burdens of achieving it must be before they become disproportionate.

Before considering that question, another benefit of feeding the comatose must be considered: namely, the benefit of caring for the comatose and maintaining solidarity with them. This consideration has been a major element in the debate about withholding food from the comatose, but it difficult to judge its exact importance.[7] I will try to clarify it.

First, caring for those who are weak and debilitated is generally a good thing to do. This value is distinct from the other goods which can be realized as outcomes of this care, as the work with the dying of Mother Theresa's sisters suggests. Frequently, the sisters can do little to help these dying patients except to be with them. Such care is important because it embodies the great goods of human friendship and solidarity.

Secondly, providing food is closely tied to elemental forms of human caring. Ordinary nursing care is one of these elemental forms. And providing food is integral to nursing care, and has important symbolic meaning in that context. So, providing food is generally a good thing to do, and, it would seem, is a bad to do only if it is harmful to the recipient, or incompatible with the ful-fillment of other exigent duties.

Thirdly, the condition of the permanently comatose does not justify treating them as if they were in an altogether special cate-gory. What seems to justify such a categorization is that the patient cannot *experience* any benefit from care. That is true, at least within this life. But it is a mistake to infer that the unconscious patient cannot be benefitted. As I noted above, unconscious pa-tients can suffer indignities and other wrongs. So, likewise, we must allow that they can be benefitted, particularly by actions un-dertaken to maintain and express their status as human. Further, even if it is impossible to demonstrate that unconscious persons benefit from the care they receive by being included within the bonds of human solidarity, there is surely a benefit to those who provide that care and to others within their communities. Maintain-ing such solidarity is not enjoyable, and the benefit would hardly show up in a utilitarian calculation of benefits and harms, except perhaps as a negative factor. But refusal to abandon the very debil-itated is surely a good thing for those who reach out to them in human friendship.

I conclude that maintaining solidarity with the comatose is a benefit of providing them with food.

V. Burdens and Benefits Compared.

So, there are benefits in feeding the comatose, and relevant burdens as well. How are we to compare them?

To begin, we might note that if the burdens, in this case the costs of feeding, were so high that accepting them would prevent caregivers from carrying out other exigent moral obligations, then they would be disproportionate to the benefits of keeping the co-matose alive and maintaining solidarity with them.

Obviously, this consideration will lead to different judgments in different circumstances. Still, it has straightforward application to families living in poverty and without access to some form of medical insurance or subsidized health care. For them the cost of feeding a comatose loved one might well be bankruptcy, or the use of funds needed to educate or feed the children. Presumably, such families would justly withhold feeding and other costly forms of care and do what they could by their own efforts to maintain solidarity with the comatose, and soon to be dying, relative.

Indeed, we have no difficulty thinking of poor societies which could not afford this kind of care for the comatose, and even for the elderly more generally. One thinks readily of primitive hunting and gathering societies in which the survival of the group necessitates the abandonment of the infirm elderly. Such a policy is surely tragic, but not necessarily immoral.

However, in social contexts within which such things as gastrostomies and nasogastric tubes are routinely used, the costs of feeding the comatose become disproportionate at a much higher level. Since these are the social contexts of the technologically advanced societies within which the decision to feed the comatose is likely to be an issue, the comparison of the costs and benefits of feeding the comatose should be addressed with their resources in mind. Even within this frame of reference there are likely to be circumstances in which some people cannot afford the treatment.

But the costs of feeding the comatose are not generally disproportionate within this social context. For the costs of inserting and maintaining a nasogastric tube, or of performing and maintaining a gastrostomy are not, by modern standards, expensive. Moreover, the cost of the food itself is not prohibitive, particularly in comparison to the costs of ordinary food. In fact, once the tube is inserted or the gastrostomy completed, the costs of feeding, in comparison to the overall costs of caring for a comatose patient, are small.[8] In short, what we need is some indication that the costs involved are in some significant way excessive, and they appear not to be, at least not generally.

Of course, the overall costs of medical and nursing care for the comatose can mount, and over time become very great. But it is not these overall costs which are at issue, but rather the costs of feeding. For if the costs we want to avoid are the overall costs of caring for the comatose, then what we really want is to stop caring for them. That is abandonment, something that is morally justifiable only under the most tragic and exigent conditions of human life—and surely not in the wealthy and technologically developed societies. Abandonment of a family member is something which we would not think even a poor family should do, and certainly something which families would have judged unthinkable when the best they could do for a very dependent relative was to provide that level of nursing care which they could muster at home.[9] Furthermore, if we withhold food from a comatose person because we have decided to abandon him or her, then it is hard to see how we are not intending that person's death: the other costs of care will disappear only when the person dies, and so, it would seem, food is withheld because it will hasten death.

VI. Concluding Reflections: A Bad Precedent?

In short, we should accept the withholding of food from the comatose, or from other very debilitated persons, as morally legitimate only when that treatment involves a burden that is plain and plainly disproportionate. In the normal circumstances of life within societies where this is an issue, there is no disproportionate burden in feeding the comatose. There can be in particular cases, but that is because those cases involve other factors than the fact that the situation is one in which feeding the comatose is called for. If the only burden involved is the miserable condition of the patient, then what we propose is intentional killing; if the burden we choose to avoid is the overall cost of caring for the comatose, then what we propose is abandoning them, and, very likely, achieving the savings by causing their death by starvation.

Needless to say, the social acceptance of the abandonment of the comatose would be a great victory for the cost cutting wing of the euthanasia movement. The rationale for abandonment is not and cannot plausibly be limited to the comatose, but necessarily has application to many other dependent persons. In fact, it applies more plausibly in those cases in which the patient can experience pain and misery. Furthermore, the category of the profoundly and permanently comatose, while perhaps conceptually clear enough, does not appear to be empirically well defined. In practice it is very difficult to identify those certainly in this category and those certainly outside it.[10]

These considerations are often overlooked by those, including Germain Grisez and myself a decade ago, who try to test the fairness of withholding food from the comatose by asking whether one would object to having food withheld from oneself if one were permanently comatose, and concluding that one would not object.[11] Our answer was much too fast: We ignored the fact that this answer put us into a much larger and less well defined class of people than we supposed, and so put many weak people at risk; that we were endorsing a brutal precedent for abandoning the weak; that the burdens we would have imposed on others by objecting were relatively insignificant; and that we were hypothetically rejecting a kind of human care which human solidarity demands. In short, it now seems clear to me that appeal to thought experiments about what we all, or what reasonable persons, would want done to ourselves if we became permanently and deeply unconscious are much less decisive than moralists often believe.

NOTES

1. John R. Connery, SJ, "The Ethics of Withholding/Withdrawing Nutrition and Hydration," *Linacre Quarterly* 54 (1987), 22–23, puts this point particularly well: "When one withholds or withdraws a means to preserve life because it is too burdensome, his intention is to spare the patient the burden somehow involved in using these means. There is no intention of bringing on the death of the patient. Even if the patient lives (as in the Quinlan case), the goal is achieved. He or she is spared the burdensome means. But if one omits some means because of the patient's low quality of life, the intention is to bring the life of the patient to an end, since this is the only solution to the problem. Presumably, the patient's condition cannot be reversed, so the only solution is the death of the patient." Fr. Connery's analysis depends closely upon Pope Pius XII's classical modern statement of the doctrine of ordinary and extraordinary treatments; see "The Prolongation of Life," *The Pope Speaks* 4 (1958), pp. 393–398; (*AAS* 49, (1957), 1027–1033). Pius states that in the justified refusal to use a respirator, there is no question of the direct disposal of life or of euthanasia, but that the cessation of life is caused only indirectly and is covered by the principle of double effect and *voluntarium in causa*. The SCDF's "Statement on Euthanasia" June 26, 1980, makes unmistakable that euthanasia can be committed by omission. Euthanasia is defined as follows: "By euthanasia is understood an action or an omission which of itself or by intention causes death, in order that suffering may in this way be eliminated. Euthanasia's terms of reference, therefore, are to be found in the intention of the will and in the methods used."

2. The Brophy case is perhaps the clearest. See the discussions of it after the trial court denied the family's petition to withhold food in George Annas, "Do Feeding Tubes Have More Rights than Patients?" *The Hastings Center Reports* 16, 1 (February, 1986), 26–28, and John J. Paris, "When Burdens Outweigh Benefits," *The Hastings Center Reports* 16, 1 (February, 1986), 30–32. See also the summary of the final decision in Pat Milmoe McCarrick, "Withholding or Withdrawing Nutrition or Hydration," *Scope Note 7*, p. 5: according to McCarrick, the Court ruled "that Mr. Brophy's family could have the feeding tube disconnected so that he could die." See also Dennis Horan, "Hydration, Nutrition, and Euthanasia: Legal Reflections on the Role of Church Teaching," *Linacre Quarterly* 55, 4 (1988) 32–46, especially 42: "Although Catholic moralists have strongly denied this, what is occurring, in

fact, in cases such as *Jobes* and *Brophy* is the purposeful death-by-design of severely impared patients through the means of death by design."

3. Perhaps the best statement of this view is Gilbert Meilander, "On Removing Food and Water: Against the Stream," *The Hastings Center Report* 14, 6 (December, 1984), 11–13. Although I think his conclusions are in several ways overstated, Meilander raises starkly the question what the intent of withholding food from the unconscious could be if not an intent to end life. It should be noted that Meilander (at 13) qualifies his conclusion in the direction I recommend below in the next paragraph. See also, Patrick Derr, "Why Food and Fluids Can Never Be Denied," *The Hastings Center Reports* 16, 1 (February, 1986), 28–30.

4. See Connery, *op. cit.*, 19 for a similar judgment.

5. See Germain Grisez, "A Christian Ethics of Limiting Medical Treatment: Guidance for Patients, Proxy Decision Makers and Counselors," in F. Lescoe and R. Liptak, editors, *Pope John Paul II Lecture Series in Bioethics: Volume II: Bioethical Issues* (Pope John Paul II Bioethics Center: Cromwell CT, 1986), pp. 43–44.

6. See John Finnis, Joseph Boyle and Germain Grisez, *Nuclear Deterrence, Morality, and Realism* (Oxford, Oxford University Press, 1986), pp. 305–309 for a fuller statement of the argument that life is a good intrinsic to the person. See also *Euthanasia and Clinical Practice: Trends, principles and Alternatives,* The Report of a Working Party (The Linacre Centre: London, 1984), pp. 37–43.

7. See Meilander, *op. cit.*; Joanne Lynn and James Childress, "Must Patients Always be given Food and Water?" *The Hastings Center Reports* 13, 5 (October, 1983), 20–21; Peter J. Ausili, "Withholding or Withdrawing Artificial Nutrition and Hydration from Terminally Ill and Permanently Unconscious Patients: Some Recent Case Law and Contemporary Catholic Theology," *The Catholic Lawyer* 32 (1978), 55–87 provides a useful summary of recent discussions of this and the entire question of withholding food.

8. See Lynn and Childress, *op. cit.*, 18. There is surprisingly little discussion of the costs of feeding in the ethical literature. I believe this is because it is not the costs of feeding which most moralists regard as morally significant, but either the patient's bad prospects and debilitated condition or the overall costs of caring for the patient.

9. The only discussion of the relationship between withholding food and abandonment of which I am aware is William May et al, "Feeding and Hydrating the Permanently Unconscious and Other Vulnerable Person," *Issues in Law and Medicine* 3, 3 (Winter, 1987) 203–207. My argument on this point and throughout is dependent on this important statement. Paris, *op. cit.*, 31 discusses the cost of feeding Paul Brophy. He does not mention the cost of feeding but the over-all monthly cost of caring for Mr. Brophy. Ronald Cranford, "The Persistent Vegetative State: The Medical Reality (Getting the Facts Straight)," *The Hastings Center Report* 18, 1 (March 1988), 31–32 discusses costs, but, again, the overall costs of care, not the specific costs of feeding.

10. See Cranford, *op. cit.*, 26–31. Cranford details the bewildering linguistic complexities even within the scientific and medical communities, as well as the diagnostic and prognostic difficulties. Even if these difficulties are solved, the fact remains that the underlying neurological conditions related to permanent unconsciousness appear to form a continuum of conditions which make decisive categorization of many patients an unlikely prospect.

11. See Germain Grisez and Joseph M. Boyle Jr., *Life and Death With Liberty and Justice: A Contribution to the Euthanasia Debate* (Notre Dame: Notre Dame University Press, 1979), pp. 269–272.

II. The Case for the Removal of Nutrition and Hydration from Those in a Persistent Vegetative State

The Reverend Philip J. Boyle, O.P.

A vocal public sentiment has emerged within the United States that the provision of nutrition and hydration to a patient in a persistent vegetative state (PVS)[1] is not morally obligatory. Those holding this view do not see any point in doing anything, especially medical therapies for patients who cannot regain the capacity to be aware of their situation. No benefit seems to be derived by the patient from living in this condition. This sentiment has taken on public sanctioning with approval by professional associations such as the American Medical Association,[2] American Nursing Association,[3] and the American Dietetic Association.[4] Moreover, state courts, with a few exceptions,[5] have permitted the withdrawal of nutrition and hydration from PVS patients who are not in a dying condition. Thus, it is fair to say that a significant segment of the population believes that the withdrawal of nutrition and hydration from the PVS patients is permissible. This widespread sentiment rejects the position which maintains that benefit is derived from taking care of these individuals and there is not sufficient burden.[6] Thus we must ask: Do sufficient reasons exist for believing the burdens outweigh the benefits of providing nutrition and hydration to PVS patients?

The practical conclusion that no benefit and grave burdens exist is supported by different lines of reasoning. For example, some maintain that the PVS patients with only lower brain stem function are dead and thus withholding food is not killing them. Others maintain that while the patient is a human being, the patient is not necessarily a person and the holder of rights, and thus withholding nutrition and hydration is not the direct killing of an innocent person but the killing of a human which is permissible. Still others argue that the expressed wills of PVS patients justify removal of nutrition and hydration. Within the Roman Catholic tradition, a position which rejects the fact that any benefit exists can be found in the writings of Kevin O'Rourke, O.P. who, unlike others with his same practical conclusion,[7] sticks very closely to the teaching of the Church. Thus, I am primarily concerned with O'Rourke's position and the family of arguments which take seriously the received teaching on the removal of life-support.

Not surprisingly, positions for and against the removal of nutrition and hydration to PVS patients are in substantial agreement. Both affirm the Eternal law and Natural law norm proscribing the direct killing of the innocent. Both positions maintain that the burden/benefit ratio is central to the moral obligations because a disproportionate burden specifies that an action is not the direct killing of the innocent, but rather the avoidance of disproportionate burdens which a patient might legitimately forego. Thus, both acknowledge that under the Principle of Double Effect not all actions which hasten death are considered the direct killing of the innocent. Specifically applied to medical care, withholding, withdrawing or refusing medical treatment is permissible if the treatment can be shown to be either futile or disproportionately burdensome.

In addition, both positions set aside as less substantive but nonetheless the vexing question of who will make the decision. Both realize the inadequacies of forms of egoism which assert that the simple choice by the correct decisionmaker to remove nutrition and hydration makes it licit.

Both positions also broadly agree on the factual situation. Medical facts indicate that it is possible to identify classes of patients who, because of the duration of the persistent state and the underlying systemic illness, have a high probability of remaining unconscious.[8] Both agree that at times provision of nutrition and hydration are strictly and utterly physiologically futile or contraindicated: i.e., congestive heart failure and gross systems failure. Both also agree that a competent patient who indicates readily identifiable grave burdens along with little benefit of nutrition and hydration could refuse it.[9] For example, a competent patient with cancer whose esophageal tumor is obstructing eating and creating aspiration and discomfort, and where death is imminent, could consider this a disproportionate burden and legitimately forego nutrition and hydration.

Disagreement remains, however, with the case of PVS patients as to what constitutes burdens and benefits and from whose perspective this is judged. For PVS patients who are not consciously experiencing burdens or benefits, is it possible to identify sufficient reasons to forego nutrition and hydration?

Nutrition and Hydration are Ineffective and Excessively Burdensome

Broadly conceived the argument for withdrawing nutrition and hydration from PVS patients denies one of two arguments that are proposed by those who favor giving nutrition and hydration to PVS patients. First, O'Rourke insists that no benefit is derived from living in this state. Second, he insists that grave burdens exist.

More specifically, O'Rourke interprets the Catholic tradition and especially Pius XII as maintaining that the prolongation of life is not warranted if the means used prohibit one from attaining the spiritual purposes of one's life.[10] Pius states:

> But normally one is held to use only ordinary means— according to circumstances of persons, places, times and culture—that is to say, means that do not involve any grave burden for oneself or another. A more strict obligation would be too burdensome for most people and would render the attainment of the higher, more important good too difficult. Life, health, all temporal activities are in fact subordinated to spiritual ends. On the other hand, one is not forbidden to take more than the strictly necessary steps to preserve life and health, as long as he does not fail in some more serious duty.[11]

O'Rourke interprets this to mean that the purposes of medicine are all "subordinated to spiritual ends" of one's life. Thus, "anything that would make the attainment of the spiritual goal of life less secure or seriously difficult would be considered a grave burden and would be considered an optional or extraordinary means to prolong life."[12] O'Rourke has a different starting point, unlike his opponents' interpretation of Pius XII who assume that a list of burdens can be identified irrespective of why the burdens are morally relevant. Since O'Rourke interprets Pius XII as saying that it is possible to estimate burdens as anything which inhibits attainment of the spiritual ends of one's life, then in the case of a PVS patient a list of burdens is unnecessary in order to realize that it is simply impossible for a PVS patient who has no cognitive-affective function to meet the spiritual ends of life. PVS patients who will never again regain cognitive-affective function have lost their ability to meet the spiritual ends of their life such as loving God and neighbor.[13]

Thus, the starting points for positions for and against are critical. Those favoring the provision of nutrition and hydration for PVS patients need a theory of estimating the burdens. On the other hand, O'Rourke does not need to estimate the burdens. With PVS patients it is simply impossible to meet the spiritual ends of one's life. Thus, nutrition and hydration are not burdensome, but ineffective.

The obligation not to take ineffective therapies is found in the Tradition and grounded in reason. No one is obliged to use useless remedies (*nemo ad inutile tenetur*). Even if something is in someway effective, it is not obligatory unless it offers a reasonable hope of checking or curing the disease.[14] Thus, Gerald Kelly citing Cardinal DeLugo deemed food and water morally dispensable.[15] For example, if a prisoner were unjustly condemned and sealed in a room to die but given a plate of food, the prisoner would not be obliged to stave off death because one need not prolong the inevitable. Moreover, justice demands that people not pursue ineffective endeavors or waste precious resources. Any person who has voluntary control of some resource, be it materials or manpower ought not to squander the resource, because in fairness that same person would not want others to use the like materials, time and talent in ineffective pursuits, especially if the resources could be utilized. In short, fairness demands that we not waste our resources.

O'Rourke's second argument maintains that grave burdens are present when providing nutrition and hydration to PVS patients. Ample fiscal evidence exists which shows that the cost of maintaining some PVS patients with nutrition and hydration by means of intravenous lines which require skilled nursing annually exceeds $100,000.[16] The total cost of care, the feeding with total parenteral nutrition, (TPN) itself being a sizable factor in this cost, far surpass the means of an average family and thus create excessive burdens. Thus, not only is the provision of nutrition and hydration ineffective, but also excessively burdensome. In cases where the PVS patient has a fatal pathology, such as the inability to swallow, the provider may, but is not obligated to, circumvent the pathology and to continue providing nutrition and hydration. In not circumventing the fatal pathology the provider is not directly killing the innocent but avoiding disproportionate burdens and letting the natural pathology take its course.

Several objections to this conclusion must be addressed. First, some argue that feeding PVS patients is not excessively burdensome. If feeding were burdensome because of cost, then fairness would demand that all patients in similar situation with similar cost should be abandoned. By and large, burdens are not placed on the family because normally the excessive cost of skilled nursing the PVS patients are absorbed by social mechanisms such as Medicaid. While at times it is permissible to abandon patients, such as in the case of triage, society's present situation is not one of extreme emergency and does not warrant abandoning PVS patients or others.

However, one need not consider the burdens from either the family's or society's perspective, but rather from the position of a reasonable person. Assuming for the moment that we know nothing about the wishes of any PVS patient, it is nonetheless possible to estimate that any person in this circumstance who stood not to gain by the situation and to create excessive cost for others, would find the cost of a skilled nursing facility burdensome. Common estimation of cost excessive of $100,000, a sizable portion from the TPN, is plausibly a grave burden. While positions for and against removal recognize steep costs to feed some PVS patients, those who favor nutrition and hydration estimate the burdens from society's perspective and conclude society cannot abandon these PVS patients. On the other hand, the position favoring removal estimates the burdens from the perspective of the reasonable person would find the cost excessive and legitimate to forego.

Second, those who favor feeding suggest that no disproportion exists because while there may be burdens, benefits to feeding PVS patients can be identified. Not only is there no direct intention to kill the innocent, but the family also receives benefit in their charitable caring for the patient. Thus considering these benefits and even with certain burdens, nonetheless disproportionate burdens are not present.

Suggesting that benefits exist for the patient is troublesome. Surely it is a benefit not to kill the innocent; however, this begs the question. If the entire argument about the withdrawal of nutrition and hydration is to determine whether this action is killing the innocent, then it is inappropriate to assume what is not yet proven. More importantly, if we too hastily adopt a position that withholding nutrition and hydration from PVS patients is direct killing, and if our argument is flawed, this could inadvertently help pro-euthanasia forces.[17] Those who favor euthanasia see no benefit to feeding PVS patients and if they show that the Catholic position is weak, we might unwisely promote public policy which we would find deplorable.

Charity is arguably another of the benefits. From a common estimation, most people who had nothing to gain and at the same time would have their bodies subjected to bodily invasions and physical indignities would find this charity questionable. More dubious is the suggestion that provision of nutrition and hydration to PVS patients is charity, hence a benefit to caregivers. However, when a family decides to take care of a patient who neither experiences any physiological or spiritual benefit, and at the same time the family is foregoing taking care of other real social needs, then this is not charity. When a family foregoes obligations of justice to others and pursues something that is essentially ineffective this is a misuse of resources and an injustice, not charity.

Finally, when one assumes at the beginning that any treatment of a PVS patient is ineffective to meet the spiritual ends of the patients life, that is, no benefit to this end whatsoever, then any burden could be considered excessive to the reasonable patient. Any amount of burden compared to ineffective means must be considered disproportionate.

While neither side of the debate would deny that the therapy from a physiological perspective is effective insofar as it keeps the person alive, all the same it seems debatable to equate effectiveness with benefit.[18] At least from the perspective of the patient, while nutrition and hydration is physiologically effective in keeping the person alive, nevertheless it is not beneficial to pursuing the spiritual purposes of life.

In conclusion, several points must be reviewed. First, the different starting points of interpreting Pius XII's statement on life-sustaining treatment must be acknowledged. While both sides would agree that life and health are subordinate to the spiritual ends of one's life, those favoring provision of nutrition and hydration would first enumerate a list of burdens and why they are morally relevant. O'Rourke on the other hand, views it is impossible to meet the spiritual ends of one's life in this PVS condition, hence the distinction between the burdens and why they are morally relevant is irrelevant. PVS patients by definition would find any therapy ineffective to meet the spiritual ends of their lives.

Secondly, not even considering the burdens from the family's or society's perspective, it is still possible to estimate that any reasonable person would find that when there is no benefit to be gained and while the costs are perceived as excessive, then anything is considered disproportionate. Interestingly, those favoring feeding seem to assume that the burdens and benefits are from the perspective of the family or the society. However, the position to remove costly intravenous feeding from PVS patients is patient centered. The benefits are not experienced by the patient. As well, any reasonable patient who stood to gain nothing but to create excessive cost in the process would be presumed in fairness not to want the hydration and nutrition.

Finally, the case for withholding nutrition and hydration from the PVS patients is plausible in some cases when one accepts that the means are ineffective and costly as in the provision though intravenous feeding administered by skilled nursing. This interpretation seems consistent with an interpretation of Pius XII and the tradition. This admission must be realistic that a tide of disrespect for life is a real threat. All have an obligation to stand clearly against any initiative which undermines respect for human life. Nonetheless, any hasty move to public policy which does not take account of accurate facts and fit squarely with the rich tradition of moral theology within the Catholic Church must be criticized.

NOTES

1. Fred Plum and Jerome Posner, *The Diagnosis of Stupor and Coma*, Second Edition, F.A. Davis: (Philadelphia, 1982), p. 6.

2. American Medical Association Council on Ethics and Judicial Affairs, (March 15, 1985).

3. American Nurses Association, Committee on Ethics, "Guidelines on Withdrawing or Withholding Food and Fluid," (January 1988).

4. American Dietetic Association, "Position of the American Dietetic Association: Issues in Feeding the Terminally Ill Adult," *Journal of the American Dietetic Association* 87 (1987): 78–85.

5. Nancy Beth Cruzan v. Robert Harmon, 760 S.W. 2nd 408 (Mo. banc. 1988).

6. "Feeding and Hydrating the Permanently Unconscious and Other Vulnerable Persons," *The Healing Ethic* 1 (Winter 1987): 2–6.

7. Thomas Shannon and James Walter, "The PVS Patient and the Foregoing/Withdrawing of Medical Nutrition and Hydration," *Theological Studies* 48 (1988): 623–47.

8. Ronald E. Cranford, "The Persistent Vegetative State: The Medical Reality (Getting the Facts Straight)," *Hastings Center Report* 10 (Feb/March 1988): 26–47.

9. Mark Siegler, and Alan Weisbard, "Against the Emerging Stream: Should Fluids and Nutritional Support Be Discontinued?" *Archives of Internal Medicine* 145 (1985): 129–31; Joanne Lynn, and James Childress, "Must Patients Always be Given Food and Water?" *Hastings Center Report* 13 (1983): 17–21.

10. Kevin O'Rourke, "Evolution of Church Teaching on Prolonging Life," *Health Progress* (January/February 1988): 28–35, esp. 32.

11. Pope Pius XII, "The Prolongation of Human Life," (November 24, 1957) *The Pope Speaks* 4 (1958): 393–398.

12. O'Rourke, Op. cit.

13. Kevin O'Rourke, "The A.M.A. Statement on Tube Feeding: An Ethical Analysis," *America* 155 (1986): 321–4; "Withholding or Withdrawing Life Prolonging Medical Treatment," *The Medical-Moral Newsletter* 23 (29–31; "Nancy Beth Cruzan Revisited," *Ethical Issues in Health Care* 10 (November 1988); With Philip Boyle and Larry King, "The Brophy Case: The Use of Artificial Hydration and Nutrition," *The Linacre Quarterly* 54 (1987): 63–72.

14. John Paris, "When Burdens of Feeding' Outweigh Benefits," *Hastings Center Report* 16 (February 1986): 30–2.

15. Gerald Kelly, "The Duty to Preserve Life," *Theological Studies* 11 (1950): 203–20.

16. Total parenteral nutrition (TPN) is administered through a central line into the subclavian vein. A patient on TPN receives two bottles of dextrose and one bottle of intra-lipid solution daily. The manufacturers costs for dextrose solution is approximately $4. per bottle, however, manufacturers charge hospitals approximately $115. per bottle for dextrose and $40 for the intra-lipid solution. The hospital charges the patient approximately $640. per day which is not inclusive of dressings and vitamins. When the patient returns home with TPN, the average monthly cost for TPN is $10,000, not including nursing services. Thus, the provision of TPN alone could be considered excessive.

17. Michael Place, "The End of Human Life: Ethical and Public Policy Questions," *Chicago Studies* 27 (1988): 257–70. Place, while admitting that it may be permissible to withhold nutrition and hydration, offers two cautions for public policy. Such a policy might be a source of confusion and widespread abuse, as well as a "slippery slope" argument favoring euthanasia.

18. Al Jonsen, "What is Extraordinary Life Support?" *Western Journal of Medicine* (Sept 1984): 358–63.

Chapter 4

PASTORAL CONCERNS ARTIFICIAL
NUTRITION AND HYDRATION—I

BISHOP: Dr. Plum, I was not sure where it was in your talk, but my table would appreciate if you could clarify for us the medical definition of a human person.

We thought that you put that together with the state of consciousness and, at least I understood that the person in the vegetative state was not conscious. So could you please comment on that?

Dr. Plum: [Item 1] I hope I correctly understand your question. I know of no medical definition of a person, although some members of the legal profession have attempted to define personhood in terms of consciousness. It seems to me that much of what we are discussing here centers on the ethical and moral dimensions of what can be considered personhood. Biologists regard human beings as persons, distinguishing them from other members of the animal kingdom which are not regarded as persons. Lawyers regard all living human beings as possessing the constitutional rights of personhood, whatever their mental status. The question we are asking today is a spiritual one: are we to consider a body which contains a brain that operates at no higher a level than that of primitive members of the vertebrate kingdom to be comparable to one which possesses a normal working human brain? Or do we believe that some element of personhood has been taken away from the brain as a result of disease? I don't know the answer to those questions. Personhood, I think, lacks precise biological definition and may mean different things to different individuals, according to their backgrounds.

BISHOP: I think the problem we had was precisely whether, from the medical point of view, in that third stage, which you were describing as permanent there was a possibility to restore consciousness.

DR. PLUM: [Item 2] Thank you. Let me turn to that question. What I said was that brain death is absolute, and that prognosis in the vegetative state is probabilistic, i.e. has an unavoidable element of uncertainty. The probabilities are overwhelmingly influenced by the extent and nature of the disease, the acute circumstance and how much time has elapsed since onset. When an unresponsive state exists that one knows to be associated with severe brain injury, the longer the unresponsiveness lasts, the less likely becomes the chance of ultimate recovery. The best statistics on this matter that I have been able to find, and I believe I know most or all of those that have been published, indicate that one should wait at least 6 months before predicting that the condition approaches hopelessness. Between six and twelve months of continued unresponsiveness, the probabilities of any recovery decline further. Youth and head trauma are factors influencing a favorable outcome. Conversely, age or cardiac arrest producing severe brain anoxia are factors which unfavorably influence prognosis. In making or maintaining the diagnosis of the vegetative state, we change a patient's category to "severe disability" if they succeed in saying as little as a single intelligible word. We must err, if at all, on trying to find favorable signs.

BISHOP: Doctor, could I pick upon that last remark of your erring on the side of generosity. I don't think that for us, permanent vegetative state is the determinant whether or not there's a person, but that's not what I'm asking. I'm asking about the identification of permanent vegetative state. I've been told that in the

Nancy Ellen Jobes case in New Jersey, you testified that she was in a permanent vegetative state.

I've also been told that two prominent neurologists, Dr. Allan Ropper of Harvard and Dr. Maurice Victor of Case Western Reserve, who, I've been told, has written a standard text in the field—Both testified that she was not in a permanent vegetative state.

Now, I guess I'm a layman here. Is the problem there a different definition of permanent, vegetative state? Is the problem that the criterion that were being looked at were different? Is the problem a difference in interpretation of criteria? Obviously, it was a matter of great significance in terms of a Court decision on this. And I'm really asking how much division is there in the field of experts on this and what is the significance of that with regard to recommendations to a Court?

DR. PLUM: [Item 3] I use the term "persistent," not "permanent," because of the probability issue. The testimony in the Jobes case was given after a period of approximately four and a half years of unresponsiveness on the part of Mrs. Jobes. Some would justifiably call that permanent, but all would recognize it as persistent. And in repeated medical examinations by people other than myself, prior to my seeing her, no medical professional was able to discern in Mrs. Jobes any glimmer of either a consistent or a recognizable form of learning or learned behavior or purposeful behavior in response to stimuli. Similarly, neither my close and experienced associate, Dr. David Levy, nor I were able to obtain any sign that she understood our words or actions or that she carried out any learned behavior. Since I wasn't present at the bedside when either Drs. Ropper or Victor examined the patient, I can only tell you what I read from the record. As I read the cross questioning at the trial itself, the responses of the doctors were sufficiently inconsistent that the Judge apparently considered their appraisal less reliable than my own. As all of us know, for better or worse doctors have feelings and these sometimes influence their otherwise dispassionate decisions. What all the things were that lay behind Ropper and Victor's considerations, I am not able to say. Other cases with similar disabilities have received conflicting diagnoses from well experienced medical experts. Medicine is not absolute when it lacks the findings of instruments to buttress its opinions. We did not have the good fortune of having performed a PET scan on Mrs. Jobes, but clinically she didn't look any different to us from any of the patients on whom we did do such scans with the results I reported today.

BISHOP: Doctor, I think you have said very wisely that it isn't in the realm of the medical profession or the field of biology in general to define what is a human person. In point of fact, though, most people in the field probably do have a definition. I think that's one of those things that works behind the scenes. It's difficult to verify. When investigators such as yourself set out in your research, you try to be as scrupulously scientific as possible. But it appears to me that, in point of fact, there probably are biases and probably clinicians and researchers do have a vision of the human person, his dignity and his destiny. Would you comment on that?

DR. PLUM: [Item 4] As a physician, my responsibility is twofold: one, to do everything possible to maintain the life of the individual; the other, to do everything possible to relieve pain and suffering. Physicians sometimes differ in the degree to which they feel they must make their entire commitment to a particular individual as opposed to spreading that responsibility somewhat so as to consider also the needs of those with whom the patient shares the available resources that can be devoted to medical care. That sharing extends to the patient's family, who are participants in the suffering that takes place in association with any serious disease. I think I've given my own philosophy, which can be stated this way: You and I are equipped with this unbelievably creative instrument, the thinking, sensing, realizing, feeling and, above all, giving and loving, brain. But if you reduce my brain to the level of that possessed by a bird, which is what the autonomic system is, then I think my essential humanity will have departed my residual body.

BISHOP: Doctor, for the patient appropriately diagnosed in the persistent vegetative state, and let's take the case of beyond the six months, where the probabilities are that there will not be any recovery. Number one, is there a way to progressively recheck the diagnosis? In other words, is the PET scan used progressively after that time to see if there's any further deterioration and can we measure further deterioration? Number two, and if we can measure further deterioration, at the present moment, is there enough of a bank of knowledge, that is, cases having been tested in this way, that you can conclude that the person appropriately diagnosed in the persistent vegetative state is, in fact, continually deteriorating despite anything? Now, what I would like to separate from this would be patients with some other pathology such as cancer or some other problem.

DR. PLUM: [Item 5] My answer, Bishop, is twofold. First, one can only assume brain worsening under circumstances where the brain is subject to a continuing disease process or to recurrent injury. Recurrent injury, for example, would be successive strokes adding onto the damage which had already taken place; a continuing process would be one of the several brain diseases such as malignant tumors which eventually can wipe out cerebral function.

Most instances, however, that would be under our consideration at present as causing a vegetative state would not be suffering a progressive disease but would be the result of a single severe head injury or cardiac arrest. Those represent by far the largest number of cases in either Bryan Jennett's large surgical series or in our medical series. Such bodies survive indefinitely, until they die eventually of pneumonia, aging or some other systemic problem. They don't die of their brain damage, as such. Longevity records in such vegetative cases include the youngster who lived 37 years after an anesthetic accident with a tonsillectomy and a grown woman who survived vegetatively for 42 years following an anoxic injury. One usually cannot plot life expectancies of patients in the vegetative state once they've survived for even a few months and are receiving total nursing care.

I may not have been clear enough about the results of the PET studies on the vegetative state. By PET analysis, every vegetative patient had a rate of metabolism in the cerebral hemispheres so low that it meant that almost no nervous tissue was working at all. What little chemical turnover was going on reflected the activity of residual supporting systems made up of blood vessels, epithelial cells and non-thinking support cells called glia. The picture resembled that of very deep surgical anesthesia, which suppresses nearly all of the functions of the working brain so as to carry out the surgical procedure. No lower state of metabolism, death excepted, can possibly affect the brain's cerebral hemispheres.

BISHOP: Doctor, you mentioned when we began this session to me that you had some comments on Professor Boyle's remarks regarding the possible burdens to a comatose patient. I wonder if you would share those now and perhaps Prof. Boyle would care to respond.

DR. PLUM: [Item 6] It seems to me that we neglect two pertinent considerations when we face discussions of this kind. First, we are talking about a problem confined to the results of medicine in the modern age, a contemporary problem in the relationship of science and society. The increasing problem of persons whose bodies survive but whose brains have become mindless is a direct result of the product of advances in technology which at the same time have had the very beneficial effect of saving many self rewarding lives and of restoring many persons to good health.

Sometimes, these resuscitative measures cannot be performed rapidly enough to save the brain at the same time. It follows that a large proportion of what we're looking at are patients who are artificially restored by modern technology. Thirty years ago at least half and probably more of such patients would have died from the absence of resuscitative measures. In the early 50's I was responsible for establishing one of the very first of such resuscitative programs. My commitment has always been to save as many lives and as many brains as nature would allow. The troublesome part is that this approach sometimes has led to unwanted outcomes for which society had no precedent.

Another social consideration is that medical care has nowadays become a public, rather than a private responsibility. When I was young, I knew many families that brought a father, a mother, an uncle, a sister or even a badly damaged child home to be cared for, quietly and soberly, until they died a few days or months later. Such dying people, because of the public assignment of medical costs, no longer go home and they often survive in medical facilities a very long time. I'm thrilled that families no longer must face the financial burden of terminal illness, but I think that the family has been socially diminished by no longer "caring" for their dying loved ones. Let me, if I may, illustrate several categories of sociological costs that the current situation has produced.

First, chronically non-competent, hopelessly damaged persons create enormous placement problems for large metropolitan teaching hospitals, .because affordable nursing homes are filled and won't take totally dependent patients of the vegetative category. As a result, such patients divert precious, medically-needed attention from our nursing staff. At the New York Hospital, I have had my acute intensive care unit closed 30% of the time over the past year because we could not transfer chronic patients to nursing homes. As a result of this, we could not provide our best care to patients with diseases such as acute subarachnoid hemorrhage, acute meningitis, acute encephalitis, or acute stroke. Yet the care of this latter group is what the tertiary medical center is designed to carry out. Secondly, the indefinite survival of a body that does not think produces huge emotional as well as financial costs. The damaged body itself does not suffer, but its related families suffer inordinately. Whole families can disintegrate emotionally as the weeks pass into months and years and body-preserving treatment goes on and on with no goal other than mindless survival in sight.

The financial costs of vegetative patients are enormous. We are diverting critically needed medical support systems and medical financing to the treatment of those who have no sense of their own suffering and whose bodies have no hope of returning to the cognitive or intelligent enjoyment of life. The most recent Public Health estimates of the costs of the neurologically totally disabled in the U.S. equals over $35 billion per year. It almost certainly will be impossible to take these large costs from any source but the health care dollar. Societies make decisions as to what they are willing to devote to the social contract. We decide how much we will grant to Medicare costs, to Social Security, to education and to medical care. When medical care costs begin to approach or exceed 10% of the gross national product, the society gets its back up and demands reductions. These reductions only can come by taking from one program if we wish to expand another. Ultimately, this last step represents a qualitative decision as to which part of medical care we most wish to invest in.

DR. BOYLE: I think the issue that we face here is, in fact, the result of the developments of modern science and the developments of artificial things of various kinds that we all need in some way and want for those we love, and so on. My concern is that we should not allow the fact that what is going on is high-tech to overwhelm our moral sensibilities and allowing us to do things that are really contrary to the kind of human fellowship and human care which we should maintain for every human being, particularly those that are very debilitated. So the problem, as I see it, is in fact, caused by modern technology. We're happy to have it. I don't think there's anything wrong with things that are artificial. But it seems to me that we have to be careful that this environment, this social context, doesn't block us from seeing the requirements of elementary care for a dying person. It seems to me that feeding and nutrition are plausibly connected to the kind of care that we owe to everybody, that we would have given fifty years ago or thirty years ago when we brought a debilitated relative home.

And it seems to me that we need to deal with the cost problems, but we also need to deal with the fact that unless we're in social conditions that are much different and much more straitened than those we face, we shouldn't simply abandon those people who are comatose and weak. That's what we're concerned with. The issue of feeding and nutrition is part of a question of whether or not we're going to stick with these folks or whether we're going to abandon them.

We shouldn't abandon people. Maybe Eskimos, in the 18th Century, had to abandon their elderly. I don't think our society's in that situation. Now, it's true that this costs a lot. It's true that people in this condition shouldn't be in the most advanced hospital wards. But it seems to me we've got to face the question: are we stopping the feeding because we're abandoning these folks? And if that's what we're doing—and it seems like it might be and I'd like to hear some reaction to this—then I think we really need to think twice about this. We shouldn't simply take those who are dying and say goodbye, as long as we can stay with them.

BISHOP: We do have a law to love others as we love ourselves. In pursuing this, are we denying primary care to lots of people who would have these nurses available and the monies available through the public sector, through grants, medicare and so forth? How do we balance the concentration on this individual when, in doing so, we are depriving others of health care that would allow them to live years of productive life, both spiritually, socially, biologically?

DR. BOYLE: If I thought the alternative really was that we were not fulfilling other exigent health care responsibilities, then I would agree with you. I think these are decisions that have to be made socially and they have to be made in a very public and articulated way, argued out the way we're trying to do it today. I think that, in fact, issues of fairness may arise. But the other worry is that we're abandoning the weak by refusing to feed them. But it seems to me we need a rational policy. There are limits. We can't spend everything. But why pick out people to whom we publicly have a serious responsibility, at least to maintain solidarity with them and care for them?

BISHOP: I have difficulty with that word "abandon" and that should be always equated with allowing God's Will to be fulfilled here. You know, as another thing, I'm apprehensive about my own death but it is coming and I'm looking forward to it in that sense, to eternity. And I would like to get it when it comes, hopefully. Well, you know, to keep the person, or myself, alive for five years, postpone my eternity simply to keep alive and I'm talking simply about the food and water bit here, I have difficulty with that.

DR. BOYLE: Well, look, there are several things. I maintained in my talk that keeping someone alive is a benefit. It's a benefit, even when we're talking about somebody we know to be in a persistent vegetative state. They're unconscious and we believe on good scientific evidence they're going to be unconscious until they die. Now, I believe that there's a benefit there. For many of us, it's hard to see this benefit. It's hard to feel this benefit.

But it seems to me that this human being is a human life. Life is a good thing. I can't see how we can block that without accepting propositions that are incompatible with our view that the person and the human body are intimately connected.

That's one issue. The issue about abandonment, Bishop, is a somewhat different question. And this is where I went fast at the end. My view is this: that there's a prima facie obligation to maintain solidarity with people, to be with them, to keep caring for them. And by abandonment, I mean a situation in which you simply don't care at all for a person. You put them away from any sort of care. And what gets me to using that nasty word, and it is a nasty word, is precisely that it seems that the costs we're talking about aren't just the costs of a gastrostomy. They're not just the cost of an NG tube or the substances that are poured into somebody's stomach or something like that. The costs that we're talking about are the costs of what we normally think of as normal nursing care, which a family in less technological situations would provide itself.

Now, if we're withholding the food so that we don't have to care for that person so that life will be over and we don't have to care of them, it seems to me, although it is a loaded word, it is reasonably descriptive here. And if you judge that what we're doing is not abandoning the person, then it seems to me the case for withholding treatment in these cases becomes much stronger. But that's what worries me. In other words, what worries me is that we ought to care for people, even the very weak, people at death's door. But an awfully integral part of that caring is feeding and hydrating. And the feeding the hydrating themselves, as a part of the overall cost of care, don't seem to be that great. So, when we stop feeding, why are we stopping the feeding? Is it the cost just to the food or the gastrostomy? I think not. And, in fact, when people talk these figures of $100,000 a year or, $13,000 a month, that's what they seem to be talking about. And that's the worry. And, you know, I was asked to state the case as best I can. That's really the best I can say.

BISHOP: Would there be a difference if a person was conscious in this?

DR. BOYLE: Oh, yes.

BISHOP: And that he would say, take that away?

DR. BOYLE: It seems to me—the irony of this situation—that it's a lot more plausible for withdrawing fluids and artificial foods from a person who's conscious. I mean, you've got this thing going down your nose. You've got something that plausibly interfering with what you're doing and your life. So it's not my position that we may never withhold food and water artificially provided.

There are situations which we can do that. My position is this: Suppose that all we know about a patient's condition is that the person in question is unconscious; that person is deeply unconscious; that person is not dying but it's permanent; and that got to feed them via gastrostomy or an NG tube or something like that. If we know only that much about what's going on, does that give us reason for saying that there's a disproportionate burden here? I say 'NO!' I think you've got to get down to the cases and look for specific burdens. I don't think it's enough to say there's a burden just because the person's unconscious, etc. and what's being done is artificial provision of food.

Obviously, a competent person can refuse treatment. Whether we think that person is acting morally or immorally, we are obliged to honor that, to go back to the beginning of your question.

DR. PLUM: [Item 7] I thank you for mentioning what, as a technologist, I couldn't introduce to this group, which is that, for those who believe that there's an afterlife, and who have lost all chance of a meaningful life here, we're depriving them of that joyous afterlife by the endless prolongation of body without mind.

BISHOP: Perhaps more a comment than a question, but perhaps the Professor might comment on it. It seems to me, as I listen to this fascinating conversation that we should never lose the question of principle. And the question of principle is that we're talking about a non-dying person.

And if we remove nutrition and hydration, are we not introducing a new cause of death? There are instances where, because of any number of reasons, if the burden becomes greater and you make a decision to cease this because it is no longer in proper proportion. But constantly, it would seem to me, what we are arguing about or discussing now is, "Is there a principle?"

And I would submit the principle is that you cannot introduce a new cause of death. That there is no brain stem death, there is still life present, and if you cease this treatment, you introduce a new cause of death. Obviously, there are circumstances, individual cases. In a particular hospital, you may have the need of people who will have to make a decision to desist because they have to take care of somebody else. But the principle, I think, is the important thing that we should remember.

DR. BOYLE: First of all, the opinion you've expressed, Bishop, is a very strong component of the strongest rejection of the position that it's okay to discontinue artificial food from permanently unconscious people. I think we should not push that too hard. I hate to say the dreaded word. I talked to you a couple of years ago about this topic, which is *double effect,* and I think you're sailing into those troubled waters.

I would want to say that we can't say that in principle, when you withhold food and water and the person dies, even if strictly speaking, the person dies in the order of nature, as a result of withholding the food and water, that therefore you're guilty of intentionally killing the innocent. But I think that worry you express ought to be there. It ought to be on the table and the concerns of very many serious people are exactly along these lines. Gilbert Milander, who writes brilliantly in the same vein as your comment, quotes Daniel Callahan. Now, Callahan might overstate, and he's not advocating this, but this is Dan Callahan's observation. He says,

"A denial of nutrition may, in the long run, be the only way to make certain that a large number of biologically tenacious patients actually die." That's the worry, or that one big chunk of the worry and I think we ought to face it.

So I largely agree with your comment.

BISHOP: This is a question with three parts. And it starts with you, Father Boyle, but I don't know if the others might not want to comment also.

But first is this: You state the need to be patient-centered in dealing with the question. And my question is, what are the implications for society in making a decision concerning the quality of human life to give it basic support. In other words, if you're simply patient centered and don't take into account the implications of that decision for society, is that really a sufficient perspective to deal with the question?

Secondly, Dr. Plum mentioned the 12,000 cases in a permanent, persistent vegetative state, I believe, is that correct? In this country?

DR. PLUM: [Item 8] Yes, the best estimate. (N.B. Post conference estimates place the number much higher, perhaps 1.5 to 2 times as many.)

BISHOP: Do you have any data on that figure—as to how many of these were resuscitated by extraordinary means where they might have been a reasonable expectation that the result of that resuscitation would not have insured recovery and full brain function?

And the third is just simply the statement that came out of our table about the relativity of extraordinary and ordinary means. It's one thing if you're talking about a remote island hospital in the Philippines and a more complex medical center in Manila, for example. And that, it would seem to us, would be pertinent to the discussion.

FATHER BOYLE: With regard to the question about being patient centered, when I was asked to give this talk, I was asked to address from whose perspective are we going to judge the burden?

Now, there's a great debate whether or not the burden ought to be judged from the family's perspective, or from the society's perspective? This is rather troublesome because often the family is not necessarily an accurate judge; they don't know enough. There's reason to question whether or not the family sufficiently understands what the patient would find burdensome.

Secondly, there are questions of social utility from the society's perspective which are difficult to evaluate and might not think of life as rather important. One solution which looks neither to the family nor to society asks the question:

Would I want food and water? If I could say it of myself or I could universalize it, that would be what the reasonable person would want. So the questions about who is making the judgement, whether it is the family or is it the society do not have to be asked. I think you can, from the perspective of fairness and justice say, "I'm the person that's deciding." We could say it of all reasonable people in like circumstances.

The ramifications for quality of life judgement I can see are troublesome. But I think if the reasonable person standard was applied to quality of life judgement, I think it would be instructive. If we could universalize our decisions across the board, and that's all I was trying to do, then I think that would be instructive for quality of life. It would tell us when we're not at least acting patently unfairly.

DR. PLUM: [Item 9] The slippery slope issue is one that faces society everyday and demands our judicious attention and debate of many important topics besides the present one. To give an example, as a nation we recently have raised the highway speed limit from 55 to 65 mph to meet commercial demands, yet we know that doing so will cost 12,000 lives a year.

We do not, as a nation (nor do most Churches), choose conscientious objection rather than send our young men and women to fight and die in far corners of the world, whatever the political view might be about the worth or non-worth of that experience. The health care system already has acted to reduce care of many acute patients who enjoy a good prognosis but are forced to leave

90

hospital before their illnesses are fully treated. Nationwide, hospitals nowadays must meet a mandated process, called disease-related guidelines, which states that no matter how old or how sick, patients must leave within a certain number of days or the hospital itself must go unpaid. Each week, I send 15–20% of our still unwell patients out of the hospital before it is ideal for their health because Medicare will not reimburse us for the number of days necessary to take full care of that patient. Imagine what happens to our costs, which we cannot recover, when we have patients with hopeless prognoses and no capacity to think or humanly express themselves. Such problems in the long run necessarily face every one of us in this increasingly complex area of meeting the social needs of not only this country but other nations which lie beyond our borders. One thing I hate to see develop is a selfishly bipolar society divided between those who wish us to afford every possible entitlement for the elderly and those who will regard the educational, health and social needs of the young as the first imperative. In these matters, the Church can have a far greater influence than medicine, but by working together, I think we can succeed better than if either of us try to go it alone.

FATHER BOYLE: Could I respond as well to the relativity of means? One last point. Surely the relatively of means is important. Obviously, Dr. Tom Dooley over in Viet Nam could only do stone age medicine. You're not obligated to do that which is impossible. Nonetheless, simply to say that it's possible, we wouldn't want to get ourselves caught up in the technological imperative because we have the possibility now, therefore we must do it.

And this question I think is debatable, that which Joseph said earlier. Joseph thinks that because it's human life and should be respected and the like, he thinks you immediately fall into a dualist position by saying, we can keep these people alive and that's a benefit.

I will admit that feeding is physiologically effective; it's doing something. But that doesn't mean to say necessarily, that feeding is a benefit. Joseph seems to think that, if it's effective, it therefore must be a benefit.

I think that's debatable. I don't think that by saying it's not a benefit, I immediately fall into a dualist position that rejects human life.

MODERATOR: Now, it will be very frustrating to Dr. Boyle if I declare the hour of lunch to have arrived. But I'm not going to frustrate him. I'm going to allow him to respond to his brother because I think fair is fair and we can all recognize when it is that.

DR. BOYLE: I think the family feud may have begun. He hasn't called me Joseph for thirty years.

Chapter 5

THE RIGHT TO DIE MOVEMENT AND THE ARTIFICIAL PROVISION OF NUTRITION AND HYDRATION

Mrs. Rita Marker

In the thirteen years since passage of the first "living will" law in California[1] the "right to die" movement has clearly moved to open advocacy of death by fatal injection. We are now assured that it would be good to kill patients as is presently being done in Holland.

In April 1988 the World Federation of Right to Die Societies held its seventh international convention in San Francisco. That convention coincided with—and was geared to—a campaign to place the "Humane and Dignified Death Act" on the California ballot.

On the evening preceding the convention, during a debate on the Death Act,[2] its co-author, attorney Robert Risley of Americans Against Human Suffering explained, "What we want to do is change the law ever so slightly." (He was referring to California's living will law.) First he reminded the audience that it is now acceptable to remove food and water and thus cause death by starvation or dehydration. He then stated, "There is a better way." The "better way" proposed was the lethal injection.[3]

Although that first California attempt failed, Risley's organization and its alter ego, the appropriately named Hemlock Society, currently are concentrating efforts to enact the Death Act in Oregon, Washington, Florida and California in 1990.[4] The Death Act would enshrine "aid-in-dying"—death by lethal injection—as a right under the law. Just as the "right to privacy," first articulated in the *Griswold* contraceptive decision[5] and later expanded in the 1973 *Roe* and *Doe* abortion decisions,[6] has enabled the extinction of 1.5 million unborn children each year (4000 each day) so, without question, that same "right to privacy" is now being expanded to include the already born "unwanted" helplessly dependent in an ever widening circle of the unprotected.

I ask you to listen carefully to the following statement:

"If we can get people to accept the removal of all treatment and care—especially the removal of food and fluids—they will see what a painful way this is to die, and then, in the patient's best interest, they will accept the lethal injection."[7]

That statement was made in 1984 by a speaker at an international euthanasia convention. It seemed extreme at the time because, in 1984, it was universally presumed that care, including food, water, hygienic care, a warm bed and compassionate nursing was due every patient.

But today, after less than five years, a crucial shift has taken place. Framed as requests made in patient's best interests, courtsand legislatures are asked to release profoundly disabled individuals from what others view as a demeaning form of existence. The release mechanism, death by starvation and dehydration, is referred to as the "right to die."

Please make no mistake about the terms of the current debate. It is not about the "right to die." It is about the right to kill.

Cases reaching the courts do not deal with those for whom the provision of food and fluids is burdensome. They deal with profoundly disabled individuals, totally dependent upon others for care—individuals whom others consider better off dead.

These cases are about euthanasia, that act or omission of which death is the intended result.

The Church has always stated unequivocally that innocent human life may never be directly attacked. But now, in 1989, the Church is being asked to sanction death by starvation or dehydration for the profoundly disabled. This step, once taken, will lead to the next inescapable step—the lethal injection. Certain death, which occurs for all deprived of food and water, can be excruciating for the victims and for others involved, including care givers, who take part in the death watch.

Once it is decided that the patient must die, it is a given that the lethal injection is quicker and more efficient and, many would assert, more humane than days of waiting for the patient to die from lack of food and water.

If there is a constitutional "right" to cause death—whether by denial of food and water or by provision of lethal injection—how long will it be before it will be demanded that this "right" be exercised for those considered better off dead or too expensive to sustain?

In the time available to me I propose to review developments of the last five years that have brought us to the present moment. I will briefly examine three illustrative court cases as well as the role played in these developments by selected organizations, prominent individuals, and perceived "Catholic voices."

Three Illustrative Court Cases
Mary Hier

Is insertion of a gastrostomy tube (g-tube) highly invasive and highly risky? Or is it a minor medical procedure? The case of Mary Hier indicates the answer may depend upon one's social status.

92-year-old Mary Hier had lived in mental hospitals for more than half her life. She thought she was the Queen of England. She was not terminally ill but, because of a non-malignant defect (an esophageal lesion), she had received food by means of a gastrostomy tube for over ten years.

When, in an unexplained incident, that tube became dislodged, the care facility sought to replace the tube but her court appointed guardian refused permission. The court, agreeing with denial of permission, stated that implanting the tube was a "highly intrusive and highly risky procedure."[8]

Just as Mary Hier's case was being reported in a Boston newspaper, another story appeared in the same paper. It concerned a 94-year-old woman who was doing well following "minor surgery to correct a nutritional problem." The surgery was performed on an outpatient basis under local anesthesia.[9]

The woman's name? Rose Kennedy.

The minor surgery? Insertion of a gastrostomy tube.

For Mary Hier—elderly, demented and without family—it was described as "highly invasive and highly risky." For Rose Kennedy—matriarch of a rich and powerful family—it was a "minor medical procedure."

Last minute intervention by Massachusetts physician Joseph Stanton and attorney Robert Ledoux resulted in Mary Hier's tube being reinserted. And, at last report, Mary Hier continues to live comfortably and happily—still signing her name "Mary Hier, Queen of England."

Nancy Ellen Jobes

The second case, that of Nancy Ellen Jobes of New Jersey, exemplifies the lack of medical unanimity among experts testifying about the medical status of patients. Board certified neurologists often disagree as to the correct diagnosis and give conflicting testimony when describing the same patient.

In June 1987, the New Jersey Supreme Court upheld a lower-court ruling authorizing the removal of food and fluids and the consequent starvation and dehydration death of Nancy Ellen Jobes, 32, who had sustained severe brain injury in an anesthesia accident during surgery.

Shortly after a $900,000 malpractice settlement was made, Mrs. Jobes' husband requested that her food and fluids, provided to her by jejunostomy tube, be stopped.

Dr. Maurice Victor, a Board Certified neurologist, professor of neurology at Case Western Reserve and co-author of a leading neurology textbook, testified under oath that Mrs. Jobes was aware and responsive. He stated, "I gave her a number of verbal requests and it became apparent the patient could hear and understand what I was saying. I said, 'Pick up your head,' ... and within no more than one or two seconds she picked up her head ... I said 'Nancy, wiggle your toes' ... and ... she made a distinct, recognizable movement of the toes."[10]

Another expert witness, Dr. Allan Ropper—an associate professor of neurology at Harvard Medical School who maintains an active practice treating patients with severe head injury—testified that Mrs. Jobes could see and hear; respond to commands; make purposeful and volitional movements; could fatigue and could feel pain.[11]

Testimony of two other expert witnesses differed radically from that of Victor and Ropper.

Neurologist Henry Liss described Mrs. Jobes as a "monstrosity."[12] "She is not functioning," he said. "She is receiving the same kind of care that we would lavish on an experimental project in our laboratory to maintain something as in an animal we are working on ... "[13]

Even if Mrs. Jobes' brain damaged state were of a higher level than persistent vegetative state, Liss said, he would still recommend her feeding be stopped.[14]

Dr. Fred Plum, Director of Neurology at Cornell University Medical College, testified, "With good care, she is in such good medical condition that she could live indefinitely," but he also said he'd stop her feeding.[15]

Nancy Ellen Jobes died on Friday August 7, 1987—only days after her food and fluids were stopped.

Nancy Beth Cruzan

The third case, that of Nancy Beth Cruzan of Missouri, demonstrates that death is the intent in withdrawing food and fluids from severely disabled persons.

Nancy Beth Cruzan was left severely brain damaged after being injured in a one car accident on a lonely Missouri back road as she returned from work in January 1983.

She is receiving no unusual or heroic medical treatment and needs no life-support equipment. As long as she receives proper *care*, doctors say she could continue to live for another 30 or 40 years.

According to court testimony, Nancy Cruzan can hear[16]; she tracks (follows) people with her eyes[17]; she sometimes smiles in response to amusing stories[18]; she seems to try to form words[19]. She has, on occasion, wept after visitors have left.[20] She experiences pain.[21]

Because of her disabilities, she is totally dependent on others to meet her needs. Her condition has been extremely difficult for the family. According to psychologist Barbara Carter, "They've had a hard time finding their places again and can't get on with their recovery because Nancy's still here."[22]

Her family requested that her food and fluids be stopped so that death could occur.

Less than two months after her accident, when she was released from a rehab unit, Nancy had been eating by mouth. The record shows she ate mashed potatoes, link sausage, eggs, and bananas. She drank a glass of juice with each meal.[23]

She now receives food and fluids through a gastrostomy tube. According to court records, the tube was implanted in her stomach to make her long-term care easier.[24] (With this type of feeding, there is less risk of aspiration and less attendant time required.)

Her ability to swallow, however, does not seem to be an issue. One expert witness, Minnesota neurologist Ronald Cranford, testified he would consider even spoon-feeding Nancy Cruzan to be "medical treatment."[25]

Cranford explained there really isn't any definition about what "artificial" feeding is. Noting that "there is a legitimate difference of opinion concerning spoon feeding" and that most groups have not yet "addressed the question of spoon feeding," he said "... it is not fair to say that artificial feeding would only characterize what we call gastrostomy and so forth."[26]

Cranford said spoonfeeding is denied in cases like Ms. Cruzan's. He explained, "... when we've withdrawn the gastrostomy, we have deliberately not attempted to do any sort of syringe or spoon feeding...," because it "would be totally inconsistent" with what was wanted.[27]

What is wanted is death for Nancy Cruzan.

News coverage has made this abundantly clear. For example, one headline stated, "Family seeks peace after '5 years of hell'."[28] The *New York Times* said, "One day soon, perhaps in a month or two if all goes as the family and its lawyer have asked, the Cruzans may be released from an ordeal that has seemed more tormenting than an endless prison sentence... "[29]

On July 27, 1988, Circuit Court Judge Charles E. Teel, Jr. approved the withdrawal of Nancy Cruzan's food and fluids with the "inevitable attendant consequences of carrying out such an act."[30] However, Missouri's Attorney General appealed the case to the state supreme court. The high court overturned the lower court decision.

In its opinion, the Supreme Court of Missouri states:

[This is a] case in which euphemisms readily find their way to the fore, perhaps to soften the reality of what is really at stake. But this is not a case in which we are asked to let someone die. Nancy is not dead. Nor is she terminally ill. This is a case in which we are asked to allow the medical profession to make Nancy die by starvation and dehydration. The debate here is thus not between life and death; it is between quality of life and death.[31]

Dehumanization of Victims

Lessons from the abortion debate that provide valuable insight into the rhetoric of the euthanasia movement have gone largely unheeded.

Before one can jettison the natural impulse to care for and protect a dependent human being, a certain dehumanization of potential victims has to occur.

From the 23,000,000 human preborn children sacrificed under a "right to privacy" we know that carefully crafted words—"blobs of cells," "mass of tissue" and "products of conception"—were skillfully used to dehumanize the tiny victims. Few seem aware, however, that the same dehumanization of euthanasia victims is now taking place.

Profoundly disabled and dependent people are referred to as "vegetables" or the "biologically tenacious."[32] In an early 1988 edition of the *Hastings Center Report,* Paul Armstrong, attorney for the family of Nancy Ellen Jobes, referred to Mrs. Jobes and those like her as "nonmentative organ systems, artificially sustained like valued cell lines in cancer laboratories."[33]

Yet often the very people who declare unborn children and profoundly disabled individuals "non-persons" advocate abortion and euthanasia as being "rights" of the unborn and the disabled. We hear of the right of every child to be "wanted," and of the right of the disabled to "die with dignity."

Role of Organizations & "Catholic" Position

The present collapse and disorder of the traditional defense of human values was anticipated in a 1970 editorial in *California Medicine*:

> It will become necessary and acceptable to place relative rather than absolute values on such things as human lives...
>
> The process of eroding the old ethic and substituting the new has already begun...
>
> The very considerable semantic gymnastics which are required to rationalize abortion as anything but taking a human life *would be ludicrous if they were not often put forth under socially impeccable auspices*...
>
> One may anticipate further development... as the problems of birth control and birth selection are extended inevitably to death selection and death control... [34]
> (emphasis added)

The "socially impeccable" auspices under which euthanasia is now set forth—support from professional organizations, prominent individuals and officials of religious institutions—has placed society at the threshhold of death selection and death control.

As the Jobes case was wending its way up to the supreme court of the State of New Jersey, the American Medical Association (AMA) Judicial Council, composed of seven doctors, issued a revolutionary policy declaring for the first time that it is ethical for doctors to remove food and fluids from a comatose patient.[35] Even though Mrs. Jobes was not comatose, the policy was cited by the court in her case. Though the full membership of the AMA was never consulted on it, the policy has had a great influence in a succession of court cases.

Another radical change in position—that of the American Academy of Neurology (AAN)—occurred in early 1988. The position states that individuals in a persistent vegetative state are not terminally ill but that food and fluids can be stopped for such patients. As in the case of the AMA's policy, the AAN position was never approved by the membership at large but was adopted by its Executive Board.[36] And, as in the case of the AMA statement, it was released at a time when crucial arguments were taking place in the courts.

In fact, the AAN position was introduced on March 10, 1988, in the Nancy Cruzan hearing, five weeks *before* the AAN executive board officially approved it.[37] While the position paper has yet to be published in any scholarly journal it is being made available to the public by the Society for the Right to Die.[38]

Also in 1988, the prestigious *Journal of the American Medical Association* (JAMA) printed, without comment, an anonymous article in which a young resident related providing a morphine injection calculated to end the life of a 20-year-old cancer patient known only as "Debbie."[39] The ensuing discussion, prompted by this editorial trial balloon, placed death by lethal injection in a far more "respectable" position than it had previously held.

The following month the American Bar Association held a conference on euthanasia to explore the possibility of model legislation regarding the practice of active euthanasia. Chairperson for the workshop was Paul Armstrong.[40] Armstrong, who served as the attorney for the family of Nancy Ellen Jobes has explained that he approached his work "as a Catholic."[41]

The Ethicist, the Theologian
& the "Catholic Position"

In his paper, "The Return of Eugenics" Richard John Neuhaus declared

> Thousands of medical ethicists and bioethicists, as they are called, professionally guide the unthinkable on its passage through the debatable on its way to becoming the justifiable until it is finally established as the unexceptional.[42]

Among ethicists guiding the unthinkable on its way to the unexceptional are Daniel Callahan and David Thomasma.

Callahan, the former editor of *Commonweal* who is founder and director of the Hastings Center for bioethics, has written that it is the task of care givers "to determine when someone has lost the capacity for *meaningful* personal life"[43] and that the costs involved in caring for such individuals may lead to denial of Medicaid or Medicare payment for such care.[44]

In his recent book, *Setting Limits,* Callahan proposes a "natural life span" described as "a fitting span of life followed by a death that is relatively acceptable in its timeliness."[45] For those beyond this natural life span, which he explains "would normally be expected by the late 70s or early 80s"[46], medical care would be "limited to the relief of suffering."[47] This would indicate that, for the 78-year-old with appendicitis, pain relievers would be given but an appendectomy would be considered inappropriate since the person has lived out a "natural life span."

Callahan has long been on the "cutting edge" of medical ethics. In 1983 he wrote:

> ... a denial of nutrition may in the long run become the only effective way to make certain that a large number of biologically tenacious patients actually die. Given the increasingly large pool of superannuated, chronically ill, physically marginal elderly it could well become the nontreatment of choice."[48]

It is Callahan's Hastings Center that is now working in conjunction with the Prudential Foundation to establish community bioethics programs across the country. These programs are "to serve as a vehicle for the development of a new consensus on health policy priorities." The impact of these projects, according to the Hastings Center "may be felt on the national level."[49]

Hundreds of thousands of dollars have been and continue to be expended for "citizens committees" which will usher in "least common denominator" morality. Such committees will have a tremendous impact on legislative and judicial decisions and threaten to oversweep the authentic voice of the Church.

David Thomasma, director of medical humanities and chief ethicist at Loyola University Stritch School of Medicine (and, what few are aware of, a director of the Society for the Right to Die) is another widely published ethicist.

In his article, "The Range of Euthanasia," which appeared in the *Bulletin of the American College of Surgeons,* he called for a change in the goal of medicine, saying:

Medicine should aim at reconstructing life sufficiently to sustain other values.

When these human values can no longer be sustained because of the physical condition of the patient, than a decision should be made for euthanasia on the basis of the patient's or surrogate's request.[50]

According to Thomasma, "inducing or bringing about death is a virtuous and moral act, especially if it is done in conjunction with the wishes of the patient."[51]

In an article published by the Society for the Right to Die newsletter, Thomasma hailed the position taken by Bishop Louis E. Gelineau in the Marcia Gray case saying that the bishop's statement was "right on the mark." To prolong life that has no meaning, Thomasma said is "a form of idolatry."[52]

Thomasma's writing would not be as surprising nor would it be as influential if it came from the pen of a Joseph Fletcher but, coming from a professor at a Catholic medical center, there is a tendency on the part of many to view it as an authentic Catholic position.

The current Illinois case of Dorothy Longeway has furthered this type of perception. The 76-year-old Mrs. Longeway is severely disabled due to several strokes. According to her physician, she is not in a coma or a persistent vegetative state. In fact, she responds to painful stimuli and seems to obey verbal commands.[53] Her family has requested that her feeding be stopped.

Representing the family is Catholic Charities Legal Services for Seniors which, in its brief and argument presented to the court by Rev. Eugene Parnisari, noted that such actions "would likely create various effects resulting from lack of nutrition and hydration leading eventually to her death."[54]

The Catholic Charities brief acknowledges, thus, that Mrs. Longeway will die of starvation and dehydration but states that removing her feeding "would be in accord with the teaching of her [Catholic] Church."[55]

It is a fact of contemporary American life that those who wear Roman collars and purport to offer "new insights" into Catholic teaching make news. Jesuit Father John Paris, and Dominican Father Kevin O'Rourke have played a prominent role in the food and fluids debate.

Paris, an ethics professor at the College of the Holy Cross in Worcester, Massachusetts, who has appeared as an expert witness in a number of major food and fluids cases argues that it is morally wrong not to withhold food and fluids from certain patients. To maintain the lives of hopelessly ill patients, according to Paris, leaves them "in a state of suspended animation halfway between life and death."[56]

Father Kevin O'Rourke, O.P., the former director of Medical-Moral Affairs of the Catholic Hospital Association and current director of the Center for Health Care Ethics at St. Louis University Medical Center, publicly condemned a position taken by the New Jersey Catholic Conference.

Speaking at a Catholic Health Association conference in 1987, O'Rourke stated that the New Jersey bishops' brief in the case of Nancy Ellen Jobes "should not be taken seriously."[57]

In his writings, O'Rourke refers to those "whose spiritual function is irreparably lost."[58] "To pursue the spiritual purpose of life," he states, "one needs a minimal degree of cognitive-affective function. Therefore, it this function ... cannot be restored or will never develop" the person "may be allowed to die."[59] "Allowing to die," for O'Rourke, includes the denial of food and fluids.

His public criticism of briefs filed to protect life gave way to more aggressive opposition when his Center for Health Care Ethics took on the role of judicial lobbyist for the removal of food and fluids by filing an Amicus Curiae brief (along with the SSM Health Care System sponsored by the Franciscan Sisters of Mary) in the appeal of the Nancy Cruzan case.[60]

The brief which used the pejorative label "vitalism" to characterize those who favor providing nourishment to Ms. Cruzan[61] and stated that, if Nancy Cruzan continues to receive food and fluids, "she will be sentenced to what may be thirty more years of a vegetative existence, a life devoid of dignity, hope or purpose."[62]

The brief concludes with the statement:

> Regardless of the continued provision of nutrition and hydration, Nancy has no hope of improvement. Instead, she may be forced to live for several decades as a prisoner of medical technology, robbed of all human dignity.
> Amici urge this Court to uphold the decision to allow the Cruzans to exercise Nancy's right to refuse further nutrition and hydration so that Nancy may die a natural, peaceful death.[63]

A strikingly different stance was taken by noted medical-ethicist, Leon Kass of the University of Chicago, when interviewed recently on national public television. "I don't see how anyone can withhold food and water and say they are doing anything other than killing the patient," Kass declared.[64]

The late Dennis Horan, in his 1987 presentation before this group, stated, "Many Catholic moralists have not only ignored the public policy consequences of these decisions, but have also offered rationales for the withdrawal of nourishment that will further undermine the public policy against euthanasia."[65]

Regrettably his prediction has come true. Some of those described as "Catholic ethicists" have had a deadly impact on medical practice and patients.

The positions taken by Thomasma, O'Rourke, Paris and others discussed above—if viewed as reflective of authentic Catholic teaching—place at risk the very lives of all who are retarded, all who are demented, all who are in that particularly vulnerable zone currently known as "persistent vegetative state."

The fact that their positions and those who reflect the same viewpoint are widely carried in Catholic health publications suggests that this trend must be addressed. This is particularly important in view of the fact that the very carefully drafted statement on food and fluids—formulated by a committee chaired by Professor William May of Catholic University and signed by over one hundred theologians, ethicists and others, including Professor Mark Siegler, Germain Grisez, the late Paul Ramsey of Princeton, Rabbi David Novak, the late Dennis Horan, Arthur Dyck of Harvard, and Rev. Richard John Neuhaus—has received little or no mention in the same publications.

Summation and Reflections

A chain of events has been put into motion. As a result, we long ago passed any discussion of extraordinary, useless, burdensome or disproportionate treatment.

Episcopal statements that "the Magisterium of the Church has not yet issued a definitive statement regarding the moral necessity to provide nutrition and hydration artificially in *all* cases to the permanently unconscious patient" (emphasis added)[66] risk totally missing the point and the clear and present danger.

Now, as never before, clear thinking and clear speaking are necessary.

The question is not, "Is it always required to provide food and fluids to all people in all cases?" Nor is the question, "Must the dying process of the imminently dying patient be prolonged?"

Instead, the question is, "Do we continue to feed the disabled, the demented, the abandoned, and the unwanted who are not dying or do we certainly end their lives by the universally effective lethal measure of stopping food and water?"

The answer to this question will determine the direction of our society.

Will emphasis be placed on the inarguable case in which feeding is truly burdensome and not indicated? If so, this will be exactly what the euthanasia proponents want.

Or will you articulate the obligations we commonly share, in justice and in charity, to respect, to speak for, and to defend the life and dignity of every person?

In his classical writings on the Holocaust forty years ago, Leo Alexander, M.D., who served on the staff of the Office of the Chief Counsel for War Crimes in Nuremberg, wrote:

> Whatever proportions these crimes [the Nazi war crimes] finally assumed, it became evident to all who investigated them that they had started from small beginnings. The beginnings at first were merely a subtle shift in emphasis in the basic attitude of the physicians. It started with the acceptance of the attitude, basic in the euthanasia movement, that there is such a thing as life not worthy to be lived... Gradually the sphere of those to be included in this category was enlarged... But it is important to realize that the infinitely small wedged-in lever from which this entire trend of mind received its impetus was the attitude toward the non-rehabilitable sick.[67]

Do we continue to travel the road that ends with death-on-demand?

Or will we hear ringing opposition to euthanasia such as once delivered by a bishop in his Sunday homily when he stated simply:

> It is said of these patients: They are like an old machine which no longer runs, like a horse which is hopelessly paralyzed, like a cow which no longer gives milk.
> What do we do with a machine of this kind? We put it in the junkyard. What do we do with a paralyzed horse? No, I do not wish to push the comparison to the end... We are not talking about a machine, a horse, nor a car... we are talking about men and women, our compatriots, our brothers and sisters. Poor unproductive people if you wish, but does this mean they have lost their right to live?[68]

The homily was given by Clemens Count von Galen, Bishop of Munster, Germany August 3, 1941. It is just as applicable today.

NOTES

1. California Natural Death Act (1976), Cal. Health & Safety Code 7185–7195 (supp 1987).

2. " 'Aid-in-Dying': The Right to Die or the Right to Kill?," sponsored by the International Anti-Euthanasia Task Force, April 6, 1988, at the University of San Francisco, California.

Speakers were Derek Humphry of the National Hemlock Society, Robert Risley of Americans Against Human Suffering, Dr. Joseph Stanton, an advisor to the International Anti-Euthanasia Task Force and Rita Marker, Co-Director of the Human Life Center. Moderator was Michael Smith, professor of law at the University of California at Berkley. Video tapes and transcripts of the debate are available through the Human Life Center, University of Steubenville, Steubenville Ohio. Audio tapes are available from National Public Radio.

3. Ibid.

4. Derek Humphry, "Active Voluntary Euthanasia," *Free Inquiry,* Winter, 1988/89, p. 9.

5. *Griswold v Connecticut,* 381 U.S.479, 85 S.Ct.1678, 14 L.Ed2d 510 (1965).

6. *Roe v Wade,* 410 U.S.113, 93 S.Ct.705, 35 L.Ed.2d 147 (1973); *Doe v Bolton,* 410 U.S.179, 93 S.Ct.739, 35 L.Ed.2d 201 (1973).

7. Fifth Biennial Conference of the World Federation of Right to Die Societies; Nice, France; September 20–23, 1984. From "Ethics Panel: The Right to Choose Your Death— 'Ethical Aspects of Euthanasia.' " Remarks by panel member Helga Kuhse, Ph.D., lecturer in philosophy at Monash University and research fellow at the Center for Human Bio-Ethics in Melbourne, Australia, September 21, 1984.

8. Anne Bannon, M.D., "Rx: Death by Dehydration," *Human Life Review,* Vol. XII, No. 3, Summer, 1986, p. 74.

9. "Rose Kennedy 'doing well' after surgery," *The Boston Sunday Globe,* July 29, 1984, p. 35.

10. "Doctors Testify Morris Woman isn't Vegetative," *Star-Ledger,* April 2, 1986.

11. *In the Matter of Nancy Ellen Jobes,* Superior Court of New Jersey, Chancery Division—Morris County, Docket No. C-4971–65E, App. Div. No. A-4087–85T5, Stenographic Transcript of Trial, Morris County Courthouse, Morristown, New Jersey, April 1, 1986, pp. 8–14.

12. Ibid., March 24, 1986, p. 124.

13. Ibid., p. 118.

14. Ibid., p. 154.

15. Ibid., p. 74.

16. *Cruzan v Harmon and Lampkins,* In the Circuit Court of Jasper County, Missouri, Probate Division at Carthage, Case No.CV384–9P, March 9–11, 1988, p. 595. Hereafter cited as "Cruzan Transcript."

17. Ibid., p. 606.

18. Ibid., pp. 599–600.

19. Ibid., p. 653.

20. Ibid., pp. 644–645.

21. Ibid., pp. 600, 617–618, 643.

22. PBS "Frontline" presentation, "Let My Daughter Die," March 1, 1988.

23. Cruzan Transcript, pp. 281–285.

24. Ibid., p. 423.

25. Ibid., p. 228.

26. Ibid.

27. Ibid., pp. 229–230.

28. Jo Ellis, "Family seeks peace after '5 year of hell,'" *Joplin Globe*, December 1, 1987, p. 1.

29. William Robbins, "Another State Joins Right-to-Die Issue," *The New York Times*, November 25, 1987, p. 41.

30. *Cruzan vs. Harmon and Lamkins*, In the Circuit Court of Jasper County, Missouri, Probate Division at Carthage, Charles E. Teel, Jr., Judge, Estate No. CV384–9P. July 27, 1988, p. 6.

31. *Cruzan vs. Harmon and McCanse*, Supreme Court of Missouri, No. 70813, November 16, 1988, majority opinion, p. 6.

32. Daniel Callahan, "On Feeding the Dying," *The Hastings Center Report*, (October 1983), p. 22. Hereafter cited as "Callahan."

33. Paul W. Armstrong and B. D. Colen, "From Quinlan to Jobes: The Courts and the PVS Patient," *Hastings Center Report*, February/March 1988, p. 39.

34. Editorial, "A New Ethic for Medicine and Society," *California Medicine*, Vol. 113, No. 3, September 1970, p. 68.

35. "Feeding withdrawal gets conditional nod," *American Medical News*, March 28, 1986.

36. "Position of the American Academy of Neurology on Certain Aspects of the Care and Management of the Persistent Vegetative State Patient," Adopted by the Executive Board of the American Academy of Neurology, 21, April, 1988, Cincinnati, Ohio.

37. Cruzan Transcript, pp. 798–799.

38. "Neurologist Adopt Stance on PVS Treatment," *Society for the Right to Die Newsletter*, Summer, 1988, p. 8.

39. Editorial, "It's over, Debbie," *JAMA*, Vol. 259, No. 2, (January 8, 1988), p. 272.

40. "Active Euthanasia Explored at ABA-Sponsored Workshop," *Concern for Dying Newsletter*, Vol. 14, No. 1, (Spring, 1988), p. 6.

41. "Theologians called key to care of terminally ill," *The Chicago Catholic*, October 2, 1987, p. 24.

42. Richard John Neuhaus, "The Return of Eugenics," *Commentary*, April, 1988, p. 19.

43. Daniel Callahan, "Vital Distinctions, Mortal Questions: Debating Euthanasia & Health-Care Costs," *Commonweal*, (July 15, 1988), p. 403.

44. Ibid., p. 404.

45. Daniel Callahan, *Setting Limits: Medical Goals in an Aging Society*, Simon and Schuster, (New York, 1987), p. 64.

46. Ibid., p. 171.

47. Ibid., p. 172.

48. Callahan, p. 22.

49. *The Hastings Center Annual Activities Report 1987–1988*, p. 34.

50. David C. Thomasma, "The range of euthanasia," *American College of Surgeons Bulletin*, Vol. 73, No. 8, (August, 1988) p. 5.

51. Ibid., p. 10.

52. "Rhode Island Bishop Endorses Removal of Artificial Feeding," *Society for the Right to Die Newsletter*, Spring, 1988, p. 6.

53. *In Re the Estate & Person of Dorothy M. Longeway, a Disabled Person*, Appeal from Circuit Court of DuPage County, Eighteenth Judicial District, No. 88 P 270, In the Supreme Court of Illinois, No. 67318. Brief of Intervenor-Appellee, Community Convalescent Center, p. 16.

54. *In Re the Estate & Person of Dorothy M. Longeway, a Disabled Person, (Bonnie Keiner, Appellant), vs. Community Convalescent Center, Appellee*, In the Supreme Court of Illinois, No. 67318. Brief and Argument for Appellant filed by Rev. Eugene P. Parnisari, Catholic Charities Legal Service for Seniors, Naperville, Illinois, p. 10.

55. Ibid., p. 15.

56. Andrew H. Malcolm, "Propriety of Withholding Food From Seriously Ill and Comatose Patients," *The New York Times,* August 18, 1986, p. Y9.

57. Rita Marker, "Catholic Health Association Conference," *The Pilot,* (Boston), February 20, 1987, p. 14. Rev. Kevin O'Rourke, O.P. was among the speakers at the CHA's conference titled, "Ethical Issues Surrounding Nutrition and Hydration."

58. Kevin O'Rourke, "Evolution of Church Teaching on Prolonging Life," *Health Progress,* (January-February, 1988), p. 33.

59. Ibid.

60. "Brief of Amici Curiae SSM Health Care System and the Center for Health Care Ethics, St. Louis University Medical Center," in Appeal from the Circuit Court of Jasper County Missouri, Probate Division. *Cruzan v. Harmon and Lampkins,* Missouri Supreme Court, Appeal No. 70813.

61. Ibid., p. 9.

62. Ibid., pp. 25–26.

63. Ibid., p. 44.

64. PBS Interview with Bill Moyer, aired on Boston area public television, December 16, 1988.

65. Dennis, J. Horan, "Legal Reflections on the Role of Church Teaching," *Scarce Medical Resources and Justice,* The Pope John Center, 1987, p. 152.

66. Press statement by the Most Reverend Louis E. Gelineau, Bishop of Providence, regarding the Marcia Gray Decision, October 17, 1988.

67. Leo Alexander, M.D., "Medical Science Under a Dictatorship," *New England Journal of Medicine,* vol. 241 (July 14, 1949), p. 44.

68. Robert Jay Lifton, *The Nazi Doctors: Medical Killing and the Psychology of Genocide,* Basic Books, New York, (1986), pp. 93–94.

Chapter 6

THE PASTORAL COUNSELING OF FAMILIES FACED WITH A DECISION REGARDING THE ARTIFICIAL PROVISION OF NUTRITION AND HYDRATION

The Reverend Joseph P. Gillespie, O.P., D.Min.

Primum Non Nocere

First of all, try to do no harm. From my earliest experiences as a chaplain at a large midwestern hospital during the summer of 1968, I was inducted into a professional healing context where it was assumed that Hippocrates' sage advice to students entering the healing arts would be respected. Unfortunately, my personal obser-

111

vations regarding medical care seem just the opposite. On many occasions, patients and their families complained that the physician and the nursing personnel were doing more harm than good.

Whether or not my own observations would warrant the conclusions to be drawn by Ivan Illich in his book *Medical Nemesis* (1976), where "clinical iatrogenesis" seemed more documentable than fanciful, I was gradually having to face some of my own illusions about health care and the professional intrusion of the healing arts upon patients. I began to observe patients, who through fear and their own helplessness, had capitulated their personal healing needs into the technological wizardry of our modern day healing centers. Gradually, however, the patients approached being healed with a kind of healthy hermeneutic of suspicion. Unfortunately, for the medical profession, many patients and their families began to recapture their own sense of lost power through the use of lawsuits. The ensuing legal atmosphere surrounding doctor-patient relationship has done little to create the necessary healing atmosphere in which a trusting relationship between patient and doctor can often be the crucial difference between a bid for life and death. Somewhere between a naive experience of narapoia (a condition where everyone seems to be out to help you) and delusional paranoia (where everyone seems to be out to get you), we are in need of a metanoia (an invitation to experience reality in a new way). Perhaps it is in the pursuit of this metanoia, that an open and honest dialogue can once again take place between the patient, the patient's family and the healing profession. Might it be miraculous to assume that Hippocrates' dictum of Primum Non Nocere might apply equally to the medical profession, the patient, the patient's family and the Church?

Function of Pastoral Care

Our point of inquiry does have a lot to do with how we help or harm patients and their families. And as we explore the pastoral care and counseling of families faced with the decision regarding the provision of artificial nutrition and hydration, we are drawn in as professional Curae Animarum. Historically, we as pastoral care persons have been charged with the care of souls and, traditionally, the Church has lifted up four century spanning pastoral care functions (Jaeckle & Clebsch, 1964; Clinebell, 1984, p. 42):

1. Healing—A pastoral function that aims to overcome some impairment by restoring the person to wholeness and by leading the person to advance beyond the previous condition.
2. Sustaining—Helping a hurting person to endure and to transcend a circumstance in which restoration to a former condition or recuperation from the malady is either impossible or remote as to seem improbable.
3. Guiding—Assisting perplexed persons to make confident choices between alternative courses of thought and action, when such choices are viewed as affecting the present and future state of the soul.
4. Reconciling—Seeking to re-establish broken relationships between a person and other person(s) and between human beings and God.

My personal hunch is that in our pursuit of being effective care givers to families who are faced with decision-making issues around our topic, we will need to employ all four pastoral care functions in the process. Primarily, however, I would like to explore the functions of Sustaining and Guiding as parameters for working with families who are experiencing decision-making in what might metaphorically be described as a family crucible. Secondarily, I would like to address Reconciling and Healing as functions which help the patient's family and the medical staff to deal with their decisions. Let us first look at what is considered to be the problem around which we experience our pastoral care functions and then address how these four functions might facilitate "more good than harm."

The Problem

George Berkeley, an eighteenth century bishop and philosopher, was quoted as saying "first we raise the dust and then complain we cannot see." Perhaps in a similar way we too find ourselves disoriented and complaining because of the ethical and legal "dust" that has been raised around the theme of the workshop. The "cause of the dust raising" may not always be clear, but the "effects of the dust settling" on relatives who are faced with a decision regarding the provision of artificial nutrition and hydration for a loved one are very clear and disturbing.

The decision on how to treat a fatal pathology (i.e., an irreversibly comatose patient or a patient who persists in a vegetative state) or when to let the pathology take its natural course has, over the years, clouded our ethical and legal sense of orientation. If we cannot see very clearly, then what direction should we take? Whose moral and legal maps do we read? Whose reading of the moral and legal compass do we trust? In re-orienting ourselves in this dimly lit area of controversy, it is with some consolation and common sense that we look not only to medical science but to our moral theologians and ethicists as hopeful beacons of light. The legal dilemmas and economic realities of court cases and precarious financial burdens on families demand that we come out of our ethical shadowland. The cloudedness of the confused and disoriented moral and social dilemma, begs for enlightenment. Our legal and healthcare systems are in need of an orientation which proclaims a living theology, one rooted in gospel values of justice and compassion. What we do not need is the dim flickering of a casuistry of means.

At present, removing a respirator from an irreversibly comatose patient who shows no sign of recovery has, for many, been accepted as standard and ethical practice in medicine. But removing artificial methods of providing nutrition and hydration when the patient is in the same condition is not so readily accepted. One has only to refer to the Claire Conroy, Paul Brophy or Marcia Gray court cases to illustrate this point.

In Bishop Gelineau's statement regarding the case of Marcia Gray, he addressed the highly complex and sensitive dilemmas surrounding a decision to withdraw nutrition and hydration from the permanently unconscious person. In consultation with Fr. Robert McManus, a moral theologian, Gelineau sought to assist the family of Marcia Gray in reaching a conscientious decision in accord with Catholic moral theology. The conclusion to withdraw the supplying of nutrition and hydration was arrived at with the "unambiguously clear" primary intention of alleviating the burden and suffering of the patient (diagnosed to be in a persistent vegetative state) and not to cause her death.

What became increasingly clear in the Marcia Gray case was that the Church's magisterium has not yet issued a definitive statement regarding the need to provide nutrition and hydration to the permanently unconscious person. Within the Church, however, at least two theological opinions are presented. The first, that nutrition and hydration can be considered extraordinary means of sustaining life in certain circumstances; the second, that fluid and nutritional support are always provided. (*Origins,* 1/21/88).

It is in this theological, ethical, legal, economic, social and emotional "dust storm" that the pastoral care and counseling with families faced with the decision regarding the provision of artificial nutrition and hydration takes place. In every case, however, the rights of the terminally ill patient need to be protected and the rights of the patient's family respected.

Sustaining

"Plus ca change, plus c'est meme chose." Most of us are all too familiar with this experience of "the more things seem to change, the more they remain the same." In fact, perhaps some of us are experts at insisting (quite honestly) that we want to lose weight (would a diet of food and water help or hinder?), quit smoking (cigars don't count!) or quit drinking (as W. C. Fields once said: "I've read so much about the dangers of alcohol that I decided to quit reading!"). But, sadly, many of us have discovered that what we said we wanted to change about our habits, had not really changed with any sense of permanence.

As we explore the pastoral care function of Sustaining, we must quite honestly deal with the reality of change. Is change possible or impossible? Essentially, the function of Sustaining is to help a hurting person (patient or family) to endure and to transcend a circumstance in which restoration to a former condition or recuperation from a malady is either impossible or too remote as to seem improbable. To inquire about a patient's wishes or the family's wishes to make decisions around what seems "unacceptable" (denial is a working reality for all of us!) or to change the "unchangeable" (that is, to see different options) is to enter into a situation that often smacks of hopelessness. I think it only fair that as we go about struggling with "life-death" decisions, we pastoral counselors must also ask ourselves when was the last time that we were able to accept the unacceptable, or to change the unchangeable situations in our own lives. To help sustain people so that they can function while decisions are being explored in light of stark realities, personal and genuine empathy is absolutely critical.

At the heart of helping families who are faced with decisions regarding the provision of artificial nutrition and hydration, is the dynamic of loss. The realization and acceptance of a radical change in any area of life is the realization of loss, an ending. What is not so easily understood or accepted is that with each ending is offered a new beginning. Oddly enough, it is often the possibility of a new beginning that is so easily rejected in favor of what was known or believed to be unchangeable. Helping a patient or family to accept the inevitable necessary losses is, in effect, inviting them into the realization of sustaining a new beginning. In my experience of counseling families who are exploring a decision around our topic, I have found that it is an invitation to a metanoia. But it is not a process that is without anxiety, guilt, depression, anger and fear. Perhaps Woody Allen described the process of metanoia a bit more realistically when he said: "The lamb might lie down with the lion, but one of them won't get much sleep."

To Exit Or Not To Exit

"The way out is through the door. Why is it that no one will ever use this exit." This old bit of advice from Confucius introduces us to the problem and the solution. However, many of us, like families of patients or medical staffs, find it difficult to address both the problem and the solution as if they might be connected. No doubt the failure to address the real problem (again, we cannot underestimate the need for denial; change is difficult!) might have something to do with our inability to get people to use available exits.

When Ludwig Wittgenstein was asked "What is your aim in philosophy?" he answered, "To show the fly the way out of the bottle." The question with regard to "our problem" is who will

116

show us out of our dilemma? Whom can we trust? How will we know we are doing the right thing? These questions parallel those of families who anxiously wrestle with what they have come to hope are not fly-by-night solutions. As leaders and symbols of a living church, we cannot absolve ourselves from the mission of guarding the sanctity of life. However, we must be bold enough to look critically at how our inability to address the real questions of those with whom we keep vigil in the hospital and hospice wards keeps us and them from real solutions to bottled-up dilemmas.

As we are functioning as Sustainers of God's presence in the midst of painful realities, how do we openly invite families to choose the "suffering work" that we also willingly undertake in the decision making process? First of all, we must take the moral dilemmas the family brings to us, and openly and respectfully explore their honest moral inquiries about solutions to real problems. Secondly, if we as church leaders are anxious and fearful and struggling to suppress questions that "should not be asked because there is no official Church policy," then I suspect that our people will stop asking questions and will view us, as they might medical staff, as people who do more harm than good.

Thirdly, I think it fair to conclude that an inability to address the real problem with real solutions will predictably lead to viewing the inside of the bottle merely from a different angle. Perhaps a more graphic metaphor might be "rearranging one's deck chair on the Titanic."

To "hear" a family's desire to forgo or withdraw artificial nutrition and hydration from a relative who is in a diagnosed irreversible coma or persistent vegetative state is both a blessing and a curse. As the "solution" is communicated and clarified (is the message sent the message received?), the "change of view" might at first appear weird, unexpected and puzzling. There is, at times, a kind of genuine relief coupled with a "why didn't we think of this before?" conclusion. In effect, what has happened is a shift in the way in which the solution is viewed. The crucial question no longer revolves around the "why?" questions (why did God let this happen?" "Why won't she get better?"), but rather around the "what?" question.

The task of the pastoral counselor is to help facilitate "why?" questions with "what?" answers. To sustain families while they struggle through the paradox of entrapment in a room with an open door, requires patient as well as gentle confrontation. All of us who call ourselves followers of Jesus and take his teachings seriously know the struggle of not wanting to "lose our lives in order to find them" or to "die in order to live." The resistance to choose the "death door", which means, to stop asking the "why" questions and move to the "what" questions, may revolve around our hidden fear that the door will only swing one way.

As pastoral care givers and counselors, we are charged to enter into the common extremes of life and death, health and sickness, joy and suffering, as well as into the inevitable awareness of what has radically changed about the life of an individual in an irreversible coma. We cannot afford to be exceptions to what it is that we are inviting families to do, namely, to help make ethical decisions regarding the provision of artificial nutrition and hydration for loved ones. In light of the fact that the Church struggles openly with this issue, we are committed to safeguarding the sanctity of human life; however, safeguarding this life-giving decision demands that we not only consider the wishes of the patient and the patient's family, but the common good of society as well.

In the process of caring for a patient's right to life, we are entering into the process of letting the patient "care for" our lives as well. The question of letting the patient's diagnosed condition (e.g. an irreversible comatose state) "speak for us" is very important. It is not the patient who is dictating the diagnosis or decision regarding future medical care, but rather it is the medical "condition" of the patient which draws the patient, the family, the medical staff, the courts and the Church into a decision regarding the provision of artificial nutrition and hydration. In providing responsible pastoral care it is more important to remember Paul Tillich's admonition to pastoral care givers: "When I hear the term pastoral care, I sometimes imagine myself to be in the situation of receiving pastoral care and imagining this, I somehow feel humiliated. Someone else makes me an object of their care, but no one wants to become an object and, therefore the person resists situations like pastoral care. Perhaps this feeling cannot be removed entirely, but it can be reduced to a great extent by understanding that care is universally human and is going on in every moment of human existence. And more important is the reason that care is essentially mutual: one who gives care also receives care" (LeFevre, 1984, p. 125).

Guiding

In the process of assisting perplexed persons to make confident choices between alternative choices of thought and action, it is well to keep in mind two important dynamics, namely collusion and resistance. Both collusion (a kind of "circle the wagons" mentality) and resistance (a kind of attitude of "I wish you could help, but I can't let you") can be major impediments to change and health decision-making. Along these lines, I'm reminded of the story about a man who thought he was a chicken. His wife was quite concerned with her husband's perception of himself as a chicken (collusion) and she got tired of his clucking about the house, so she called a psychiatrist. The doctor recommended that her husband be hospitalized at once. After much hesitation, the wife finally concluded that she could not commit her husband to the hospital just yet because, after all, she still needed the eggs (resistance).

As the pastoral counselor listens to the presenting problem, it would be a false assumption to presume that, because persons say they would like to change a situation (e.g. to forgo or withdraw nutrition or hydration for a loved one), it is what they really want to do. This, I hope, is not an invitation to not take seriously a patient's or family's request for change. My only caution is all of us do need our eggs and until we can honestly let go of needing the eggs there will be no metanoia. Many of the family dynamics which make decision-making so difficult exist precisely because all the members are not in agreement to give up the eggs. Awareness of the emotional dynamics surrounding family members' lives and relationships is critical in guiding people into the process of healthy decision-making. We can make all the decisions we want in our minds, but in reality we have to live out those decisions in our everyday lives.

The decision pastoral counselors struggle with around this topic must be made within the context of mutually caring relationships with the patient and the patient's family. As pastoral counselors we are concerned not only with the Church's teaching, but also with the blunt reality of our patient's condition and the condition of the family. However, with or without an explicit knowledge of the patient's view regarding the provision of artificial nutrition and hydration, we must minister with other family members who have personal agendas. The decision to either sustain, forgo or withdraw artificial nutrition and hydration is the point around which the family, the medical staff and the Church must dialogue. It is important to keep in mind that the pastoral counselor is not value free in this area and must be aware of his or her own agenda regarding the family's decision. There is no such things as a neutral observer. I think it fair to conclude that a family can turn to the Church or to pastoral counselors in their search for clarity in helping to make the "right decision." I think it also fair to assume that the family or various members of the family can be terrifically angry or confused by the Church's "unofficial" position regarding this whole matter of sustaining or withdrawing artificial nutrition and hydration. What is of critical importance is that pastoral counselors know the teaching of the Church as they continue to dialogue with the family's struggle with an ethical decision.

Crisis: Opportunity Riding on Dangerous Winds

When we explore the crisis that is being presented to the family, it would be well to keep in mind that a crisis can be understood not only as a sign of danger (change or loss), but also as an opportunity for growth. Hence, the old proverb "crisis: opportunity riding on dangerous winds." Whenever we have the chance or opportunity to fly, we also risk the possibility of crashing. Who among us is not a frequent flyer these days? The curious fact about a crisis is that it cannot be avoided. Crises, like stress and pain, are realities that we must learn to live with in life. How we react to our seems to make all the difference between maintaining or losing our health or the relationships that are valuable to us.

In exploring any family decision to "do the right thing", we are entering into a family system—a labyrinth of sorts—that requires some basic but accurate cognitive maps. In realizing the complexity of family decision-making, one friend of mine concluded that "every damn part is connected with every other damn part." In actuality, this is not a bad understanding of the dynamics of any system. In its most basic definition, any system (human or otherwise) might be understood as the interrelatedness of individual parts operating with some goal (purpose). Implied, of course, in a family system is a sense of purpose or we might conclude, agenda. Along with purpose we need to be conscious of the self-esteem (individual and familial), communication (clear or confused), the flexibility or rigidity of a family's rules, roles or rituals as well as the family sense of connectedness with other systems (open or closed).

Of all the family therapists whose work inhabits our planet these days, I have repeatedly gone back to Virginia Satir (1987), to Frank Pittman (1987) and to Edwin Friedman (1985) as helpful guides in understanding how and why decision-making can be so difficult for families. A special recommendation would be Friedman's book entitled *Generation to Generation—Family Process in Church and Synagogue* (1985). In this book, Friedman helps us as pastoral counselors to understand our own connectedness to multiple systems as we struggle professionally and personally to help others examine their own family systems and dynamics.

In trying to guide a family which is in the process of facing a crisis, it is important to have some sense of normality of what is going on. Often when the counselor can help to "bracket the family's anxiety" and places their decision within a "larger anxiety system", then this allows the "smaller family anxiety system" to function with an appropriate sense of loss. In my years of doing family therapy (regardless of the presenting problem), this "bracketing of anxiety" (i.e. producing a "safe zone") is critical. Without it, the system tends to either "dig in its heels" or to explode into pieces. The "safe zone" is a necessary but difficult place to be in, crises or move towards solving problems that are presented to us for this zone is charged with multiple emotions all of which, in my observation, have much to do with the twin dynamics of collusion and resistance.

People in crisis are, by definition, emotionally upset. They are unable to solve life's problem in their usual way. My thumbnail definition of a crisis is when "the old magic doesn't work anymore." In attending to the decision-making process surrounding our topic, many family members go into a crisis state because of a feeling of powerlessness to deal effectively with the potential loss of someone who is considered essential and important in their life. In many cases the real dynamic does not revolve around the decision to forgo, sustain, or withdraw hydration and nutrition, but rather the individual family member's perception of how life will change as a result of this decision. To ignore the anticipation of a grieving relationship is, in my estimation, promoting more of a crisis than attending to the decision making crisis at hand.

Grief: a Normal but Bewildering Experience

One of the more common sense understandings of grief is that "it is the normal but bewildering cluster of ordinary human emotions arising in response to a significant loss, intensified and complicated by the relationship to the person or object lost" (Mitchell and Anderson, 1983, p. 54). Grief is anything but a systematic process. Emptiness, loneliness, isolation, fear, anxiety, quiet, shame, sadness and despair are some of the predictable emotional dynamics which complicate a human decision regarding the provision for or the withdrawal of artificial nutrition and hydration.

To forgo or withdraw artificial nutrition or hydration from a loved one, or to even participate in what might be construed as a decision to let a loved one die, is to evoke the loss of a role, a perception of self with a living, historical source of personal continuity. The resistance to forgo or to withdraw treatment is understandable in light of one's confusion, fear, guilt and perceived threat of disconnectedness. To seemingly let go of what medical technology can and has been able to preserve may appear to many family members not only a precipitous decision, but a sacrilegious one as well.

It is critical for the pastoral care counselor to understand the types of losses and the variables surrounding these losses for the family members. At the heart of the loss is *Relationship Loss*. Relationship loss is the ending of opportunities to relate oneself to, talk with, and otherwise be in emotional and/or physical presence of a particular human being. *Intrapsychic Loss* is the experience of losing an emotionally important image of oneself, losing the possibilities of what might have been, abandonment of plans for a particular future, the dying of a dream. *Role Loss* is the letting go of a

122

specific role of one's accustomed place in a social network. And *Systemic Loss* has to do with the change of interactional patterns (rules, rituals, roles) which have defined our lives and families. Also, the pastoral counselor must be prepared to sort out how the individual family members are perceiving "loss" with regard to decision making. Is the "loss" avoidable or unavoidable? Temporary or permanent? Actual or imagined? Anticipated or unanticipated? And most important, are the family members viewing the decision in light of leaving or being left (Mitchell & Anderson, 1984, pp. 37–50)?

In many ways, collusion and resistance can manifest themselves throughout this grief process in a kind of stubborn chorus of "better the devil you know than the ones you don't know." Or perhaps in somewhat of a more analogous relationship to the topic at hand, the old limerick goes:

> There was an old widow named Price
>
> who kept her late husband on ice.
>
> She said it's sad since I've lost him,
>
> But I'll never defrost him.
>
> Cold comfort, but cheap at the price.

Stages of a Crisis

In all honesty, the role of the pastoral counselor in a family's anticipated grief dynamic is an important one and, I suspect, one that will facilitate or complicate the decision-making process regarding our topic. In effect, the pastoral caregiver is not only a guardian of the Church's moral and ethical teachings, but also a grief and crisis counselor. Helping to explore the normality of the crisis, its stages and emotional characteristics could very well be the most important components in helping the family to be at peace with the decision-making process.

One author who is making more and more sense to me these days is Robert Veninga who wrote a book entitled *A Gift of Hope* (1985). In his analysis of a crisis, Veninga describes five stages that I think bear worth repeating.

First Stage: *the bombshell* is characterized by shock, an inability to make decisions, to carry on meaningful conversation and it generally filled with anxiety. Generally speaking, the survivors in this crisis situation do not want a lot of advice.

Second Stage: *deliberate activity* is just that, a lot of activity. Initial symptoms of grief are put on hold and the basic objective is to stabilize one's life in the midst of this newly perceived crisis.

Third Stage: *hitting rock bottom* is the gnawing realization that the loss is permanent. Dominant feelings are anger and a growing fear that the loneliness will only get worse. Generally speaking, each family member will need to explore this heartbreak as a solitary experience and plot out their own coping defenses.

Fourth Stage: the *awakening* seems to be characterized by a desire to imbue one's life with meaning. The conclusion might be the first real signal that healing is taking place.

Fifth Stage: *acceptance* seems to be predicated upon a kind of healthy stubbornness which survivors exhibit. A stubbornness that allows one to forgive the "injustice" of life and one's predicaments (Veninga, 1985, pp. 12–41).

I suspect that Veninga as well as someone like Kubler-Ross would be the first to advise caution on the rigid application of his model. However, I have found his model helpful as I enter into the complexity of any family system where decision-making around life and death issues prevails. In the process of sustaining and guiding family members as they explore their options regarding the legal and moral ramifications of their decisions, it is important to orient them in time and place relative to the process of their own personal and systemic crisis. I think it fairly obvious to conclude that family members and their experience of grief within the crisis may vary considerably in terms of particular stages. It seems that the primary task of the pastoral counselor or caregiver is to help address the emotional, and spiritual dilemmas which cluster around each family member's particular stage. In effect, the pastoral counselor enters into a process of facilitating reconciliation and healing within the family.

Reconciling and Healing

A not-so-famous moral theologian by the name of Groucho Marx was quoted as saying: "I would not dream of belonging to a club that would be willing to have me as a member." If this sounds a bit paradoxical, then I think we are on the same track. On the one hand, I am not sure that Groucho's dry wit doesn't capture the dilemma that so many families must struggle with as they (we) yearn to belong to clubs where the "good life" (one without anguish, fear, loss, rejection and decision making) is a part of our innermost thoughts. On the other hand, could we possibly want to accept an invitation to belong? Guilt, fear, pride and confusion can keep us from even thinking about joining.

The resistance to make decisions around the provision for or withdrawal of artificial nutrition and hydration for loved ones is, for the most part, a hesitancy to accept an invitation to a human process (a rational club, of sorts) where one can think through the ambiguities and anguish of the moral dilemmas. The major step in any area of reconciliation is being able to "let go" of what one thinks he or she "needs" to hold onto. Mature decision making must address the realities of alternatives. I can think of children (grown) who are still mad at their parents (now dead) and will not forgive them for the wrong (imperfect) decisions they made.

The invitation to "let go and let God"—a life-working philosophy coming out of Alcoholics Anonymous—does in some way help families to commend into God's hands and care loved ones who are in permanent vegetative states or irreversible comas. Being able to see the problem in terms of living solutions is not always an easy one for families who are operating in enmeshed (i.e. very close) family systems. Traditional roles, rules and rituals are such that "blessed are the ties that bind" and damn the member who thinks outside the family club. Misplaced loyalties and misperceived demands for non-change, can become the basis for stagnation and no-exit for the comatose patient and for family members. Hidden anger and silent prayers for a "natural death" begin to quietly erode the persistent calm of no action.

In effect, the function of Reconciliation seeks to re-establish broken relationships between a person and other persons, between a patient in a vegetative state and vigilant family member who yearn for a living connection. Helping families to examine their "impossible demands" upon God, to explore their human anger, guilt and depression is one way of inviting them into a healing of memories and to an exploration of dutiful perceptions. The Healing function aims to overcome the impairments of human relationships by restoring the person(s) to wholeness by leading them to advance beyond their previously stuck conditions. In the process of helping families to address the realities of decision making, we are inviting them to experience a sense of wholeness even amid the blunt realization of loss, separation and change.

The prospect of "belonging to a club that would have me as a member" need not be viewed as selling out one's moral integrity. To explore alternate views regarding the provision for or withdrawal of nutrition and hydration does not of itself draw one into the "slippery slope ethical club." Faithfully exploring moral choices in light of the Church's traditional teachings, does invite all of us into a "club" where abundant life must be understood as a source of saving grace. Jesus invited all of us to "live life, life more abundantly." Helping people to openly and honestly struggle with life giving solutions to real problems, can do much to restoring health and reconciliation within families crippled by fear and indecisiveness.

Conclusion

My observations around the topic of counseling families faced with the decision regarding the provisions for or the withdrawal of artificial nutrition and hydration must be understood as being framed within the moral context of pastoral care. I have not tried to be an ethicist, for I am not. Rather I have tried to focus on what I believe to be an important area of concern, namely how to approach a family system and its decision-making process. Trying "not to harm" a patient or the patient's family is of paramount importance. However, helping a patient or family to genuinely confront as well as to understand appropriately some of the normal dynamics that accompany a crisis is very necessary. To help bracket the family's bewildering emotions and fears within "safe zones" and with the aid of some realistic cognitive maps, is to bring that family to the possibility of regaining health even in the midst of decision-making around a caretaking crisis.

Acting responsibly within the four historical functions of pastoral care—Healing, Sustaining, Guiding, and Reconciling—the pastoral counselor needs to find effective means of sustaining a family as it sorts through the medical information, ethical considerations and invitation to decision-making. Helping to guide families in addressing the necessary losses (anticipated and real) as well as the unpredictable emotions surrounding events which explore the normal illusions of life, will be a necessary pastoral challenge. The need for personal and family healing and reconciliation can be fairly natural consequences stemming from a willingness to sustain and guide a family in crisis.

Almost without exception, those who survive crises often give credit to one person who stood by them or supported them throughout the process. For many families that one person could very well be a sensitive pastoral care counselor. The realistic pastoral care counselor is one who can help family members to "survive" a family crisis by helping them to understand the magnitude of that which they have lost. Also, that pastoral counselor can draw families into creative reconciliation experiences by helping them transcend their guilt by offering the family an ethical process by which to make a decision. In the final analysis, then, people seem to survive the crisis of decision-making only when they are able to find a reason to live as they begin the process of letting go (Veninga, 1985). It is their hope, this belief in transcendent values that human life has meaning which offers people the ability to make sense of the decisions that they have made. More often than not, in the moral context of the pastoral care setting, this hope begins to speak loudly and clearly, not only to families who have struggled through a decision, but to the institutions in which these decisions are being made.

127

In conclusion then, I want to share with you an old proverb that has made sense to me as I have explored and continued to examine this area of crisis and decision-making:

A crisis makes you think.

Thought makes you wise.

Wisdom makes a crisis bearable.

It is my hope that in the combined wisdom of the Church's moral teaching, the advanced medical technologies of science, the legal protection of human rights through our court systems and through the perceptive pastoral counseling insights that we can truly understand how best to help the patient and the family faced with the decision regarding the provision of artificial nutrition and hydration. It is my hope that we can always end up doing more good than harm. Primum Non Nocere.

References

Clinebell, H. J. (1984). *Basic Types of Pastoral Care and Counseling.* Nashville: Abingdon Press.

Friedman, E. H. (1985). *Generation to Generation: Family Process In Church And Synagogue.* New York: The Guilford Press.

Illich, I. (1976). *Medical Nemesis.* New York: Pantheon Books.

Jaeckle, C. & Clebsch, W. A. (1964). *Pastoral Care In Historical Perspective.* New York: Jason Aronson.

LeFevre, P. (1984). *The Meaning of Health.* Philadelphia: Westminister Press.

Mitchell, D. R. & Anderson, H. (1983). *All Our Losses, All Our Griefs: Resources for Pastoral Care.* Philadelphia: The Westminster Press.

Pittman, F. S. (1987). *Turning Points: Treating Families in Transition and Crisis.* New York: W. W. Norton & Company.

Satir, V. (1987). *The New People-Making.* Palo Alto: Science and Behavior Books, Inc.

Veninga, R. L. (1985). *A Gift of Hope: How We Survive Our Tragedies.* New York: Ballantine Books.

Chapter 7

PASTORAL CONCERNS ARTIFICIAL NUTRITION AND HYDRATION—II

BISHOP: To Father Gillespie. First, our table had a sense of disquiet because we thought we perceived a Rogerian, non-directed approach and we weren't altogether comfortable with that.

But then, we felt that it really wasn't so non-directed. At least, it seemed to presume a decision to remove the means of hydration. And then, we focused finally on what was perhaps the nub of our problem and its question:

Is the statement, Father Gillespie, in your outline, when there is no definitive Church statement, an adequate statement of the Church's teaching on this matter? Is it not true to state the traditional medical-moral teaching would affirm nutrition and hydration as ordinary means of sustaining lives, means which become extraordinary only because of extenuating circumstances such as the breakdown of tissues, making the insertion of a tube a difficult and burdensome procedure? Is not artificial provision of nutrition and hydration ordinary in today's medical-technological world?

FATHER GILLESPIE: I would agree with you. This response ought to dispel the Rogerian non-directive approach!

I think the term "ordinary means" has, at times, been used in the conference to err on the side of the rights of the patient and attempting to preserve life at all costs. In pastoral care and counseling, the moral dilemma I enter into with families and medical staff is around the question of letting a "normal death" occur when there is no real life that can be lived apart from extraordinary means of artificial support.

Perhaps the unspoken question that needs to be asked is "Cui Bono?" In the midst of advanced medical technologies human bodies can be preserved for an extraordinarily long time. Indeed, the teaching of the Church is clear regarding the reverence for life. However, the Church must be knowledgeable about when death has occurred and be willing to assist families and medical staff in the decision making process.

BISHOP: This question is addressed to Mrs. Marker. May I put this in the context of your paper, which I will read for those who may not yet have a copy of it. It is as follows: "Instead, the question is! Do we continue to feed the disabled, the demented, the abandoned and the unwanted who are not dying or do we certainly end their lives by the universally effective lethal measure of stopping food and water."

Our table wanted to know whether or not there was any exception to this? Do you envision any exception to this?

MRS. MARKER: Well, first of all, in Father Gillespie's talk, I think there was something in there—I'm answering your question by referring to his, as well. There seems to be a misperception that there are only two possible positions, one that views food and fluids provided by tube feeding or such, as being something that is dispensable. And the other side, so to speak, says that you never remove food and fluids, that you must always provide food and fluids for all people. I think that's an inaccurate portrayal of the situation. I think we have to recognize that there are times when it is either not possible or, in very unusual cases, could be excessively burdensome.

Again, we have to look at the situation very carefully. The Vatican Declaration on Euthanasia very clearly gives, in Part IV, a clarification of what is "burdensome".

130

So if we looked at something we said: Is this method of providing food and fluids extremely burdensome, extremely painful and so forth, certainly, it would be permissible to remove a particular means of providing food and fluids, with the intent of removing something that is itself extremely burdensome or painful, not with the intent of taking the life of the patient. So, yes, there are cases when food and fluids could be removed but the intent in those cases is not to kill the patient.

BISHOP: The second question that our table had was, and perhaps this is unfair to address this to you, but there were those who wanted to know the cost of the G-tube package in the home, do-it-yourself in the home? Would you have any idea?

MRS. MARKER: I'm glad you asked. I even have one with me. I always carry artificial feeding tubes along. I happen to have two types, although there are more. Here is a jejunostomy kit. By the way, for those of you who assume that tube used for feeding looks like a garden hose, you can see it's very, very small. Here is a nasogastric tube. I carry a spoon along too, since that's considered artificial feeding by some people. The tube, itself, is very, very inexpensive. And if anybody would like to look at it closer, I'll have it up here.

The food that goes in it—I had planned to go across and buy some so that I would be able to show it to you but couldn't find my way across the freeway last night—is approximately $1.19 for one can. It provides total nutrition. And, in fact, you can take it orally. I've suggested it to my oldest son who is a very thin police officer and needs a little extra meat on his bones. It comes in chocolate and vanilla. And I can see why they feed it through a tube because it doesn't taste very good.

We're talking here about something that is inexpensive. To be totally accurate about it, feeding someone by means of a tube in the home is less expensive than the normal family diet. The people about whom we were talking today were the ones in the Court cases. Every one of them could have been cared for at home. That's not to imply that their families abandoned them because they weren't caring for them at home but, as far as the possibility of doing so, it could have been done. When we say $100,000, that's if we put people in intensive care units. These people don't need intensive care units. They need care, food, water, a warm bed and that's it.

131

BISHOP: I'd like to thank Mrs. Marker very much for her talk. I've been at all of the sessions here for eight years and that talk was more useful to me than any of the others that I've heard throughout the whole of that time. So I'm very grateful for that.

I don't have a question. I'd like to make kind of a brief statement. I had discussed this with Bishop Maida and Mons. Klister last night. I think many of you are probably aware, there's been a public complaint over three of the speakers and over holding a debate on the issue of nutrition and hydration from unconscious patients. This has come from some anti-euthanasia societies, especially from one called CURE. It's headed by a West Virginia woman whose husband has been in a coma for eight and a half years and has been cared for at home, and her son, who is an aide to a Senator in Washington. They were joined in their protest by many people who are prominent in the pro-life movement and associations for the disabled. A lot of the names, there are more than eighty, are very well known. Many of these are people who offer a great deal to the pro-life movement. They expressed a fear that this session would be used as a propaganda vehicle for stopping the feeding of the dying, the beginning of a continuation of euthanasia.

My own reaction is, there is no way that would happen in the light of Mrs. Marker's talk. They are upset that priests have testified in court cases in favor of stopping feeding and, I suspect, they have a suspicion that Church officials may waffle on this issue, as many of them, rightly or wrongly, feel that we have waffled in leadership on abortion. That's really where they're coming from and the people who feel that way feel it very strongly. They suggested, I think you know, that the Pope John XXIII Center cancel the three speakers and, if they didn't, they suggested the Knights of Columbus withdraw sponsorship. Neither of those things has happened. I don't agree with the protest on there being no debate on this matter in this closed circle. It seems to me the issue is important. It's urgent. It needs an airing. And I think the Pope John XXIII Center has made a real contribution by facilitating that this week.

I guess—I mentioned this to Bishop Maida—I would have preferred that there be another physician in addition to Dr. Plum because most of us are not physicians. We're not in a position to criticize positions that come from there. We can handle the theologians ourselves. The physicians are a different kind of a problem. I disagree with the positions of Dr. Plum and Father Boyle and Father O'Rourke. I feel sure that the Church will formally exclude those positions in its future teachings. And, from my own point of view, the sooner the better, but I'm not sure how soon that will come. But I would just ask all of us to be sensitive to the concerns of good people in this regard.

Many people are upset because they feel we didn't effectively teach *Humanae Vitae* for twenty years. They feel we've allowed abortions to go on in our own country at a million and a half a year without a strong and effective response. I'm not sure what a strong and effective response would have been. I'm not sure anything we could have done would have changed it. But there's a sense of failure in terms of almost 25 million having died and we still haven't reduced the number there at all.

There are people who are fearful and suspicious of a weak Church response on starving disabled babies and on euthanasia for the old and the disabled. And they expressed that. They left 200 packets with me, about ten pages. They contain strong statements of what I've just said, stronger in language. They're angry statements with regard to the three speakers. I'll give a copy to any Bishop who asks for it. I would hope that would be more useful than copies of those packets would be a copy of the talk that Mrs. Marker has given, which is much more useful and on a better level. I spoke to Bishop Maida and to Mons. Klister simply about saying this, not attacking the three speakers, but I think we have to be very conscious of the public impact of what we do and say on people who have very vital concerns in this area.

MODERATOR: Thank you, Bishop. Bishop Maida, did you have anything you'd like to say at this time?

Since Bishop Vaughan took the occasion to bring up something extraneous to our concerns and had discussed it with you, I thought perhaps you might like to have some reflection on behalf of the Pope John Center.

BISHOP MAIDA [Chairman of the Board, Pope John Center]: Well, every diocesan Bishop here, I'm sure, has been faced with the same reality in his own diocese. We have people who want us to listen to some people and not to others. And yet, in a Church which is always seeking understanding guided by faith, we have made the decision in this matter.

We're grateful for all the speakers who came and we hope that through their efforts we are all enlightened. And so I think that's the position of the Pope John Center. I want to reiterate with all my heart and my mind our fidelity and loyalty to the Holy Father, to the Holy See and to the Magisterium. We are here to be deepened in the knowledge of what our Magisterial teaching is.

I'm a lawyer in my roots, a civil lawyer, a canon lawyer, and I know that in the argument of debate, issues are focused and truth is ultimately then appreciated. Judgments are easier to make. And so, in this context of highly intelligent and interested and devoted Bishops, I hope that this opportunity is a good one for all of us and I want to thank all of you for being here and for supporting us.

BISHOP: I was wondering, Father Gillespie, it seemed to me that you might have been advocating a neutral position as far the priest/counselor or the counselor. And I guess I'm looking for clarification. It seems to me that the counselor does have right and an obligation to insert his conviction about Church teachings into the process. Now, I appreciate a lot of the things that you said, so I'm not trying to say he forces families to comply.

In fact, somebody at our table said you were looking an internalization of their decision. If that's so, it clarifies it. But it seemed to me that you weren't advocating the priest/counselor giving the benefit of the Church teaching, especially the presumption of life as hope.

FATHER GILLESPIE: I appreciate the question. I think that was part of the time constraints. We are beholden to official position. We are, whether it has to deal with the issues we discovered or talked about last night with regard to *Humanae Vitae* or whatever, it is very important to be able to reiterate the Church's position. I think that sometimes it is difficult, not because the counselor, pastor or care person doesn't have access to that. It is simply trying to hear what appears to be the dilemmas that are internalized and, to some extent, may be coming out for the very first time. It isn't a question of trying to agree with them. It's simply a question of trying to give them some kind of safe zone, as I've indicated in my paper, in which that can be discussed.

I think from that point of view it is very clear that, as a representative of the Catholic Church that I have to clearly state, as best I can, as it is presented, what the position is.

BISHOP: First of all, Mrs. Marker, I would like to commend you for the first part of your talk. It's the second part that kind of confuses me and it triggers a concern that's been floating for a while among some persons who think and feel as I do. I'd like to hear your response to my comment. My comment is this: That the typical theological process whereby persons who disagree with one another do the thing the scholarly way, point by point. What I see here emerging, what I heard this afternoon, and what my colleague had said about the letters that many concerned people have about either Bishops or theologians, we have two separate genres existing.

One, the highly reasoned, the well thought out theological attempt at trying to give a position on the one hand, and on the other hand, a mode of disapproval using guilt induction, persuasive communication, that could be very well used in the public forum but not in academic circles.

And so, it appears to me that we're missing the middle ground. You have concern and a theologian, Father O'Rourke, had a reasoned approach. I may not agree with it; that isn't the point. But it seems like we're missing each other. And I don't know that we get much from missing each other.

MRS. MARKER: I'm not sure that I understand what the question is.

BISHOP: It's not so much a question; it's a comment. Ordinarily, in the theological process, if, say, Father O'Rourke offers out an opinion, his colleagues in the field will comment on the strengths and weaknesses of the points that he is offering out, as well as bring in, we'll say, past Magisterial statements to shed some light on whether or not there's some validity or lack of validity to his position. What's emerging, it appears to me, is we're kind of obviating that process by bringing a political pressure on someone such as that. And we don't get his theological question addressed point by point in the more traditional way in which the theological process and debate is worked.

MRS. MARKER: I think there are several ways to deal with your concern, related to the specific discussion here. I used a particular method in the presentation because I had been asked to explain the relationship of the food and fluids issue with the right to die movement.

My purpose was to show how various statements, made in particular by Catholic spokespersons, had dovetailed with what is happening. I agree with you that addressing this from a scholarly perspective is also very necessary. But I also have a concern that this has not been confined to a scholarly debate. If we were talking merely about a theologian having raised these issues in a scholarly context, we would be dealing with something very different.

And with all apologies to Father O'Rourke since his name has been brought up, I'll use that as the example. I realize he has some time tomorrow to respond to that. Father O'Rourke has not confined his remarks to the academic arena. His positions have played on the front pages of papers, on television programs, in court rooms and in *amicus* briefs. This has been tremendously influential. It has not been from the standpoint of academia. And so that was my purpose in addressing the issues in the way I did. I will be very glad to deal on an academic level, point by point, bringing about an understanding of the Magisterium and its teaching within that context. But I think we need to deal with this issue on all levels where it has surfaced and recognize that there is a clear and present situation facing us. The gates have been opened. We are no longer dealing with a discussion contained within the realm of scholarly debate.

BISHOP: I think it probably is partially addressed to a comment that Father Gillespie made. At the end of this morning's session, and once again, Father Gillespie's comments, we seem to give too much accession to the will of the patient. The choice or the will of the patient does not become an absolute. The choice of the patient may well be a wrong moral choice. Just because the patient voluntarily offers that choice, doesn't make it a compelling moral norm, either for physicians or for pastoral ministers or for us. Leon Kass, in an article in the current issue of *Public Interest,* raises this particular point. He says that the autonomy of the patient does not become the compelling norm. I think that we should be careful as we proceed through these discussions that we don't give almost unlimited validity to the will of the patient.

136

PART TWO

THE BISHOP AND CATHOLIC HEALTH FACILITIES

Chapter 8

ETHICS COMMITTEES IN CATHOLIC HOSPITALS: RELATIONSHIP TO THE LOCAL BISHOP

The Reverend Monsignor James P. Cassidy, Ph.D.

Introduction

It is a great honor for me to be here to speak to you about the topic of Ethics Committees in Catholic Hospitals. As a priest and as a psychologist, I speak to many groups; sometimes very large and important groups, but certainly I have never spoken to any group as important as you Bishops gathered here in Dallas. I am keenly aware of your tremendous responsibility, and this tremendous opportunity for the Church of Christ.

I've been asked to talk about ethics committees in hospitals and health care institutions. It could be simple to talk about them;

to be specific, to speak from experience, and give you some rules of thumb and some quick and easy answers. But, I feel it's really impossible to give a presentation about the place of the ethics committees in hospitals unless you understand Catholic hospitals in the United States, how they are set up, and the role of health care in the Church. Therefore, it is necessary to give some background in order to place ethics committees in their proper perspective in health care.

Christ's Command to the Church to Heal

In St. Luke's Gospel, the ninth chapter, second verse, Christ sends out his Apostles and commissions them to preach the Kingdom and to heal. Two things—to teach and to heal. Healing has always been a part of the Church of Christ, even though at times we may feel that it's not as important for the Church to stay in health care. The Catholic Church today is the single largest provider of health care in the world. Most of our health care institutions are in the third world. It seems as we become more civilized, we seem to lose more and more control over health care institutions; while in the third world, Catholic influence seems to grow stronger and stronger. It is important that the Church observe the command of Christ to be involved in health care.

It is more important today than ever before, because most of the moral and ethical issues that face the Church today arise from health care. They are very basic issues—death, birth, development of life. So, we are involved in problems with euthanasia, abortion, in vitro fertilization, and new technologies which effect life itself.

Some people in advertising have pointed out that 70 percent of the advertising that we see is somehow related to health care, because health is so important to people. It's more important today than ever before because people are living longer and better lives. Very often people say that the costs of health care are too much, but you've got to realize that one of the reasons for the increasing costs is due to the fact that people are living longer, therefore, increasing the need for health care. If you want to consider the alternative (death), then you might say you want to do away with health care. Health care is basically important to life; and the supernatural is always built upon the natural.

Church's Responsibility in Health Care Today

In many ways it is very difficult to stand up and talk about moral and ethical problems in health care if we are not involved in health care. The Church must stay in health care because one of the great problems in our time, as many have said, is the depersonalization of life. We have become more like robots; we have lost the human touch, which is most obvious in health care.

When you go for health care, you loose your identity. I remember the story of a priest taking his father to the hospital for the first time. When his father was registered, they put an armband on him and they gave him a number and said, "Well, now your number is 09145." The old man looked up and said, "My name is John." They take your name and identity away from you. Look at those stupid pajamas they give you. As a patient in the hospital, you are reduced to infancy. They put you into bed, and they put a babysuit on you, and they expect you to act like a child. They take away your whole personality. You don't even have a name. They give you a number on the door of the hospital room. The nurses and others may refer to you as the "bad appendix" or the "hot AP in Room 345." They identify with the disease rather than with you as a person, and your identity as a person is lost.

Governments in many different countries, and in the United States are getting more and more involved in health care. However, it is still very necessary that the Church remain in health care and teach people how health care should be rendered. Health care is for the whole person—body and mind and spirit—not for a part, the diseased part. It should be given to the whole person with the deep awareness that when dealing with the whole person, you are dealing with a person made in the image and likeness of God, who should be treated with dignity and respect. There is always going to be the need for the Church to set a model for how health care should be given, with a deep awareness of the sacredness of the human person.

Past history of the Catholic Church of the United States in health care has an effect on us in the present situation. It seems that in the early days of the Church in the United States, the Bishops were more involved in education, and so we have the tremendous educational system. They really weren't involved in health care. Many of the bishops didn't even know, or ever cross the threshold, of the Catholic health care institutions in their own dioceses.

This work was done by religious women who came to the United States from many different countries, bringing with them skills and techniques in order to set up hospitals. I have always been fascinated when I look at the state of Michigan. Practically all of the hospitals in the state of Michigan are Catholic. You see this throughout the whole country, the great history of religious women in the United States and the tremendous contribution they have made to health care.

Now, health care delivery is one of the largest industries in the United States. It has become more important for the Bishop to be involved in health care. Health care has become very much involved in politics. Someone once said "health care is politics, and politics is health care." It is really impossible for a single, small Catholic hospital to survive by itself in the United States today. It has to have the support of the Catholic people; it has to have the support especially of it's local Bishop. He has to take positive action and be involved, or it will not be able to survive.

The other particular thing that has happened in health care in the United States is that health care is not just a mission and a commitment as it was in the past, it has also become a big business.

Now, I know my Cardinal does not like me to use these terms—talking about health care as big business or the second largest industry in the country—but that is a fact. Twenty, thirty or forty years ago, the religious community could run a hospital with no problem. The sister, who was the administrator, had no big financial problem, money was made for the many other good works of the religious community. Health care has changed, with the advent of Medicaid and Medicare, health care has become "big business." That doesn't mean the Catholic Church should abandon it, but we should realize that it is a big business. Probably by 1990, it will be the largest industry in the United States, employing the largest number of people.

When we look at our own Archdiocese of New York, we see our 18 Catholic hospitals, with a budget that comes to over a billion dollars a year. The rest of the different services in the Diocese, do not come close to that financial cost. I can take even the smallest hospital we have in the Diocese, which is maybe 80 to 100 beds, and that hospital will have a budget of over ten million dollars. It is a tremendous problem because of the tremendous amount of money involved and the amount of expertise that is necessary to run a good hospital.

Besides health care becoming a big business in our time, there has been a decrease in the number of religious in health care. Ever since 1960, more than 65 percent of the religious in health care have left the health care field. It is interesting to look at the figures. Before the 1960s, almost everyone of the administrators in Catholic hospitals were religious. Ten years ago, about 50 percent of the administrators were religious. Today, the number of laity as administrators in Catholic hospitals is much higher. In our own Archdiocese, we have at least five hospitals owned directly by the Archdiocese, run completely by lay people. I think these hospitals are just as Catholic as they ever were. It is necessary to use more lay people because of the tremendous drop in religious in this field, and also because of the greater need for technology, knowledge, skill and financial administration that are necessary to run a hospital today. I think it is rather difficult to look at a small religious community of a couple of hundred people, and feel that in that religious community there is somebody who has the expertise to be able to run a big business in today's world.

There are two basic problems in Catholic hospitals in the United States. First of all, if you lose a Catholic hospital, if a Catholic hospital closes in the United States, there will probably never be another opportunity to set it up as a Catholic hospital again—not in our time. Secondly, looking very carefully at the history of Catholic health care in the United States, I have yet to find a true merger between a Catholic and non-Catholic hospital where the Catholic hospital hasn't gone out of existence within three years. Take the example of Kingston, New York. You have a Catholic hospital, and a local voluntary hospital—Benedictine Hospital and Kingston Hospital. Maybe health planners will say that town doesn't deserve two hospitals—"We don't need two; merge the two of them." If this happens, you've got to realize that the Catholic hospital is going to go out of existence because they will not do abortions and sterilizations. Many people are still striving to see if it's really possible to have a merger without the Catholic hospital going out of existence. I have yet to find one in the history of the United States that has been able to do it.

A large number of Catholic hospitals have been closing in the United States—20 in the last three years, seven within the last 12 months. More will close because it is very difficult to deal with hospitals in this present day. The economy is such that everybody is trying to save money in health care and there are stricter more difficult regulations on the hospital. It is a great problem for them to be able to survive.

Structure of the Hospital

In the United States, most of the hospitals are set up as independent and separate corporations, as they should be. The hospital is an institution by itself, so that legally within the law it is set up as a corporation. Now, that corporation can be owned by shareholders, it can be owned by members, but the ones that are really responsible for the running of the hospital legally are the board of trustees or the directors. They are the ones who are really responsible for running the hospital. The person who is a member of the board of trustees has a tremendous responsibility. They are responsible for the running of the hospital, for the quality of care that is given there, for the quality of doctors that are practicing in the hospital, and for its financial survival. More and more state health departments are looking at the boards of trustees of hospitals because these are the people who really run the institution. The administrator may be responsible for day-to-day operation, but the people who set the policies are the board of trustees.

If there is a Catholic hospital or health care institution in your diocese, I think it is very important that you have somebody on that board of trustees as your representative. You can have observers, but one of the most important things is to have your own person on that board of trustees, whom you hold responsible and reports to you about the condition of the Catholic health care institution.

I would not suggest that you go on the board of trustees by yourself. No one would be doing you a favor by putting you on a board of trustees. Sometimes people say "we'll make the Bishop (or the Cardinal) the Chairman of the Board!—What greater honor can we give to him." These well-meaning people could really be making life difficult for you, because you become too vulnerable to local and state health departments. In our diocese, we try to see that the Cardinal is the honorary chairman of all these boards, but that one other priest sits on that board as his representative as a member of the board of trustees. He has a right to the information and the data of what's going on in the hospital. It is his responsibility to see that it's mission is carried out.

To be able to have some observer who has no legal right, isn't much help. You have got to have someone on that board of trustees. When we look at ethics committees, we know ethics committees are only advisory. They should only advise the administrator and the board of trustees in a particular situation. They really have no power by themselves. It is good to have them in case there is some legal problem, but the responsibility of the hospital lies with the board of trustees. The ethics committee is only advisory.

Now, in every hospital it is important that there be an ethics committee. It has the responsibility of keeping the Catholic identity of the hospital. Situations come up that require very difficult decisions, which demand the support and understanding of people with some expertise to help and advise. In most dioceses, it would be most helpful if the Bishop had one good theologian whom he assigns to work with the Catholic hospitals. Theologians, however, can get into all kinds of arguments or discussions about particular points. People in hospitals don't have the time to do a lot of philosophical thinking. They want and need safe, straight answers. They are not looking to go into all the possibilities in a certain situation. They are dealing with the reality in a Catholic institution that is very much open to the public. They have to have answers that are in keeping with the Church and on time, not two years later after the problem has gone away.

145

Back in the years of Cardinal Stritch in Chicago, he set up a group throughout the country of what were called the Bishops' Representatives in Health Care. This is a group that still meets, but has changed it's name over the years. Each Bishop is still being asked to appoint somebody, now called the Diocesan Representative for Health Care. Those Diocesan Representatives still meet, and they report to the USCC—United States Catholic Conference. Somebody may have this position as a full time job in a large diocese. It may be a part time job somewhere else. They have meetings usually once a year, and this has continued over the years. They usually meet in some warm clime—Florida, New Orleans, some other place in the south, or California—usually during the month of January each year for three or four days. They discuss the latest things in health care, latest finances and the latest technology. When the Catholic Health Association has their big congress in early June, they usually go to it and have one meeting among themselves. I feel that role has sometimes been neglected by many of the Bishops. It would be very helpful for each Bishop to appoint someone as his Diocesan Representative for Health Care to help him to see what is going on in health care in his diocese. He could also help with the theologians that are involved in giving direction to Catholic Health Care Institutions and Pastoral Care Directors.

Theologians assisting in health care must not only know their theology well, but also they must know health care. Sometimes a good theologian may know nothing about health care, or what the latest technology really does, and therefore, can make mistakes. We always try to have our theologians who are involved in health care on the boards of trustees of several of our hospitals, so that they are really involved and have access to the doctors to be able to ask questions.

Besides the theologian and the Diocesan Coordinator for Health Care in the diocese who help the Bishop in this role as a leader in health care, the ethics committee itself must be set up with representatives on different levels within the hospital, and with different levels of expertise.

One of the problems with most ethical committees is that they are set-up mostly with doctors. Most Catholic doctors in the United States today, I can assure you, have never had an ethics course in their life. Anybody who graduated from Medical School less than twenty years ago in the United States, has probably never had an ethics course on moral and ethical issues in medical school.

There are four Catholic medical schools in the United States. All of the medical schools, except for the one I come from, are Jesuit medical schools. I have had people from our medical school go to Georgetown and say to them "Well, now what makes a Catholic medical school?", and have the head of that medical school and the doctors tell the person, "Well, people think we're a Catholic medical school—we're not a Catholic medical school," I think you can say that for all of the others—for St. Louis, for Creighton, for Loyola in Chicago, as well as Georgetown. They will tell you themselves that they really don't feel that they're Catholic medical schools.

Within the Archdiocese of New York, we were very fortunate when about ten years ago one of the medical schools was in financial difficulty, and we were able to take over that school. We are trying to make it more and more Catholic. We now say we're a "medical university in the Catholic tradition." We see as a matter of policy, certainly, that the medical school is not involved in anything that is contrary to the teaching of the Catholic Church. Doctors today, and we have been dealing with this in the medical school, have not had any ethics training. The problem is that the doctors, whom I guess, are sometimes like young priests, think they have all the answers. You'd be surprised, as I was, at the number of doctors who've never had an ethics course. Some of the old timers have had some ethics training, but this is not true of younger doctors today.

At New York Medical College, Cardinal Cooke had set up an Institute for Human Values in Medical Education, which is an institute for teaching ethics. At the present time, we are really making an effort to do that. Now, we have a director of this institute who is a priest with a doctorate from the Angelicum in Rome, and has been involved in health care. He is also a lawyer. We found out in our largest Catholic hospital in our Diocese, when we tried to set up an ethics committee, our moral theologian had to educate the doctors and nurses, as well as other professionals at the hospital, on what ethics was about. At the present time, this year, we are developing ten tapes on basic moral and ethical issues, and how we arrive at a moral and ethical decision. Doctors try to give the impression that they know all about morals and ethics, and what should be done, without ever having had a course in ethics. Setting up an ethics committee is not something that can be set up just overnight. Very often you are going to find that when you question people who appear to be good candidates for an ethics committee, you will find that they have had no moral or ethics training. You will have to educate them yourself in order for them to be able to fulfill their role as a member of the ethics committee with any sense of responsibility.

Even then, ethics committees can only recommend. They cannot make the decisions. The final decisions rests legally, and every other way, with the administration and the board of trustees of the hospital. That is why it so important for every Bishop to have a representative on the boards of trustees of every hospital and health care institution within his diocese.

Conclusion

With an understanding of the Church's mission in health care, the structure of health care in the United States, the structure of health care institutions, and the Bishops' responsibility, we can then deal with ethics committees in hospitals. As we said before, the people who are chosen to serve on those ethics committees, are very important.

I can remember an ethics committee in a hospital outside of our own Archdiocese, in the State of New York, where many people felt they had a problem with the moral theologian. Several of the sisters who ran the hospital were trying to make the moral and ethical decisions. The Catholic doctors in that diocese got up in arms with some of the decisions that were being made, especially the allowing of the tying of tubes in sterilizations. When they say "tied the tubes", you know they don't tie tubes, they cut the tubes and they insert the ends of them into the muscle tissue so that they can never be repaired. Once in a while, they can try to repair them, but it is a very difficult operation. I find very often that the doctors, many of them, are the ones who really have the best understanding of these moral and ethical issues. They see the implications in a broad sense, rather than some people who are just so narrowly involved with the situation that they lose perspective. This happens on some ethics committees in the United States. These ethics committees are used—just to avoid the teachings of the Church—to find exceptions. The ethical directives are not observed, because every thing is an exception. With that approach then they can allow sterilizations, and things very close to, and including abortions, in Catholic hospitals. They talk about abortion—maybe they don't do anything that's put on the record as being an abortion—but very often, in some D&C's where they go in and remove some material from the womb, it really is an abortion. The doctor knows it, and the others know it, but they are doing it under another guise. There are other things, too, that are done, and then written up in technical terms. It is also interesting to find out, in Obstetrics all across the country, the number of cesarean sections that are being done. It is probably performed four times as much as it was ten years ago. Why? Because the doctors are worried about malpractice. Doctors are getting lazy; they want to do things their way. Natural childbirth, or anything that takes too much time—they do not want to do. It is so much easier to bring the patient to the hospital and induce labor, and do a C-section, then they don't have to worry about it anymore. Then, if they don't do a C-section, natural childbirth may be a greater risk for the doctor being sued for malpractice. In most states, of course, if something happens to the child in childbirth, doctors may be sued up until after the child becomes 21 years of age. Many people sue their doctors because of something they think may have happened at childbirth.

It is important to have people in health care who know what they are doing; who are aware of the medical terms and what their implications are. Doctors, as a group, are very protective of each other. Even though a doctor may be a very good Catholic himself, he's not going to speak out when he sees other doctors doing something wrong. It's fascinating to watch. Doctors may not always give good health care to priests, or other patients. I know a priest who was having some medical problems. Well, I know his doctor is a very nice guy, and he goes to Church every day, but other doctors and nurses know, that you wouldn't send a dog to that man for treatment. But, because he's such a nice person, and he goes to Church every day, Father thinks he's a great doctor. He's a good person, dresses well, goes to Mass in the chapel every day, receives Holy Communion. The Sisters all worship at his altar, but if you went to his office for treatment, if you didn't see his old Irish nurse, you could not be sure of what kind of treatment you were going to get. This went on for years, but nobody said a word about it.

Now, quality assurance in many states, especially in New York, is really cracking down on what doctors are doing. Many say "Doctors bury their mistakes." What bothers me more, is that doctors support each other, even when things are not right. Doctors may be doing something wrong in your hospitals, and the other Catholic doctors are not going to talk about it. One of the problems we face is that among the staff of Catholic doctors in your hospital, in OB/GYN particularly, a doctor may abide by the Catholic directives in your hospital, but go down the road to his own office, or another hospital, and perform abortions. Many of the Right to Lifers get very upset, and we all get upset about it. Legally, there is not much you can do about it. We've gone through that one; we've tried. When you have a person on your staff, and he's doing abortions somewhere else, if he was on your staff before the abortion law went into effect, he may continue· to do abortions, but not in your hospital.

The credential committee of hospitals, and the boards of trustees, before they approve somebody, especially in OB/GYN, should check that this person is not doing things contrary to the teaching of the Church somewhere else. You really can't turn them down for that, but other means can be found for turning them down. You can find that he doesn't fit in with the spirit of the hospital; he doesn't practice medicine with the same sense that the other doctors in the hospital do. You would be able to take care of that situation becomes it blows up into a problem. As you can see, there are many problems which can arise in Catholic health care institutions, and it very important that the Bishop is aware of his role in health care. That he does have the support of people who are knowledgeable, and upon whom he can trust, and who are really loyal to the Church.

Health Care is going to grow. It will be the largest industry in this country. Health care is so important to the development of

every human person that the Church be involved. Even though it does become a high tech business, the really important thing is that people have the opportunity of making a choice of using a Catholic health care institution. For the good of the country, and for the good of health care, it is important that Catholic health care survive, and that it grows in the future. I think it is a tragic thing to look at a country such as the United States, and to look at our whole Church, and realize that real leadership in health care throughout the world is coming from the United States, and in the United States, we don't really have a "Catholic" medical school.

One of the great evangelical tools to advance civilization is health care. No matter where you go, whether you go to the Dominican Republic, or to Haiti, or to Ghana in Africa, people and governments are looking for health care. They will accept the Church in health care because they know the Church is going to help. The Church will use health care to give service to these people. The Church doesn't threaten the government as when you just send a group of preachers or missionaries to a particular area. Everybody needs health care.

I think about the tragedy that happened about five years ago. In all of Iceland (which is one percent Catholic), there were four hospitals. All four hospitals were Catholic hospitals. The impact that had on the population was outstanding. Today because of the drop-off of nursing sisters, the government has taken over all of those hospitals. That whole opportunity for the Catholic Church has been lost.

I think of Seoul, Korea, and the growth of the Church there. It is growing by leaps and bounds. Catholics are supposedly only 10 percent of the population, but Buddhism and Confucianism are not really religions. They are cultural identities, but they are not things that are practical or real. The leaders of South Korea are mainly Catholic, and they have a superior Catholic medical school and a Catholic medical center. It was fascinating to go to Mass there on Sundays because the churches were crowded, especially with young people. In the compound, there was the cathedral sitting on the top of the hill, to one side there was the school, then there was a hall, then the priest's house. On the other side, there was a large Catholic hospital. I think that image of the Church being identified with service and care of the sick and the poor, is a good image. I think it impacts the people of Korea, and that it gives a sense of the Church as always being at the service of the people.

I think it is a good thing for us in the United States to have a similar image. The Catholic hospitals don't discriminate, and just take Catholic kids like our schools have to. Catholic hospitals take everybody, no matter who comes their way, they take care of them. In New York, many people will gladly go to a Catholic hospital, especially when they get older, than go to any other place else, because they know there will be a sacred respect for their life. No one in a Catholic hospital will take their life away quickly. They are aware that in a Catholic hospital they are going to be treated with an awareness of the dignity and sacredness of human life and of the human person.

Chapter 9

ETHICS COMMITTEES: THEIR ROLE IN CATHOLIC HEALTH CARE FACILITIES

The Reverend Kevin D. O'Rourke, O.P., J.C.D., S.T.M.

Introduction

When the words "ethics committees" are mentioned, people usually think of committees in the hospitals or long term care facilities. While ethics committees in health care facilities are important, there are two other types of ethics committees which influence Catholic health care; ethics committees in Catholic health care corporations and ethics committees in individual dioceses. At present, there are approximately 600 Catholic hospitals and about 700 Catholic long term care facilities in the country. About 75% of the hospitals have ethics committees and another 13% have expressed the intention to establish committees in the immediate future. About 30% of the long term care facilities have ethics committees and another 20% indicate the intention to establish committees. Catholic health care corporations or systems come in all shapes and sizes. For the most part, they are composed of health care facilities sponsored by one religious institute, but a few corporations are sponsored by several different religious institutes united to form one corporation. At present there are over 50 Catholic health care corporations (or systems), some of them numbered among the largest not-for-profit systems in the United States. Though each Catholic health care corporation does not have an ethics committee properly so-called, each one does have a Mission Effectiveness Committee. As we shall see, Mission Effectiveness Committees consider the same issues as ethics committees, so most Catholic health care corporations have the equivalent of an ethics committee for the whole system. Finally, there are also some dioceses and archdioceses which have ethics committees. The number having committees is difficult to determine, but most seem to be located in larger dioceses or archdioceses which have a number of health care facilities.

I. Relationship and Purpose

How are these various ethics committees related to each other? Catholic health care is a ministry of the whole Church; of individuals and institutions; of families, parishes, and health care facilities. This truth is stated in the Pastoral Letter of American Bishops on Health and Health Care[1] and was the main principle of the year long study of the Commission on Catholic health care sponsored by the USCC, the CHA and the Catholic health care facilities.[2] This study entitled: "Catholic Health Care: A New Vision for a New Century," stated that the ministry of health care is the responsibility of the whole Church, but it also pointed out that because of advanced technology we have concentrated our ministry of health care in institutions. While families and individuals in non-Catholic health care facilities are involved in the ministry of health care, we tend to identify our Catholic health care ministry in the

154

USA with our Catholic hospitals, long term care centers, our Catholic health care clinics and centers.

The concept of Catholic health care ministry contained in the Pastoral Letter and the document developed by the Commission on the Future of Catholic Health Care Ministry helps us understand the relationship of the various committees. The *diocesan ethics committee* will be concerned with health care ethics for the entire diocese, but will consider helping institutional ethics committees a primary responsibility. Thus, the diocesan ethics committee might publish recommendations for all people in the diocese concerning the Living Wills but would also be concerned with questions referred to it by ethics committees in Catholic institutions. But system committees would also seek to energize and guide ethics committees in local facilities.

The *ethics committee of a Catholic health care corporation* would be concerned mainly with ethical issues of the corporation; for example, what norms to follow for joint ventures in business with non-Catholic corporations; but it would also help the ethics committees in individual institutions. But system committees would also seek to energize and guide ethics committees in local facilities.

The *ethics committees at local Catholic institutions* will be concerned with helping the institution fulfill its mission. Because our ministry in health care is centered in institutions. The institutional Ethics Committees (I.E.C.) will constitute our main interest in this study. The mission of Catholic health care facilities may be summarized as the offering of quality health care in accord with the teaching of the Church.

Clearly, achieving the mission of an individual health care facility involves medical ethics but it also requires attention to *"institutional ethics."*. By institutional ethics I mean those issues of social and personal justice which arise in any organization which serves the public. Thus, in order to accomplish it's mission the institutional health care facility will be concerned about establishing policies for issues of medical ethics; e.g., obtaining informed consent from patients, for allowing families to offer proxy consent for their loved ones, for removal of life support systems, for the declaration of death using brain function as the criterion, for orders not to resuscitate (DNR), for refusing recommended medical treatment, for leaving the hospital against medical advice, and for many other issues which fit under the general heading of medical ethics. But at the same time, the Catholic health care facility, in order to accomplish it's mission, must be concerned about such issues as: are employees treated fairly, do they have grievance procedures as well as fair wages and retirement benefits, does the Catholic health care corporation work in cooperation with other Catholic facilities, and are sincere efforts in place to help the poor gain access to health care?

In the traditional view of ethics committees in health care facilities, the matters considered by the ethics committee is usually confined to "medical ethics."[3] Indeed, the need for establishing ethics committees arose because of recommendations of the New Jersey Supreme Court in the Quinlan Case, certainly a case which concerned "medical ethics." If the ethics committee of a particular health care facility, corporation, or diocese confines its consideration to medical ethics, well and good, as long as some other group is concerned with the ethical issues which fit under the broad title, "institutional ethics." However, if matters of "institutional ethics" are not considered adequately by another committee, experience demonstrates that these issues will surface during the discussion of the committee supposedly devoted only to medical ethics, even if strictly speaking they are not on the agenda. For example, at one hospital procedures for treating indigent patients in the emergency room had to be changed. Most of the indigent patients in the inner city were using the emergency room of the Catholic hospital as their primary care center because the city hospital had moved to an area not convenient for their access. While the Catholic hospital was able to treat 5 or 6 indigent patients in the emergency room each day without interfering with emergency cure or causing serious financial loss, when the number grew to 40 to 50 patients, it became impossible for the Catholic hospital continue allowing its emergency room to be a regional primary care center.

Many of the staff became upset when new policies to limit primary care for drop-in patients had to be instituted. One nurse told me that she worked at the Catholic hospital because she wanted to serve the poor. Developing a method to explain the realities of health care financing and the shared responsibility for caring for

156

the poor became an issue for the ethics committee of the hospital. The care of the poor in a particular area is the concern of all persons and social organizations in the area, not only the concern of the Catholic hospital. To think that the sole institution responsible for the care of the poor is the Catholic hospital is shortsighted and will lead to insolvency for the hospital. Catholic hospitals must do their share in caring for the poor, but they cannot do everything. In order to handle the ethical concerns of the staff at the hospital in question, the ethics committee conducted some in-service education programs concerning the economics of health care and the shared responsibility of providing access to health care for the poor.

In the immediate future, diocesan ethics committees will be able to help individual Catholic health care corporations and facilities in the issues which seem to be more institutional than medical. Not only the issue surrounding financing, but also the programs needed to insure continued Catholic sponsorship of health care facilities and the formation of the laity in the theology of Catholic health care comes to mind.

II. The Function of Ethics Committees

The function of Institutional Ethics Committees (I.E.C.) is often misunderstood. In a recent empirical study of ethics committees, one hospital executive said that the ethics committee could be put forward to explain any actions on the part of the hospital which were unpopular, such as laying off employees or reducing services.[4] Thus, the ethics committee was considered part of the public relations department. Another mistaken impression is that ethics committees make decisions. The picture is often presented of an ethics committee acting as a jury, deciding whether life support systems should be removed, or whether the criteria for brain death have been met. The view that committees are to make ethical decisions, whether concerned with medical or institutional matters, is just as irrational as looking upon them as agents for public relations. The nature of ethical decision making requires that decisions be made by individuals. In medical decisions for example, ethical considerations are an integral element of the physician-patient relationship. As Leon Kass has observed, medicine of its very nature is a moral endeavor. The physician utilizes scientific knowledge, but the knowledge is applied to a particular human being who has a particular value system. While this matter of ethical decision making being the responsibility of individuals need not be considered further at this time, let us realize that fulfilling the mission of health care facilities is accomplished in individual acts. Thus, while lofty statements of purpose are perhaps helpful, the actualization of these statements depends upon the virtue of individual health care professionals.

The proper function of the ethics committee is education.[5] Though individuals make ethical decisions in medical and institutional affairs, each person needs help in making good ethical decisions. Providing this help is the role of the ethics committee. The committee offers education at three levels; through formal courses, lectures or seminars (at our hospitals medical rounds and ethics for lunch offer our best opportunities for teaching ethics); through formulating policies which will outline ethical behavior, and by consulting with individuals who wish help in making difficult decisions. Policies formulated by the ethics committee must be approved and implemented by the trustees of the institution. Individual consultations need not involve the entire committee. Recently in one of our hospitals an elderly woman was admitted with gangrenous legs. Her son, her legal guardian stated that his mother would rather die than have her legs amputated. But her physician realized that mother was competent to decide about her medical care, even if she could not manage her finances. At the request of the physician, two members of the ethics committee visited the patient and quickly discerned that she thought she "had another ten years" and would not "miss my legs cause I haven't been able to walk for five years."

The first priority of ethics committees should be self education. This is especially true in Catholic hospitals which have a definite ethical code to follow. Too often people in Catholic hospitals know the content of the Directives but have no idea of the reasoning and theology which underlies Church teaching. If we present Catholic teaching as mere rules, it seems to be authoritarian and not related to the good of individuals.

158

Because of its educational role concerning Catholic ethical teaching, the ethics committee is an administrative committee, responsible to the trustees of the institution usually through the CEO. To be more specific, the ethics committee, even if its interest is confined to medical matters, is not a committee of the medical staff. While physicians should play a prominent role on the ethics committee, the body ultimately responsible for ethical policy whether medical or institutional is the board of trustees. In too many hospitals, the medical staff holds the trustees in bondage. Hence, the importance of insisting that the ethics committee is an administrative committee and is responsible to the board of trustees.

III. Composition of Ethics Committees

Ethics Committees for dioceses and Catholic health care corporations should draw from a qualified cross section of people. Usually, the committee should not have more than 8–10 people. If issues beyond the competency of the committee arise, other people can be consulted or recruited on a temporary basis. Because the issues handled by a diocesan ethics committee often concern the application of Church teaching in disputed matters, I would suggest that three, four or five theologians be members of the committee. The ethics committee of individual facilities (I.E.C) should be composed of 10–14 people. Many committees have more people, but too many members impede effectiveness. The track record of health facilities' ethics committees is not impressive, and I would contend that too many ethics committees spend time soliciting opinions instead of facilitating education. More people of the facility may be involved in the ethics committee if sub-committees are formed to consider particular issues. In one hospital concerned about the uncontrolled introduction of innovative surgeries, (i.e., heart transplants for infants) a sub-committee composed of one administrator, one pastoral care person, one nurse, and three surgeons was able to formulate a reasonable policy within a week. The larger committee would have taken six meetings to complete the same task. At another facility concerned with research using fetal tissue, the topic was discussed for four months; after a sub-committee presented a definite program we were able to agree on a plan at one meeting. Health care professionals, especially physicians, are results oriented; wisely, they do not like to spend time in meetings. However, given a problem, they will devote their energies to solving it and will usually produce a workable solution.

The literature on ethics committees recommends that ethics committees should be broad based and have members from the "lay community" as well as "representatives of administration and professional staff."[6] However, members of the "lay community" do not become apt members of an ethics committee simply because they are outside the institution. The main qualification for an ethics committee member, whether the person serves on a diocesan, systems wide, or individual health care facility committee, is an acceptance and understanding of Catholic teaching in regard to health care ethics. True, our Catholic health care facilities exist in a pluralist society and there exists a great deal of pluralism inside the facility insofar as administrators, professional staff, and patients are concerned. But a Catholic health care facility will not fulfill its mission if it confuses Catholic ethics with the ethics acceptable by all in a pluralistic society.

Some may remark, in response to my contention that the main qualification for membership on ethics committees in Catholic health care facilities is acceptance and understanding of Catholic teaching, that such a plan would limit Committee membership to Catholics. Realize however, that all who accept and understand Catholic teaching will not necessarily be Catholic. Many of the Catholic ethical norms are common to people of other churches, and even to the unchurched. Many of the more sensitive ethical discussions in which I have participated have been led by persons not associated with our Church. Finally, within the realm of Catholic teaching there is room for discussion and disagreement. Thus, some enlightened people on these committees on which I serve agree with me that artificial hydration and nutrition is an ineffective therapy for those in permanent vegetative state (p.v.s.), but some benighted souls disagree as vigorously. Some of my colleagues consider T.O.T. and G.I.F.T. as methods of generation which complete the marital act and therefore acceptable from the view point of Catholic teaching.[7] On the other hand, I would consider these methods as not in accord with by the Instruction on Procreation issued by the Holy See in March of 1987.[8]

The literature on Catholic ethics committees usually states that each ethics committee should have an ethical or moral theologian.[9] While this recommendation has merit, there is always a danger that the ethicists will become the guru of the group. The ethicist or theologian should help others be familiar with the sources and explain Church teaching when necessary, but the ethicist does not make decisions which all others feel compelled to accept. Perhaps we will understand the role of the ethicist better if we reflect upon the role of a neonatologist or surgeon on an ethics committee at a childrens' hospital. The neonatologist may be called upon to describe the medical prognosis for an anencephalic infant, so an ethical policy in regard to retrieving organs for transplant may be developed. In like manner, a pediatric surgeon might be asked to predict the success rate of surgery for conjoined twins and the prognosis if surgery is not attempted, so that a family consulting with an ethics committee concerning options of ethical treatment for conjoined twins may be fully informed. In these latter cases the physicians offer information essential for good decisions, and do not dictate the decision. The role of the ethicist is similar.

Conclusion

Are ethics committees worth the effort? At the diocesan level there is limited experience and it seems too soon to determine their worth. At the corporation level and at the local level, from comments I have received I gather that they are not a raging success. At the local level, they depend for effectiveness, on the energy and interest of the local CEO. If he or she is not committed to having a worthwhile ethics committee, then no matter how much encouragement comes forth from the corporation or from the diocese, there will not be a successful ethics committee. Why are some CEO's not enthusiastic about ethics committees? Because they are immersed in the every day problems of survival. The pressure upon CEO's from reduced government funding, from business firms desiring a lower rate for services, from physician groups desiring to have the latest equipment and to permit the latest medical procedures development without consideration of ethical evaluation, is staggering.

But let us rise above the contemporary difficulties of health care facility management and look to the future of the Church's ministry through institutional health care in order to find another justification for ethics committees. In the past when the ministry of health care flourished, three assumptions governed the presence and behavior of the Church in the field of institutional health care. These assumptions were:

1) Catholic health facilities have committed Catholics as sponsors, administrators, medical and nursing staff; thus there was little need for education and formation in Catholic teaching.
2) Catholic hospitals would be able to care for poor as sign of their Christian ministry, through cost-shifting.
3) Catholic health care facilities would be able to survive without much support from an integration with the rest of the Catholic community.

I submit that all three of these assumptions are no longer operative. But each assumption enunciates an important need of Catholic health care, which now must be fulfilled in a different way. Thus if Catholic health care facilities, are to survive in the future, as the Commission for the Future of the Ministry declared, there must be an effort at integration into the diocesan community, an effort to educate and form administrators and staff in Catholic ethics and social theory, and there must be new methods to help the poor to gain better access to health care. In short, there must be a renewed effort to accomplish the mission of Catholic health care. I suggest that the forum for discovering and implementing new methods of formation, new initiatives to serve the poor, and innovative methods for integrating health care facilities into the diocese should be the ethics committee. I am convinced then, that if Catholic health care facilities have any chance of survival as Catholic in the future that there must be integrated system of ethics committees which will provide the spirit, formation and ecclesial coherence needed to accomplish the task.

NOTES

1. USCC, "Pastoral Letter on Health and Health Care," *Origins* December 3, 1981 vol. 11, n. 3 p. 396–402.

2. Commission on Catholic Ministry, *Catholic Health Ministry A New Vision for a New Century,* Farmington Hills, MI, 1988.

3. Cranford, Ronald; Doudera, A. Edward; eds. *Institutional Ethics Committees and Health Care Decision Making,* Ann Arbor: Health Administration Press, 1984.

4. Bernard Lo, "Behind Closed Doors," *New England Journal of Medicine,* July 2, 1987; vol. 317, n. 1; p. 46.

5. Brodeur, Dennis; "Toward a Clear Definition of Ethics Committees," *Linacre Quarterly* 51(3):233–247; August, 1984.

6. A.M.A. Judicial Council, "Guidelines for Ethics Committees in Health Care Institutions," *Journal of American Medical Association* 253(18):10 May, 1985.

7. McCarthy, Donald; "Tots is for Kids;" *Ethics and Medics,* vol. 13, n. 12; December, 1988.

8. Sacred Congregation for the Doctrine of the Faith, "Instruction on Respect for Human Life in Its Origin and on the Dignity of Procreation," (March 10, 1987) *Origins* vol. 16: n. 40, March 19, 1987.

9. Kelly, M; McCarthy, D. *Ethics Committees, A Challenge for Catholic Health Care,* St. Louis: Catholic Health Association, 1984.

Chapter 10

PASTORAL CONCERNS
ETHICS COMMITTEES IN CATHOLIC
HEALTH CARE FACILITIES

BISHOP: It's a very bleak situation, as I see it. My question is, can you give me any hope?

MONSIGNOR CASSIDY: There's always hope in the Church of God. I think that it's very important that the Bishop take his rightful place in health care. A historical problem with the American Bishops has been that they have had so many other problems that they dealt with that the Catholic hospitals developed without much input from the Bishops.

Now, when the Bishop asks to take an interest, some of the people who have been running the Catholic hospitals sort of resent it. I don't think that's good. But I think it important that the Bishop does take a real interest in what's going on.

Even if you don't have a Catholic health care facility, I think the Bishop still has a responsibility to see that people are getting good health care and that we try to lift the standards of health care even in non-Catholic or other organizations.

But it does look bleak. But this is a great opportunity because leadership in health care in the world is coming from the United States. If the United States can make a contribution in that area, it really will have an effect on the whole world.

I think the greatest tool for evangelization is health care. Governments are very happy if the Church gives them health care. But I think it's important that the Bishop take his role in health care and doesn't pass it off to other people.

A Catholic hospital is a Catholic hospital because the Bishop says it's a Catholic hospital, or it's not a Catholic hospital. The local Bishop has the main responsibility. That's the bottom line. It's important that the Bishop realize his role.

FATHER O'ROURKE: I would like to say that the situation in Catholic medical schools is so desperate that the Jesuits have Dominicans teaching! I really don't agree with everything that Monsignor Cassidy said. While there are four Catholic medical schools, at least in our medical school we've been working for ten years to establish a program of ethics. At the present time we have three full time people working in that and we have organized at least 35 physicians and nurses and hospital administrators who help us in our classes. For all four years of medical school and for the years of residency and for the years of nursing and hospital administration we have programs in ethics.

Having said that, however, we must realize that a medical school, like every other institution in our society today, is a pluralistic institution. If the Church is going to be alive in these pluralistic institutions, it will not result from an authoritarian stance.

We know that the development of communities is a very difficult, time-consuming effort. But I believe that Bishops are called upon to help develop Catholic communities in those institutions.

If the approach is authoritarian, it will not succeed. I know that it is not easy to suggest another approach, and that's why I used in my talk the word "coordination". I believe that it is important for people in positions of responsibility and authority in the Church to look upon their efforts, their role, as calling forth from people of good will, and of baptismal character, their best community effort.

The changing times, as illustrated by some of the documents in the Second Vatican Council, do call for a type of management that is different from an authoritarian type. Monsignor Cassidy was talking about physicians not having an ethical education, but that's true of everybody in society. You can say the same thing about people in business. So let us realize that we live in a society where ethics is very weak as a discipline and as an ideal. We may seek to supply the need for ethics through educational activities. That's part of it, certainly, but it's not the total answer. Ethics also demands that people have an affection for the good. We only develop an affection for the the good in a community of like-minded and like-hearted people who are dedicated to bringing out the good from their activities.

I think of the book, *Habits of the Heart, Individualism in America Society;* Father Sullivan of Villanova had a commentary on that book. He was part of the group that wrote that book. I think this book offers the most incisive study of our society in the last twenty years. It points out that people have friends, but they don't have any community, they're not willing to bond together to accomplish something difficult. I believe that's the inspiration of the Bishop, to bring people into community so that they bond together to accomplish something difficult. Being an ethical, Catholic community is a very difficult thing, whether in a school or in a hospital.

BISHOP: How do you deal with the case situations in the public forum? Bishops are always caught in the position of interpreting how we deal with the case situation in the public forum.

FATHER O'ROURKE: I think I'll be able to speak to that question through some practical examples. I want to speak especially to the diocesan ethics committee as it advises the Bishop. The effort has to anticipate some of the issues that will arise. The diocesan committee should advise the Bishop before the issue arises. The advice should be positive. It shouldn't be just negative in the sense of, no, we don't like that.

For example, I'm not in favor of living wills. I don't think that they accomplish the goals for which they are designed. On the other hand, the Catholic community or the Catholic Bishop, in response to a desire for legislation in regard to living wills, has to say more than, well, no, we're against them. The ethics committee has to give some positive advice beforehand.

166

A good thing happened in Missouri before the Cruzan case went to court. The Bishops called together a group of people, among whom I was one, to talk about the issues. I came up with an opinion that which emphasized the principle of double effect. The Bishops listened very respectfully but they didn't follow my opinion. Now I thought that was a reasonable approach.

They had all sides represented. But they didn't take what I was presenting as answering the case in question. That's about what happened. I thought that was a very beneficial way of meeting that issue. Then, when the case went to the Supreme Court, I was able to put in a private opinion but the Catholic Conference of Missouri put in a public opinion. That's the type of thing that I think has to be done. You have to anticipate and it has to be positive. You have to give some reasons for what you're doing.

BISHOP: In the Philippines we have very good medical schools and nursing schools, but our problem is that the students, after they finish their education, they go to the United States and other parts of the world where there is more economic opportunity. But our health care facilities are really very low standard. So the ethical question that arises is this: What could be the obligation of the First World, especially of the United States, in helping out Third World countries, such as my country, with their health care facilities?

MONSIGNOR CASSIDY: In the United States the Philippine doctor can't get a job now. Philippine doctors who come to the United States, especially to New York State, are much better if they stay home. It's almost impossible now to take somebody who is educated out of the United States and get them a job in a hospital in the United States.

I agree that the United States has a great obligation to help out. In our own diocese, we're helping out in the Dominican Republic, in Haiti and in Ghana. We have the facilities, I think, and the people. In our medical school, we're trying to make it a rule that every student before he graduates spends a rotation in the Third World. I think this is one of the things that we really should do more of because we do have the facilities and the opportunity to do so.

FATHER O'ROURKE: The problem you bring up is part of a larger problem about the lack of priorities in regard to health care

167

in the United States. At the present time the priority for physicians and for those directing large medical centers is to have high technology and to engage in the latest medical developments, such as transplants and heart catheterizations and things of that nature. That establishes the medical center as being first class.

However, there are 35 million people in our society without health insurance. This means 35 million who are not covered by Medicare, by private insurance, or by Medicaid.

Our priorities are really askew. We go for high technology instead of caring for the needs, the primary care needs especially, of the greater number of our society. In regard to foreign countries, the First World and the United States is not only exploiting these countries in regard to health care, but in regard to science, as well.

In the United States last year, 54% of those who received Ph.D.'s in science were from foreign countries. Only 6% of those who received Ph.D.'s in science last year were from minorities in from the United States. We're building a society which has many levels, and at the top economic level, we're utilizing the services of people from other countries to run our scientific programs and even to run our medical centers.

In the St. Louis area there's an association of doctors from the Philippines with two hundred doctors in that society. There is a brain drain and the thing that contributes to it is the lack of planning in the American system and the idea that high technology is the epitome of good medicine.

I think that the epitome of good medicine that we have to work toward establishing is that we care for those who are in need. That should be the highest priority we have in our health care system. I agree that there is a problem and it's because in the United States we don't look upon medical care as something that should be shared in our country and throughout the world. We look upon it as something that develops high technology.

BISHOP: In Canada we do have universal medical care and hospitalization. The poor do not have to pay the premium if they are below a certain annual income. The provinces, the ten provinces, have the control over medical care and education. Each province is autonomous but the Federal Government gives monies in order for grants to the hospitals. Catholic religious orders and communities still own certain hospitals, although they get grants from the Government and capital grants expand. They still have the controlling interest and they still also sit on the Board and they appoint the administrative officers. This, we foresee, of course, is not going to last forever because the religious communities no longer have the members to be able to assure continuity.

We are faced with a question how do we, Bishops and as dioceses, assure the continuing Catholicity of these Catholic hospitals? The question that is being posed to us is do the dioceses buy out the hospitals? Do we incorporate them in such a way that we will assure a Catholic continuity? Or are there other methods?

MONSIGNOR CASSIDY: Yes, this is certainly a big problem. It's important that you can keep sort of some basic control by being able to pick either the Members of the Board of Trustees or the administrator. If you can do that, I think you can keep your Catholic identity.

It's going to be very difficult to be able to do it. I think we in the United States have been fortunate in that we have been able to keep our identity, even though we do get grants. It's a battle, the government will give you this, they won't give you that. For example, you are told yon't give complete services if you don't give abortions. There's an awful lot of subtle difficulties. But I think it's worth fighting for survival and I think you just have to strive to find some way to succeed.

FATHER O'ROURKE: I would endorse that. I would also suggest that sponsorship must involve accountability to the Bishop and to the Church, because that's the way our Catholic Church is established. It is in the nature of the Church that there be accountability to the Bishop.

What bothers me is that hospitals might go the way of Catholic Universities in regard to the accountability to the Church and to the person of the Bishop. Many of our universities say they are a Catholic university in the sense that they are dedicated to Catholic values and Catholic teaching. But there's no accountability to the local diocese. We look to these universities as though the only thing constituting Catholic identity is the theology department. But how about psychology and how about economics? How about the literature and the arts?

In many Catholic colleges, the model of their success is not that they instill or create a Catholic community but rather that they imitate Harvard or Princeton. And Harvard and Princeton *were* religious universities seventy years ago. So if we look down the line and don't see accountability to the Church in the person of the Bishop, I fear for Catholic institutions. I fear for Catholic hospitals also, unless they have that bond of accountability. So ownership is the beginning of a bond. If you can't do it through that, as Monsignor Cassidy said, you've got to find other ways to do it.

BISHOP: Father O'Rourke, your name was mentioned several times yesterday in regard to the withdrawal of nutrition and hydration from persons in a persistent vegetative state. What is your opinion and why?

FATHER O'ROURKE: I have put together a list of points in regard to the use of hydration and nutrition. I think we can agree on some of them others need to be discussed further. Some terms were used in yesterday's discussion which don't help the discussion.

I believe everyone will agree on the presumption that is stated in the U.S. Bishops Pro-Life Committee in June of 1986 that artificial hydration and nutrition are presumed to be applied to those who need it in order to survive, unless this is ineffective or a grave burden. We have to consider what constitutes ineffective care or therapy and what constitutes a grave burden? Notice that care and therapy are the same thing. The goal of both is to exercise stewardship for ourselves or for others in regard to human life. When we talk about what is ineffective there may be some disagreement.

I believe that effectiveness has to take in account the spiritual destiny of the person. Others say that care is ineffective only if it will not prolong life. So that's a point of disagreement.

A second point of disagreement is in regard to the term, "grave burden". Many people will interpret this as applying only to physical pain, and in some cases, to economic burden. I believe that we should include here not only pain and economic burden but the psychological burden and spiritual burden.

In considering the use of hydration and nutrition we realize that we're applying the principle of double effect. There's no disagreement on that among the people who spoke here yesterday. We have to realize that we're not killing people when we make this decision, but we have to make sure that the decisions we make truly are in accord with the notion of what is ineffective or a grave burden.

A third point is the realization that the terms "ordinary" and "extraordinary" are used in many different ways and that's why the document on euthanasia from the Church in 1980 said that perhaps it is better to use the terms "proportionate" and "disproportionate".

Personally, I would rather stay with the terms "ordinary" and "extraordinary", provided we make the proper distinctions. Two distinctions should be made: First, that there's a medical meaning and a moral or an ethical or a theological meaning for these terms.

For the medical meaning, "ordinary," means that it's tested, it's standard, and it's the type of care you always give. For example, antibiotics for pneumonia are standard care now.

What's extraordinary care in medicine? That's experimental or innovative care. We have a process that we use for children now. It's called "Ecmo". When they can't breathe or they seem to have trouble, doctors put their blood in a machine and purify it and put it back in the child. It's a type of dialysis, but it's not exactly that. Ecmo is certainly experimental.

From the ethical or theological point of view, if you say something is ordinary, that means there's a moral imperative to do it. If you say something is extraordinary, it means it's optional. So we have that one important distinction. The second important distinction between ordinary and extraordinary is that you don't make that moral determination until after you know the circumstances of the patient. That's what Pope Pius XII said in 1957; that ordinary care is determined in accord with the circumstances of time, place, economics and things like that.

In other words, from a moral perspective, you don't make general statements about something being ordinary or extraordinary care. Rather, you follow through a process of investigating the condition of the patient, and then the conclusion is what is ordinary or extraordinary care for this patient.

That's why I am stressing that these decisions have to be made about particular people. In my writing, I've made a mistake in speaking about people in a persistent vegetative state as a class of people. The reason I've done that is because, as a class of people,

171

they are not able to chew and digest or act in a purposeful manner as the American Academy of Neurology stated in January of 1989. But I think that I have befuddled the issue by speaking of a group of people that should be treated or not treated in a certain way, rather than saying, let's look at the condition of this individual person in the persistent vegetative state, and determine what is ordinary or extraordinary for this individual.

The last thing that I wanted to say is that we don't solve the issue by citing court decisions. We don't improve our theological, ethical position by citing the decision of these courts in the United States because the courts use an entirely different manner of determining the issues than we use in the Catholic tradition. We follow not only the natural law tradition but, as the Vatican Council says, we make judgment in moral matters by analyzing the nature of the person and the acts of the person.

When the courts follow are legal norms or precedents. We can't say the Brophy case was in our favor and the Cruzan case was against us or vice versa. In the Cruzan case in Missouri, for example, after they said no, you can't remove hydration and nutrition from Nancy Beth Cruzan because it would lead to her death, the Supreme Court said, of course, if the legislature changes the laws, then we'll be able to remove that life support. This shows a positivistic concept of ethics.

The statements of the courts are positivistic. They follow not what we would think of as the nature of the person and human actions and human dignity but rather what has been called the constitutional right of privacy. We have a hard time tying that in with our Christian concept of individual and community because we do not have "a right to privacy" as Christians. We have an obligation to develop ourselves in community, and that's the way we work out our salvation, in conjunction and community with other people. What I'm saying is that the court decisions don't help us to solve the ethical issues that we're probing.

BISHOP: Are there ways to stress the importance of personal and interpersonal responsibility which so often is missing in the very kind of difficult cases we've discussed? Can we also press the importance of family in health care? Just as earlier this nation indicated that the parish could be the locus for education, I wonder if

172

there aren't new ways in which the parish can be the locus for health care.

MONSIGNOR CASSIDY: I think it's so important to realize that if the Catholic hospitals are to succeed in the United States, one of the things that has to be done is that they have to be very much integrated into the dioceses and into the parishes.

It's fascinating to go to Germany and find out that some parishes actually own hospitals. But I think it's been a failure in the United States system that the hospitals have never really integrated themselves into parish life.

The Bishop should be the first person informed and be involved in and merger because he's the one who decides whether it's going to be a Catholic institution or not. That's the bottom line. Authority is not a bad thing. We're in a Church that is an authority. I agree, very often we ought to coordinate. But my problem is, I think Catholic hospitals go down the tubes and Catholic medical schools go down the tubes because we haven't really stood by our faith and what's involved. In our society, you cannot use the authoritarian point of view and say this is it. But there does have to be a bottom line and I think our faith is involved in it.

FATHER O'ROURKE: The Pope says in every talk on medicine or research or experimentation we have to look to the nature of the person. In the United States, that becomes—To look to the individual—and there's too much individualism in our country. That's why I mentioned that the thing I try to get across is that you don't have a community unless you have a task to which you're devoted.

In that article I mentioned by Father Sullivan of Villanova, he uses St. Thomas's definition of community; what brings people together is pleasure from each others' company, a common goal, common values, and then a common task.

Many people in the United States have friends in the sense that they share what they call values and they have pleasure in one another. But they are not devoted to a common task. But they don't realize that that's the way you really establish yourself as a human being, as a person.

Secondly, the system of health care in the United States came into question when you talked about developing parishes. Not only is our system of health care in the United States organized toward high tech medicine, but also toward acute care hospitals. I mentioned those people who have to come to acute care hospitals for primary care. There should be clinics in their home neighborhoods where people who need that kind of health can go to get help with their aches and pains, especially their high blood pressure.

That's one of the great killers in United States, and if medicine has learned anything in the past thirty years is that high blood pressure kills people. And yet, there's no primary care system that meets the need of poor people who have high blood pressure. They think they'll go to an acute care hospital, the emergency room, when they get a cold or when they get deep pneumonia. But there's no preventive help for them before that. So we have not only a system that's out of control in regard to financing, but we have a system that's out of control in regard to purpose and in regard to care for the poor.

Chapter 11

CATHOLIC IDENTITY AND HOSPITAL MERGERS

Sister Margaret John Kelly, D.C.

I. Preliminary Observations

This presentation, which I would like to sub-title "Where conviction and pragmatism meet", will have to be introduced as both tentative and extremely important. It is tentative because it deals with an issue for which there is no established data base. While the universe of examples is growing quickly it is now relatively small. The presentation is also made somewhat tentative and difficult because of the lack of both unanimity and consistency in defining the terms "Catholic Identity" and "Merger."

Despite the preliminary and tentative character this presentation must assume, the subject is of increasing importance to all of us in Church and demands the "prudence and boldness" the United States bishops called for in their 1981 pastoral on "Health and Health Care." Just as healing was central to Jesus' ministry, hospitals have traditionally been central to church service in the U.S., but in the past decade we have seen dramatic changes in the sponsorship of Catholic facilities. As Religious Institutes experience decreasing membership and aging personnel, they must determine if they desire to or even can continue sponsorship. Communities of women now sponsor over 90% of the Catholic hospitals in this country and their membership has decreased over 30% (almost 70,000 sisters) in 20 years. In those two decades, the number of Catholic hospitals in the U.S. has de-creased from over 900 to just over 600 and 20% of these hospitals are sponsored by congregations with less than 100 members and with a median age of 65.[1]

On a positive note, in this decade of the 80's, the sponsorship of at least 30 Catholic hospitals has been transferred from one religious institute to another religious institute or to a diocese/archdiocese. In that same period, the number of Catholic multihospital health systems has doubled and the 60+ health systems now encompass over 2/3 of the 613 Catholic hospitals in this country. In that period, there has also been a significant growth in collaborative sponsorship within the Catholic hospital ministry.

While sponsorship in some cases can be controlled within church, some major changes occurring in the health care field are out of Church control. The complexity of both the financing and delivery of health care continue to increase. Hospital utilization has decreased dramatically because of new technologies and the greater reliance on outpatient services. Furthermore, the growing number of uninsured and the subsidy required for the institutional care of the aged have caused some Catholic hospitals to close, others to file for bankruptcy, and has threatened the fiscal viability of virtually all but a few hospitals. These changes and challenges have caused some forecasters to project the closure or merger of up to one-fourth of the almost 7,000 U.S. hospitals by the mid-1990's. That shocking projection seems more realistic when we consider that from 1980 to 1984, 20 U.S. hospitals closed per year but in 1986, 71 closed; in 1987, 79 closed; and in 1988 81 closed (half of which was not-for-profit)[2]. In Chicago alone 10 hospitals have closed since 1984, seven in medically underserved areas. Further more, this subject of Catholic identity and merger grows in importance when one considers that the two historical bases of our religious hospitals: first amendment rights and not-for profit status, can be jeopardized by mergers and collaborative arrangements. Aware of this, the National Commission on Catholic Health Care Ministry in their final report published this past year called for the development of criteria to guide mergers and consolidations so as to safeguard the future of the Catholic health ministry.[3]

This topic "Mergers and Catholic Identity" then seems to focus on three complex and interrelated questions:

1. Are Catholic hospitals necessary today?   Necessity
2. What makes a hospital Catholic?   Identity
3. How does one assure Catholic identity?   Integrity

These questions need to be answered as part of the ongoing commitment articulated in the U.S. bishops' pastoral *On Health and Health Care* to maintain and develop a Catholic institutional presence within the health care field.[4] While the research reported here is limited to Catholic hospitals in the United States, the material and conclusion are relevant to any country which has a blend of Catholic and other sectarian and non-sectarian hospitals and which is experiencing economic constraints in its health care budget.

Research Method

It is important at the outset to identify the fact there is no central information source that provides an all inclusive list of Catholic mergers in the United States. The data presented here has been derived from consultation with a commercial research firm, the American Hospital Association, the Catholic Health Association and personal experience. 24 cases (including two from the 1970's) are included. The Catholic party in each of these situations completed a questionnaire about the merger process and most submitted their corporate documents.[5] All but two of the church entities requested anonymity in this presentation and that will be respected.

Objectives

With those preliminary observations, let me present my objectives for this presentation. First I would like to create a typical merger scenario; secondly, I will give an overview of the profile and the results of the 24 mergers studied; thirdly, I will present working definitions of "merger" and "Catholic Identity" and explore the complexity of both terms; fourthly, I will describe the effects of "mergers" on "Catholic identity" and finally, I will present some conclusions.

II. Inter-hospital Collaborative Relationships

A. Typical Merger scenario
To put our discussion into a context, let us for a few minutes, consider a situation which could generate the need for a Catholic hospital to consider a merger or some type of collaboration with another facility. Charity Hospital, a Catholic, not-for-profit corporation, is located in Liberty, a city with a Catholic population of 20% and with one other community hospital. The Charity sisters, a public juridic person in canonical terms, founded the hospital in 1872 and still serve as the canonical stewards of the hospital. The Charity sisters sponsor three other hospitals in two other states and have 150 sisters with a median age of 64 (the median age for all women religious in the U.S.) Five sisters, a sister-administrator and four sisters in pastoral care, now serve at Charity, whereas in 1965, there were 24 sisters. Charity Hospital has a two tiered not-for-profit corporate structure of a Membership and a Board of Directors. The Board of Directors of Charity, composed of a majority of lay persons with a few Charity sisters, is responsible for general governance of the hospital. The Members, the leadership of the Charity sisters, (in fact, the General Superior and her council) *reserve* to themselves "sufficient corporate powers" in a civil sense to exercise their canonical faith and administration obligations and to act as Church steward of the mission and the assets. These powers perceived as essential to assuring the Catholic identity of the hospital are:

178

1. Changes in the Articles of Incorporation and Bylaws
2. Changes in the mission or philosophy of the hospital
3. Appointment of the Board of Directors of the hospital
4. Approval of the lease, sale or encumbrance of the corporate real estate of the hospital
5. Approval of merger or dissolution of the hospital Corporation

Through these five powers the sisters, as a Catholic church entity, *control* the corporate structure, corporate mission and corporate assets of Charity Hospital. In addition, a recent chapter of the Charity sisters developed a sponsorship statement which details what they describe as further *Catholic identity* requirements for hospitals they sponsor such as maintenance of a pastoral care department and a certain level of charity care.

Hope Community Hospital, a non-sectarian, not-for profit facility, established in 1936, is within two blocks of Charity and is governed by a Board of Directors. Each of the hospitals has about 240 beds and for three years each has had an occupancy rate below the national average of 60%. There is a great deal of overlap in the medical staffs of the two facilities.

The administrator of Hope Hospital recently approached the Sister administrator of Charity and suggested that they work out some kind of a collaborative arrangement before both facilities fail. Both administrators realize the need for a long-term care facility but neither wants to sacrifice being a hospital to become that facility. The Catholic hospital has recently been renovated and is a much better physical facility than Hope, but Hope has some very successful specialized programs. The hospitals have similar ethical postures. Both have taken public stands against euthanasia and abortion and have special programs for the poor although Charity has a much higher level of free care. Hope, however, does some male and female sterilizations.

When the sister administrator of Charity approached the congregational leadership and the Membership of the Charity Hospital Corporation, to ask about Charity collaborating with Hope Hospital, the sisters raised the following issues:

1. The initial hospital was built through the labors and donations of the congregation so the congregation has

economic interest in the facility as well as moral responsibility for it. Will collaboration diminish their control of the hospital as part of their apostolic work and the Church's patrimony?

2. Should the hospital continue? Which is a higher value: the continued presence of a Catholic hospital or decreased health care costs for the public through consolidation? Should the sisters just withdraw from the ministry and let Hope Hospital serve the people since Catholics are in the minority anyway?

3. If the two hospitals do cooperate, is it right for the Catholic facility to impose the *Ethical Directives* and the bishops' teaching authority on physicians who do not belong to the church? But if they are not imposed, will the sisters be giving scandal if procedures contrary to the Catholic ethic are performed.

4. Would it be possible and/or appropriate to maintain religious symbols and a Catholic chapel if the two facilities were merged at one site?

5. Could a legal structure be developed which would allow the sisters to protect their investment and retain the Catholic identity even while they took advantage of joint efforts and economies of scale?

6. Would affiliation with.a Catholic multi-hospital system give sufficient strength for the Catholic hospital to be the survivor if just one hospital can survive in the competitive environment? Should the Sisters compete aggressively to be the surviving hospital? How does a Catholic hospital compete in the health care marketplace and still practice the Christian value system.

7. If Charity became the needed long-term care facility, would reimbursement be sufficient to cover the capital indebtedness?

While this scenario and these questions relate to fictional Charity Hospital, they are the questions raised by the leaders, the bishop and the public in the 24 Catholic hospitals included in this study. While fictional, the case is typical. Independent of size or location, the facts are similar. Hospital mergers have occurred and will continue to occur principally because of *excess capacity* and the need to shrink the hospital system as a way to reduce spiralling health care costs.

B. Overview of Results

Having considered briefly that fact situation which generates consideration of a merger, let's take an overview of the 24 cases included in my study and then, we will do some specific analysis.

1. 21 of the 24 occurred from 1981–1988 with 18 occurring in 20 months of 1987–1988. This acceleration reveals the impact of the 1983 change from a retrospective payment system to a prospective system. Most of the mergers were developed over *several* years and with lengthy negotiations.

2. The bed size of the hospital seems to be unimportant as the 24 cases include small hospitals of well under 100 beds to several in the range of 200 and 300 as well as one 800 bed facility. (The average Catholic hospital in 1988 had 260 beds while the average non-federal hospital in the nation had 165 beds.)

3. The collaboration trend is not localized but has occurred in 16 states coast to coast with 3 in two states and two in another state and in 18 different dioceses and archdioceses.

4. The arrangements have involved 20 different Catholic sponsors including 17 institutes of women religious.

5. The results varied: we can plot the results of these 24 situations on a continuum of Catholic *influence* to Catholic *control* of the surviving entity. Beginning with no Catholic influence, we move through some Catholic influence to some Catholic control to complete Catholic control. This final point of the continuum (complete Catholic control) correlates with those reserved powers we mentioned before and provide for church control of corporate documents, corporate mission and philosophy, corporate assets and corporate Board.

No Catholic influence remained in five cases or 21% of the situations studied; the Catholic character disappeared and the Catholic entity was in fact secularized. In those cases a Catholic Hospital and a community hospital were merged, (such as Charity and Hope) and the non-Catholic entity prevailed. At the next point on the continuum, *some* Catholic influence remained in two cases (8%) which occurred a decade apart. In these cases, the Catholic influence remains through agreements to maintain such things as a Catholic chapel, Catholic chaplaincy services and prohibition of elective abortions. In ten situations (42%) *some degree of Catholic control* remains and later we will look at some of these models very closely. In seven situations, (29%) the Catholic institutions prevailed and when the two hospitals were merged, the Catholic remained.

At the extremes of the continuum, we have true mergers in that two institutions came together and one institution prevails. In summation (five) Catholic hospitals were absorbed or lost in the mergers while at the other extreme, in seven cases the Catholic corporation survived. In the other twelve situations, we have consolidations or modified mergers with two parties continuing to influence the corporation. It is important to note that in the cases where the Catholic entity prevailed, the Catholic party entered the negotiations with a list of non-negotiables and the local ethic was very consistent with that of the Church.

6. The majority of these collaborative arrangements were motivated by a need to assure fiscal viability or economic *survivability* of the institution.

7. As far as the individuals or groups initiating these mergers, one finds that it is most frequently local boards, local administrators or physicians, and infrequently the sponsors, who begin the dialogues. In one of the cases, it was the major employer in the city who suggested the merger as the way to reduce health care costs.

C. Corporate Models—Definitions, Structures and Effects

1. Definitions—Legal Structures

Before we look more closely at the dynamics and the effects of these mergers and collaborative arrangements, it seems important now to clarify the terminology "merger" and "Catholic identity". I noted at the outset that there is not consistency in the use of these terms. For the remainder of this presentation, I will distinguish "merger", "consolidation", and "collaborative relationship".

> *Merger* is the act whereby two corporations are brought together so that only one entity survives. (a + b = b)
> *Consolidation* is the act whereby two legal entities pool their resources and a third new entity emerges. (a + b = c)
> *Collaborative arrangement* is the act whereby through contract or through corporate documents, a non-Church corporation commits itself to Catholic values in some operational areas or is bound to a Catholic entity in certain restricted activities. (a + b = b + a/2) or (a + b = c + a/2)

As I indicated before, the true mergers are very straightforward but the collaborative arrangements are quite varied and quite complex.

2. Definition—Catholic Identity

During the last thirty years, a great deal of time and activity has been spent in isolating the elements contained in the concept "Catholic Hospital", but there is no consensus on its meaning. Let us consider some of the perceptions and definitions. For many persons, particularly in the pre-Vatican II period, and for some even today, "Catholic" means the visible presence of religious men or women in the facility. For others, "Catholic" is perceived in negative terms as what Catholic hospitals do not permit such as abortions, sterilizations and euthanasia. Others, particularly those who want to cut health care costs, see Catholic hospitals as the place where the poor should go to receive free health care. At the risk of over-simplifying a very complex phenomenon, I would like to describe four historical emphases which have marked discussions of Catholic Identity within the health care ministry.

a. **Pre-Vatican II and pre-Medicare/Medicaid Period**— "Catholic" was perceived here principally in the visible presence of religious at the operational level. The Catholicity was conveyed through the dominance of religious on boards and in key management positions and was transmitted through the large numbers of nurses trained in the hospital schools of nursing conducted by the sponsoring congregations.

b. **Late 1960's to late 1970's**—Emphasis in this period was on ethical issues and Catholic identity was weighed heavily on the ethical posture of the facility. In 1971 the Bishops of the U.S. had approved the *Ethical and Religious Directives for Catholic Health Facilities* in which they provided a rather broad and comprehensive interpretation of "Catholic".[6] However, this document subsequently was reduced by many to prohibitions in gynecological services. This limited interpretation is understandable because hospitals were then experiencing increased pressure to perform both sterilizations and abortions because of the more permissive sexual environment as well as the legalization of abortion in 1973.

c. **Late 1970's**—While the Maida-McGrath controversy had begun earlier, in the late 1970's it received more publicity and focused attention on the legal aspect of Catholic identity. As the two canon lawyers debated what church property was and who actually "owned" Catholic hospitals and other institutions, they drew attention to the legal basis of Church "sponsorship" and "stewardship." These two terms entered the vocabulary and documents of religious congregations. The relationship of mission to corporate structures became central and sponsorship discussions focused on being Catholic in spirit and in truth, in church law and in civil law.

Many began to recognize that the freedom to assume a Catholic moral posture is conditioned by the existence of a civil law structure which secures that right.

At the same time, some sponsors were expressing the view that in the spirit of ecumenism and pluralism, we should label our facilities Christian and not Catholic. This heightened awareness explains why the Catholic Hospital Association's 1977 survey of its members revealed a need for national clarification of Catholic identity so that Catholic health care facilities could "evaluate their effectiveness as ecclesial organizations."

d. **1980's**—In the 1980's we have witnessed broad interest and heavy emphasis on both the corporate structures and the personnel formation aspects of Catholic identity. Various theologians and health care practitioners explored the various aspects of being Catholic in a pluralistic, highly technologized society and a plethora of essays emerged.

Catholic Health Association published in 1980 *The Evaluative Criteria for Catholic Health Facilities* which detailed eight principles for measuring Catholicity and educating to mission.[7] This document included ecclesial, corporate and operational standards. Having revoked that document in 1985, in 1987 Catholic Health Association published *The Dynamics of Catholic Healthcare, A Working Document* which was to again respond to the questions: "What does it mean to be Catholic?" and "Does being Catholic make any difference?"[8] This publication focuses on the sacramental aspects of Catholic identity.

In the 80's, the burgeoning Catholic health systems as well as many local hospitals made the spiritual formation of their boards and their management staffs a priority. The staff positions of mission effectiveness and mission services grew in importance at both the hospital system and local hospital levels. At the same time, interest in the canonical aspects of sponsorship was heightened by the issuance of the new canon law in 1983.

During the 80's as well, the Catholic Health Association had to redefine its membership criteria and protocol because of evolving relationships and changing corporate structures such as mergers and consolidations. In addition, some state Catholic Hospital Associations have considered new affiliate membership categories to take care of some of the Catholic identity "anomalies" that have been created by mergers and consolidations.

For the purpose of this presentation and to assist us to work through the various models of collaborative arrangements and the manner in which they relate to Catholic identity, I will propose my own definition of Catholic identity which has three elements: A Catholic hospital is one which has the *legitimate Church mandate, the legal character (or civil standing),* and *the moral and social vision* which make the facility a *recognizable participant* in the health mission of the Catholic Church. To simplify that

a. A *legitimate church mandate* refers to the legal tie-in with the institutional church. For an institution to be Catholic in spirit and in operations, it should have its foundation in Church. At the most basic level then, to be Catholic requires some Church tie-in whether it be the traditional public juridic person status of a religious congregation or diocese or the two new experimental lay sponsorship models of private juridic person and private association of the Christian faithful.[9] In addition, the bishop has the right to determine if the apostolic work is integrated into the mission of the Church.

b. The *legal character or civil standing* refers to the civil documents which establish the first amendment rights of the facility and protect its corporate conscience. In short, there must be a basis in civil law for the Catholic character of the hospital as well as for its very existence as a service corporation.

c. The *moral and social vision* refers to the operational realities which reveal that Catholic, Christian values permeate the organization. This may also be considered the institutional or corporate culture which is recognizable as Church-based and Church-oriented.

I have presented that definition as a backdrop because some of these collaborative arrangements do, indeed, include and stress one, two or three of the elements. We are certainly not a monolith and both *conviction and pragmatism* are carving out the details of these arrangements.

3. Structures and Effects: Church Influence or Control

Because of the varying emphasis on either the corporate or operational realities of being Catholic, it is understandable that the inter-institutional collaborations that will be discussed here will show a broad range of interpretation of what it means to retain institutional Catholicity. To maintain canonical control, some sponsors have decided to retain all reserved powers or hold sufficient seats on the board of the consolidated corporation. Some chose to keep intact their Catholic corporation but to establish a parent corporation; some have negotiated sponsorship contracts; others have established management corporations to perform management functions for merged operations but have retained corporate identities. To better point up these differences and to work through the maze of corporate structures, I would like to return to my original continuum and divide my comments into the two specific designations of institutions with church *influence* and church *control.* We have already noted that 12 or one-half of the 24 cases included in this study were true mergers in which one institution lost its identity with the Catholic identity being lost in five mergers and maintained in seven others. These cases will not be elaborated on here except to say that in the negotiations, "The Ethical Directives" became a central focus of the discussions. Of the remaining twelve situations two arrangements resulted in some "Catholic influence" being retained. The remaining 10 cases allow for Catholic controls and will be discussed through a review of the matrix.

Catholic influence continues after the collaborative arrangement has been effected when the Catholic party has some legal-power to effect compliance with church values in a circumscribed area. In one situation, the Catholic party has been able by contract to gain a prohibition against abortions and has the power: to ap-

MATRIX—Elements of Control in Collaborative Arrangements

	IOTA	KAPPA	DELTA	GAMMA	LAMBDA
Powers Maintained by Church Entity	Sponsorship Board	Sponsorship Corporation	Catholic/Community Hospital—not-for-profit stock corporation 2 share holders	Catholic/ Community Hospital consolidation	Civil Trust "Catholic presence"
1. * Control over Hospital Articles of Inc.	Articles on sponsorship only	Sponsorship powers only	vote of 10 required + approval of both shareholders	2/3 vote of both Members and Directors	Trust
*Control over Hospital Bylaws	Sponsorship Elements only	Sponsorship powers only	vote of 10 required + approval of both shareholders	2/3 vote of both Members and Directors	Trust
*Control over change in hospital mission and philosophy	Yes	Yes	vote of 10 required + approval of both shareholders	Unanimous vote of 3 church members and 4 Directors	Trust

*Powers generally considered necessary to be controlled by Catholic entity.

**Pure mergers have been excluded from this matrix because the philosophy/control of the surviving corporation, whether it be Catholic or not prevails.

	IOTA	KAPPA	DELTA	GAMMA	LAMBDA
2. *Sale, Merger or Consolidation, Dissolution of hospital corporation	Yes	Yes	vote of 10 required + approval of both shareholders	Unanimous vote of 3 church members and 4 Directors	
Debt			vote of 10 required + approval of both shareholders		
Approval of transfer of stock of other shareholders			yes		
*Control of Assets Share of Assets upon Dissolution		yes	yes (leased to stock corporation)	yes (25 year lease) appropriate share	
3. *Control over hospital board appointments			7 out of 15	4 out of 9 + 1 by agreement	3 out of 23
Participation in Hospital Membership				3 out of 7 plus 1 by agreement	1 out of 2 corporate member
Participation of Hospital Board of Directors		6 out of 12	7 out of 15	4 out of 9	3 out of 23
Recommend items for Board Agenda	yes				

MATRIX—Elements of Control in Collaborative Arrangements (continued)

	IOTA	KAPPA	DELTA	GAMMA	LAMBDA
4. *Appointment of CEO	consultation		vote of 10 required + approval of both shareholders		
5. Compliance with Ethical and Religious Directives	yes	yes + Ethics Agreement	yes (Corporate bylaws)	yes	yes—1 site no—1 site
Interpretation of violation of Ethical & Religious Directives				religious superior	Bishop
Prohibition of Abortions	by Ethical & Religious Directives	by Ethical & Religious Directives	by Ethical & Religious Directives	by Ethical & Religious Directives	yes
Prohibition of Euthanasia	by Ethical & Religious Directives	by Ethical & Religious Directives	by Ethical & Religious Directives	by Ethical & Religious Directives	yes
Prohibition of sterilizations	by Ethical & Religious Directives	by Ethical & Religious Directives	by Ethical & Religious Directives	by Ethical & Religious Directives	

	IOTA	KAPPA	DELTA	GAMMA	LAMBDA
Sterilizations in separate facility			yes		yes, in the non-Catholic location
Natural Family planning					yes
Ethics Committee	yes	yes		yes	
Place on Ethics Committees	yes			yes	
6. Staff Position for sponsorship	yes				
7. Pastoral Care Department	yes	yes			yes
Catholic Chapel	yes	yes			
Catholic Symbols	yes	yes			
Use of Catholic Name	yes	yes		Name change	Name change
Projected Catholic image	yes	yes	yes, but ecumenical	no	no
Projected Christian image				yes	
8. Right of Bishop or episcopal option to assume sponsorship if congregation cease	yes			yes	yes

point three of the 13 hospital trustees; to set standards for care of the poor; to maintain an ethics committee; and a pastoral care department; to use Catholic religious symbols and continue the Catholic name. In another situation, a convenant appears in the revised bylaws of the new consolidated corporation. This convenant, in place for 13 years now, requires that at the former Catholic site, no elective abortions be performed and that a Catholic chapel and Catholic chaplain be maintained "throughout the existence of the consolidated corporation."

Because of the complexity of the legal relationship in the *Catholic control* situations, it seems most beneficial to present examples through the matrix which identifies the controls that allow for various elements of Catholic identity to be lived out. On the vertical axis of this matrix, you will see 8 categories of Catholic control:

1. Corporate documents—mission and philosophy
2. Sale, merger, consolidation, assets
3. Board appointments
4. CEO appointment
5. Ethical issues
6. Sponsorship issues
7. Catholic symbols
8. Episcopal role

On the horizontal of the matrix you see five different models with the powers that have been retained by the Catholic party in the relationship. These five models are representative of the 10 situations in which the Catholic sponsor retained some control.

The first two models are sponsorship-oriented but they differ in the scope and means of corporate control. In the first (Iota), the assets have not been retained by the Catholic party, whereas in the second (Kappa), control over the assets has been retained along with other corporate powers. The delta model provides for a two shareholder not-for-profit consolidated corporate structure. The Gamma model is a true consolidation with a Membership and Board of Directors providing a two tiered governance structure. In both of these, the Catholic control resides in the majority or unanimous vote requirements and in both the assets have been leased by the sponsoring congregation to the new corporation. The Lambda model is unique in that it relies upon a civil trust to preserve the Catholic elements. This final model has caused a great deal of discussion in canonical circles because it required alienation of the assets and in fact created a non-sectarian facility. The architects of this design prefer to call it "Catholic presence" rather than Catholic control.

We can now and later in your table discussions review the matrix to see the specific control points that are perceived to be constitutive of or contribute to Catholic identity. You will note that the *Ethical Directives* by reference guide four of the five models while the fifth model identifies specific ethical postures on abortion, euthanasia and natural family planning.

III. Conclusion

The following conclusions appear justified from the study of this diverse, accelerating and complex issue of "mergers" and "Catholic identity."

A. Because of the continuing retrenchment occurring in the acute care field, the number of "mergers"/"consolidations" and "collaborative arrangements" will probably increase and will continue to affect hospitals of varying size throughout the nation. Catholic hospitals in two hospital cities or in over-bedded areas will be particularly vulnerable.

B. Catholic identity is now perceived as based in legal and moral control rather than in the physical presence of religious but there is still much discussion about the essentials of being "Catholic."

C. A variety of patterns of church *control* is evident with mission, philosophy and governance issues apparently of greater importance than control of assets.

D. Adherence to *Ethical and Religious Directives* appears to be central to Catholic identity and is the most consistent factor in these arrangements. Ability to proscribe abortion, at least elective abortion, is present in most arrangements but there is some difficulty in limiting sterilizations. Arrangements for pastoral care also appear to be of major concern to those sponsors who remove themselves from direct governance responsibilities as in the sponsorship and trust arrangements.

E. Move is toward greater involvement of Bishops in the merger and consolidation process with bishops entering into the process during negotiations as well as assuming future responsibility through some corporate documents.

This period of history and this issue will force the church in the United States, particularly the episcopal leadership, to respond to these questions with "the boldness and prudence" called for in their 1981 Pastoral on health:

1. Is the institutional health ministry still integral to the Church's services. **Necessity**
2. What are the essential elements for Catholic identity? **Identity**
3. How will the integrity of Catholic institutions be assured in a period of overall retrenchment? **Integrity**

When I began, I subtitled this talk "Where Conviction and Pragmatism Meet." May our prayer be that conviction about Church mission and pragmatism in response to a retrenched market will meet successfully and happily so that in the words of the pastoral, Catholic health facilities will "maintain and deepen their identity and exercise a penetrating influence in the health field." May these collaborative ventures be conducted in such a way that they will be a response to the challenge Pope John Paul II offered Catholic healthcare provides during his visit to Phoenix that they be a Christian force in forming the moral and social conscience of the nation.

NOTES

1. Edward J. Mally, *Health Care Handbook.* St. Louis: Catholic Health Association, 1962, pp. 20–21.

2. American Hospital Association Statistical Reports, Chicago: American Hospital Association, 1988.

3. *Catholic Health Ministry: A New Vision for a New Century.* Commission on Catholic Health Care Ministry. Farmington Hills, Michigan, 1988, p. 17.

The commission recommended that criteria include: shared participation in ownership or governance, a formal commitment to common values, and a substantive relationship to some official structure.

4. *Health and Health Care: A Pastoral Letter of the American Catholic Bishops.* Washington, DC: United States Catholic Conference, 1981, p. 10.

5. The questionnaire was submitted to a corporate officer or a member of the sponsoring congregation of each of the Catholic entities involved in the collaborative arrangements. The questionnaire included the following areas: motivating factors for the merger; initiator of the merger; description of the corporate structure which existed prior to new relationships; corporate structures which currently exist; composition of and appointment to board of new corporation (s); description of powers or controls reserved to Catholic entity; place of *Ethical Directives;* presentation of new entity as Catholic, Christian, etc. and the role of the diocesan bishop. In most cases, copies of the corporate documents were forwarded to the author, but anonymity was requested by all but two of the respondents.

6. *The Ethical and Religious Directives for Catholic Health Facilities* were approved by the National Conference of Catholic Bishops in 1971 and slightly revised in 1975 and are currently under study. A brief history of the document is presented in *Catholic Identity in Health Care: Principles and Practice.* Boston: Pope John Center, 1987, pp. 1–19.

7. *Evaluative Criteria for Catholic Health Facilities.* St. Louis: Catholic Health Association, 1980.

8. *The Dynamics of Catholic Identity in Healthcare.* St. Louis: Catholic Health Association, 1987.

9. Catholic Health Association focused on "New Horizons: Alternative Sponsorship" in its September, 1987 *Health Progress.* In September 1985, *Health Progress* had focused on the challenges of traditional sponsorship models. These two sections provide an overview of the very complex issue of sponsorship of Catholic Facilities in the 1980's.

10. *Health and Health Care.* p. 11.

Chapter 12

PASTORAL CARE PERSONNEL IN CATHOLIC HEALTH CARE FACILITIES

The Reverend Gerald R. Niklas, M.Div.

In 1964 I went to the Catholic Chaplains' meeting in Milwaukee. At that time it was a division of the Catholic Hospital Association and had about 400 members. The most memorable aspect of this meeting was that only priests attended and only they were "allowed" to attend. At one point, as the speaker was about to begin, two sisters dressed in full garb came in and sat down in the last row. Immediately one of the priests went over and asked the two sisters to leave explaining that this was just for priests. I would like to see a priest try that today!

Presently, the organization of Catholic Chaplains is called the National Association of Catholic Chaplains and has been in existence for 24 years. The full membership totals 3,309 as of March, 1988 and 15% of them are laity, 28% priests, 53% religious sisters and 3% permanent deacons.[1] This means that all the various people who come together to form Church are involved in this ministry.

A survey performed by the Catholic Health Association last year indicated that 97% of the directors of the pastoral care departments in our Catholic facilities are Catholic while 3% are protestant ministers. The same survey revealed that 54% of the directors are women religious, 30% are priests, 3% deacons, 11% are lay people and 1% are religious brothers. In 1984, 45% were priests which means that in just four years there has been a 15% decrease in the number of priests directing pastoral care departments. The future seems to indicate that there will be fewer and fewer priest-directors and priest-chaplains in our institutions. Another development is that the directors of pastoral care are hiring Protestant chaplains to minister to the needs of Protestant patients. Presently 12.3% of the chaplains are Protestant ministers.[2]

In another aspect of pastoral care, we might note that the facilities are becoming more and more business oriented. Twenty-five years ago the titles of the leaders of the hospital were administrator and assistant administrator. Today they have adopted business titles, too. For example, at Good Samaritan Hospital in Cincinnati we no longer have a personnel department, but have a human resources department, no longer a housekeeping department but an environmental services department. Fifteen years ago when I was chaplain at Mercy Hospital in Springfield, Ohio, a 300 bed facility, there were three people full time in administration: the administrator, an associate administrator and a medical director. Today, because of many new demands, administration includes a president, a few vice-presidents and several assistant vice presidents. Administration has also created several new departments including marketing, mission effectiveness, quality assurance, out-patient care, development fund director, physician relations and planning department. Their budgets have grown by leaps and bounds to the extent that presently the Good Samaritan Hospital has an annual budget of over $150,000,000. Whenever you deal with that kind of money, it is big business and must be managed in a responsible and just manner.

Roles of the Pastoral Care Department

With this introduction to modern health facilities in mind, I would like to concentrate on the first question I've been asked to address: What are the roles of the pastoral care department in a highly technical Catholic health facility?

A Catholic health facility is a vital part of the Catholic Church's mission, especially to the poor and the underserved.[3] Often it bears the name of a saint and usually has a picture of the Pope and the local Bishop in the lobby. I say "usually" because in 1987 Cardinal O'Connor told the participants of the Catholic Hospital Administrative Personnel Program otherwise. He mentioned that he visited a Catholic hospital in his archdiocese in the evening after the visiting hours were over. He discovered that the front doors were locked and he had to enter through the emergency unit. In continuing his story he noted he had a very difficult time finding the patient he wanted to visit. In his travels through many long corridors of that building he never did find a picture of himself or the pope in the lobby, outside the chapel, or any other place.

In addition, the orientation brochure for new patients clearly states that they have entered a Catholic facility and a brief summary of the mission statement and the philosophy of the institution is given. All the new employees are told in their orientation program during the first days of work that the facility is Catholic and an explanation of the mission and philosophy is shared with them. Periodically the mission effectiveness and pastoral care departments remind the employees of these ideas in various ways e.g.: a Fall Festival of Faith; monthly employee-management meetings; annual awards dinner for employees; prayer before the monthly department directors meeting; the celebration of the Eucharist and/or a prayer service on the occasion of the feast day of the health facility; a weekly religious bulletin written for the patients, their families and the employees.

Members of the pastoral care department minister to patients and their families as well as to hospital employees. As they do this, they are participating in the pastoral ministry of the local bishop. This is just one role of the members of the pastoral care department and a significant role because in a 600 bed hospital in a period of one week there are likely to be 1,000 different patients,

3,000 employees and 8,000 other people coming through the doors of that institution as visitors, doctors and students in various health professions.

Another role of pastoral care is the traditional one of celebrating the Eucharist and bringing the sacraments to the sick. This can be done in a very perfunctory manner, or it can be enhanced greatly by appropriate preparations and participation of family members. A valuable contribution to the patients is closed circuit television from the chapel allowing the patients to participate in the mass daily and especially on Sunday. This system can be used for a prayer service in preparation for Communion when Communion is distributed publicly. Other benefits of this inhouse communication system are: the rosary; stations of the cross; value oriented programs produced by organizations like the Christophers. Related to this function, the chaplains are leaders of prayer and organize the personnel of the hospital to pray a morning and evening prayer, a reminder to the personnel, visitors and patients that the facility is indeed a Catholic Christian institution.

Related to the liturgical and sacramental role is one which includes reading the scriptures and praying with the sick. It's not appropriate to do this with every patient, but pastoral persons need to be perceptive to hints in the conversation and to personal belongings of the patient (bible, prayer book) to discern those who would appreciate a scripture reading and/or a prayer and those who would not.[4]

Another traditional role is that of walking with the sick at their pace. Henry Nouwen expressed this idea when he said that the best compliment any patient can give a pastoral person is, "He really understands me and as a result I feel comforted." He went on to explain in detail that the role of pastoral visitors is to be compassionate in our ministry by manifesting our human solidarity as we cry out with those who suffer, by emphatizing with patients through our understanding of the wounds of their lives and by comforting them by pointing beyond the human pains to glimpses of strength and hope.[5]

Hospital chaplains are teachers, too. They explain some of the changes of the Church as they minister and answer questions that are raised. They have the opportunity of explaining each sacrament to the patients and families before it is administered so that the sacrament is truly an encounter with Christ. As part of their orientation to the hospital the nurses are taught the essential elements of the sacraments so that there is an understanding of what is taking place when their patients are receiving Holy Communion, the Anointing of the Sick or a baby is Baptized. Another aspect of the teaching role is to promote programs within the hospital explaining the sacraments or some teaching of the Catholic Church to the personnel. At the Good Samaritan Hospital we have monthly "brown bag lunches" where the employees bring their lunch to a private dining area to hear a speaker address an appropriate topic. Usually the topics are medical in nature, but pastoral care has reversed the topic for the month of March (Lent) so that we might present some teaching of the Church. One year I explained Baptism of babies, noting the circumstances when a baby should be baptized and others when an infant should not. One of our struggles is to update nurses trained before Vatican II who are inclined to baptize stillborn babies even though they are clearly dead. Last year I explained the document on AIDS that the bishops published. AIDS is an extremely vital issue in a hospital. Appropriate care must be given to the patients and the employees must be protected so they do not contract AIDS.

Most hospitals have ethics committees whose purposes are to educate the people in the institution about ethics, develop policies concerning ethical procedures, be available for consultation and interpret procedures and surgical operations to ensure that they conform to the Ethical Religious Directives of Catholic Health Facilities. Usually a pastoral care person is a member of this committee and an important one because of his/her knowledge of ethics and practical experience in a hospital.

In addition, pastoral people are members of other committees, like the Mission Effectiveness Committee, the AIDS Committee and Management-Employee monthly meetings. Finally, they sponsor out-reach programs for the community at large. Some chaplains present programs to parishes giving indepth explanations of the sacraments, especially Baptism and Anointing. Others give a series of talks explaining simple communication techniques to parish communion distributors to enhance their effectiveness when visiting the shut-ins or their hospitalized parishioners. Others lead programs of bereavement to assist the bereaved in working through their grief.

Finally, the pastoral persons are a vital link between the patients and their parishes. This begins when the pastoral care department informs the parish that one of their parishioners is hospitalized. It continues by assisting the parish visitors in any way possible when they come to minister to their sick people. It concludes by informing the parish of any spiritual, social and emotional needs their parishioners might have as they are dismissed. With shortened hospital stays planning for ministry to the sick and the frail elderly in their homes has become very significant.

Assurances for Continuance of Catholic Practices

Now for the second question: How to assure that Catholic practices are adhered to in a Catholic facility? One way is to urge the hospitals to hire persons who are certified by the National Association of Catholic Chaplains (N.A.C.C.). The United States Catholic Conference (U.S.C.C.) has collaborated with the N.A.C.C. to set up guidelines for certification of chaplains. This offers a great assurance that the pastoral care personnel in a Catholic health facility are prepared to participate effectively in the pastoral ministry of the Catholic Church. These standards require that the candidates for certification give evidence of personal, theological and professional competencies.[6] The personal competency demands that the pastoral care givers possess personal integrity, an awareness of their personal and ministerial strengths and weaknesses and how they use them in ministry. It is expected that the pastor of the candidate or the religious superior writes a letter recommending a person for ministry stating that he/she exhibits the basic virtues of our faith. The supervisor also has some awareness of the personal integrity of the candidate after twenty weeks of training. In addition, it is essential that ministers know their limitations. I supervise students who are in training to become pastoral persons. One of these students, a married man; had a difficult time saying "no" even to unreasonable requests. A woman patient at the hospital had the habit of calling for a chaplain every night even though the chaplain had seen her during the day. This student-chaplain was off-duty at home at 9:00 p.m. on a Sunday night when this patient called for him. Even though she was not critically ill and was not going to surgery the next day, he struggled to deny her request. One of his characteristics was to gain acceptance from others by meeting all their expectations and not giving adequate attention to his own needs. He benefited from learning to set limits.

The candidates for certification are also expected to be emotionally mature and aware of how their feelings, attitudes, values and assumptions about life and other people affect their ministry. One woman student gradually learned during the program that it wasn't effective ministry to attempt to cheer-up patients every time they spoke about some anxiety in their lives. When one young widower who had two daughters under fourteen years of age, expressed some fear how his future wife would relate to his daughters, this student quickly told him, "Everything will work out fine so stop worrying about it." Her assumption was that anxious people are helped by focusing on happy thoughts, instead of inviting them to share the basis for their anxiety.

Theologically, the chaplains are expected to be competent which means that they have a basic understanding of contemporary theology in ten different areas, but especially in sacred scripture, moral theology, ecclesiology, general and medical ethics, the meaning of suffering and the sacraments. Meeting this requirement allows chaplains to minister effectively in a health care setting as they meet various situations. Obviously, some patients ask chaplains, "Why is this happening to me?" It's important that pastoral care persons know how to respond to this question and others that patients, families and personnel ask from time to time.

In addition, pastoral persons need to possess a knowledge of the sacraments so they can prepare patients for a deeper religious experience. This assumes they understand the sacraments and strive to give some instruction as well as some spiritual preparation to the recipient in order to achieve the greatest effect. For example, a lay pastoral person explains the effects of the Anointing of the Sick and offers a prayer with him/her as they wait for the priest to come to administer the sacrament.

Professional skills, the third competency, requires that pastoral care persons have basic listening and communication skills; are able to carry out effective intervention in acute situations; initiate appropriate referrals and understand the role of chaplain versus the roles of other professionals in the institution. This means that they know how to minister effectively after a death. Instead of trying to quiet a grieving family by telling them "be strong" or "it's God's will" or "God will take care of them", the chaplain encourages the family to ventilate feelings. In this instance, ministry is mainly by his/her concerned presence rather than by empty words. As a professional, pastoral persons must possess a solid pastoral identity, knowing who they are personally and as pastoral persons. This enables them to refrain from entering the medical field by giving medical information or from doing the work of a social worker by discussing a transfer to a nursing home in detail.

In other words, before chaplains are certified they are expected to demonstrate that they have the ability to be companions of sick and needy persons on their journey and to walk with them at their pace. In order to accomplish this task a Clinical Pastoral Education Program enables the participants to:

1. understand themselves by getting in touch with and celebrating their inner selves,
2. to understand others by discovering the art of communication and listening,
3. to experience the meaning of life by evaluating and clarifying their values and goals,
4. to experience the world by deepening their awareness of the persons and things that daily touch their lives.
5. and to experience God by exploring new ways to a closer relationship with him.[7]

There are two associations which provide training enabling pastoral care givers to achieve these standards: one is the National Association of Catholic Chaplains and the other is the Association of Clinical Pastoral Education. Throughout its history the N.A.C.C. has placed great emphasis on the development of professional standards for the certification of the members and the accreditation of the training centers. By maintaining these standards, it has made significant contribution to the quality of pastoral care rendered in Catholic settings. The A.C.P.E. which was originally a union of four different Protestant pastoral education groups, began educating Catholics about twenty-five years ago in their education centers because we had none of our own. At that time some of these centers placed a heavy emphasis on psychology with little or no attention given to theology and spirituality. Today A.C.P.E. generally blends psychological education with theology and spirituality. Last year at a regional meeting in Detroit, Michigan there were three periods of ten minutes of prayer during the day and a half workshop mainly attended by supervisors of this association. Further, at the conclusion of each verbatim where the student writes what the patient said and how they responded, there is a space for theological reflection. Here the student is urged to discover some theological meaning of that ministerial event. Presently there is an excellent working relationship between N.A.C.C. and A.C.P.E. to the extent that A.C.P.E. has given the N.A.C.C. assistance in incorporating psychological insights into its programs while the N.A.C.C. has urged A.C.P.E. to return to their spiritual heritage as they impart pastoral education.

In order to be certified, candidates must be a member of the N.A.C.C. and have completed at least two basic units in an accredited C.P.E. program. These programs contain a minimum of three students and a maximum of six. The training unit consists of at least 400 hours of supervised training for ten or eleven weeks with a blending of the actual practice of ministry with didactic presentations. Three other requirements for certification are: the candidates submit materials to support their claim that they have achieved the standards set down by N.A.C.C., formal approval for ministry by the local ordinary, his delegate or a major religious superior; finally, successfully meet an interview team of three or four people.

All of the theological competencies that the N.A.C.C. requires cannot be obtained in two basic quarters of training of only twelve weeks. Candidates need to verify in their certification materials that they have taken courses in the required subjects at the seminary, a Catholic university, a lay pastoral ministry program or have participated in mini courses for six weeks, possibly sponsored by the education department of the diocese. The N.A.C.C. not only certifies persons as chaplains, but also accredits pastoral care departments as meeting standards developed for them by the N.A.C.C. and the Catholic Health Association. These standards insure that pastoral care departments have adequate staff for the size of the hospitals, provisions for meeting the sacramental needs of the patients, provisions for meeting the ministerial needs of patients on the 11:00 p.m. to 7:00 a.m. shift, adequate office space and sufficient budget to support these services.

In addition to health care facilities hiring certified chaplains and accrediting departments, the bishops can assure themselves that these developments are carrying out the practices of the Catholic Church by maintaining contact personally or through a representative. Through this contact the chaplains are offered support by reminding them they are members of the healing arm of the Catholic Church. We in the health ministry need this so that we don't feel isolated as we engage in our specialized ministry. Possibly when the bishop visits a hospitalized patient, he might stop by the chaplain's office to extend greetings.

Not only do the chaplains need the bishops' support, but Catholic hospitals themselves require this as one looks to their future in the next decade. The Commission on Catholic Health Ministry which is supported by the Congregation and Diocesan Sponsors, the National Conference of Catholic Bishops and the Catholic Health Association indicated last year that many of them will not survive nor will the Church's practice of ministering to the sick poor continue without the bishops' support. Catholic hospitals certainly meet some of the health needs of the poor. At Good Samaritan Hospital, 1.5% of net patient service revenue is budgeted annually for charitable care as differentiated from uncollectibles. This amounted to $1,800,000 last year at Good Samaritan. Unless the bishops offer a helping hand, this amount of care for the poor will probably decrease. The bishops are urged to involve the whole ecclesical community to play an important role in initiating, evaluating and coordinating health services. Where the services of Catholic institutions and agencies overlap, or when there are unmet needs, he may convene the sponsors of the health facilities in order to promote better planning and use of Church resources. Obviously this is delicate because the bishops' support is needed, but they must not interfere with the specific responsibilities of the trustees and administrators of the institutions, nor deny the charisms of individual congregations.[8]

Finally, to maintain Catholic practices, certain basic expectations of the bishop or his delegate need to be shared with each Catholic health facility in his diocese. If these expectations are not communicated, how is the pastoral care director expected to know what the bishop wants? The following are some expectations that the bishop might want to share with the president and the director of pastoral care of each Catholic health facility in his diocese:

1. That the priest-chaplain not be assigned to the hospital but rather be hired by the hospital in collaboration with the personnel office of the diocese so that he realizes he is an employee of the institution and must abide by the same policies that all of the other employees of the institution must adhere to. In this way the priest-chaplain is included as a member of the pastoral care team rather than as an outsider who formulates his own policies which at times are contrary to those of the pastoral care department.

2. That the hospital give preference in their hiring practices to pastoral care people who are certified by the N.A.C.C. and U.S.C.C.

3. That before hiring a person for pastoral care work, the hospital consult with his/her pastor or religious superior concerning the person's integrity, relationship with God and practice of prayer.

4. That Catholic pastoral care persons participate in the Eucharistic liturgy on a regular basis.

5. That Catholic lay chaplains and volunteers who distribute communion be enrolled as Eucharistic ministers according to the diocesan policy for special Eucharistic ministers.

6. That some guideline be expressed concerning the hiring of resigned priests and lay people who are married outside the Church for positions in pastoral care.

7. That the Eucharist be celebrated frequently at the hospital. I know of one Catholic hospital where there is a priest-chaplain on the staff but he never celebrates

Mass at the hospital on "company time" because the director thinks that the personnel should go to their own parishes and the patients can watch mass on a public TV channel. In my opinion, an aspect of our Catholic identity is that the Mass be celebrated for the patients who can attend, for others on closed circuit television and for the personnel who are working twelve hour shifts and find it difficult to go to their parish.

8. That Holy Communion be available daily and that the Anointing and the Sacrament of Reconciliation be available when it is reasonably requested as far as possible.

9. That parishes be urged to provide the Anointing for their own parishioners before they enter the hospital since some facilities do not have a priest chaplain always on duty.

10. That since some Catholics are dying without being anointed because of the shortage of priests, parishes instruct their people that the Anointing of the Sick is not necessary for salvation.

11. That the hospital pastoral staff be prepared to offer appropriate prayers for critically ill Catholics when a priest is unavailable to anoint them.

12. That pastoral care departments build close relationships with local parishes so that they form a team in meeting the spiritual as well as the social and emotional needs of the patients.

13. That the needs of the Protestant patients be appropriately met, either by having a Protestant chaplain or some relationships with Protestant churches in the area.

14. That pastoral care persons be encouraged to become an integral part of the hospital by becoming members of various committees in the hospital to enhance its Catholic Christian identity.

In conclusion, the pastoral care persons in Catholic health facilities have very significant roles to fulfill. They make a tremendous contribution to the life of the Catholic Church. Their contribution can be enhanced if the bishop supports them and shares with them his expectations concerning their ministry.

NOTES

1. Daniel J. Gatti, S.J. "The National Association of Catholic Chaplains" *Journal of Pastoral Care*—Fall, 1988 p. 241.

2. Lawrence G. Seidl—*Pastoral Care in Catholic Health Facilities—1988 Survey Report*—Catholic Health Association, St. Louis, Mo. p. 2, 3.

3. Justine Cyr, C.B.S., *Catholic Health Ministry: A New Vision for a New Century,* The Commission of Catholic Health Care Ministry, Farmington Hills, Mi. 1988, p. 12–14.

4. Gerald R. Niklas and Charlotte Stephanics, *Ministry to the Sick,* Alba House, New York 1982, p. 23–30.

5. Henry Nouwen, "Compassion: Solidarity, Consolation and Comfort", *America Magazine* 1976, p. 195–200.

6. *Standards For Certification,* National Association of Catholic Chaplains, Milwaukee, Wisc. 1987, p. 1–2.

7. John Powell, S.J. *Fully Human, Fully Alive,* Tabor Publishing, Allen, Tx. 1976.

8. Justine Cyr, C. .B. S., idem. p. 13.

Chapter 13

PASTORAL CONCERNS
CATHOLIC IDENTITY

BISHOP: I was interested in Father Niklas's suggestion that we should be using dispensed priests or, at least, considering that. Now, unless I misread this, I understand that. Now, how would that work out? Would you like to expand on that a little bit?

FATHER NIKLAS: All I said was that some guidelines should be established. I did not suggest what those guidelines should be for resigned priests and people married outside the Church. I think in your wisdom, you could see that!

BISHOP: I'd like to address a couple of questions to Sister Margaret John. First of all, with reference to what you said about maintaining the Catholic identity in a merged or collaborative situation. I can't recall whether you said it was easier with two sites or one site?

SISTER MARGARET JOHN: When you begin to move towards a consolidation of facilities, then the more restrictive moral code will be challenged if the non-Catholic facility has permitted procedures contrary to the Catholic teaching.

BISHOP: Is there a single Board of Directors?

SISTER MARGARET JOHN: It depends upon the model. If you take a look at that Gamma model, that truly is one site and that is one Board. In the Delta model, that's two sites and two shareholders with one operating Board.

BISHOP: Don't you have a problem with that, Sister, with reference to the ethical implications? It's sort of difficult for me to imagine that you're getting around the obvious dilemma. If there's a single Board, an unethical practice or procedure is certainly being done in the name of that single Board of Directors. I would have a problem about that with a Catholic Board.

SISTER MARGARET JOHN: Well, it certainly raises the issue of material cooperation. In the Delta model, the sterilizations are under a corporation separate from the other corporation and that is the only activity under that Board. This was done as a compromise when the parties could not agree. Perhaps the thinking in some of these areas is, to use a rather mundane image, that a half a loaf or a quarter of a loaf is better than none. Perhaps some of the Bishops who are looking at this evaluate the local situation and see that process as a higher good than having no facility.

BISHOP: My own opinion, however, is that if it's under a single Board of Directors, all are responsible. If it's an unethical procedure, I would have a problem with it.

SISTER MARGARET JOHN: That is the local diocesan Bishop's judgment and responsibility.

BISHOP: Sister, you mentioned on more than one occasion and with some emphasis, calling it to the attention particularly, of the United States Bishops, that the *Ethical and Religious Directives* are so important. But I couldn't tell from the way you were talking, whether or not you considered them helpful or a bit of an obstacle?

SISTER MARGARET JOHN: The message I'm getting to you is that these *Directives* written in 1971 and slightly revised in 1975 are perceived by the sponsors and the Boards of Catholic hospitals as central to Catholic identity. I think if we did not have that particular document, we would have very little to guide our hospitals. So, I'm making a bid that you review and revise it and I know the Committee on Doctrine is doing just that it is about all we have to look at in terms of First Amendment conscience rights. The corporate documents in these mergers and consolidations specifically reference the *Ethical Directives*. This has become the only document that people look to as actualating the Catholic position. That document has many, many good things in it, but I fear that it has been reduced in the minds of many as only containing prohibition in the reproductive areas.

The Preamble has a beautiful image of why we're in health care, the value of physical, spiritual health, the transcendent meaning of suffering, and the intrinsic value of persons. The book that the Pope John Center did, *Catholic Identity in Health Care: Principles and Practice*, by Monsignor Orville Griese, has the history of those Directives in it. For the younger Bishops, who were not part of all that history, it's a helpful story to read because it appears that some of the initial controversy is still raging.

My plea is very strong. If you throw out *Ethical Directives* or fail to revise that document, the Catholic health care facilities will have no objective and consistent ethical posture. It's the only thing in print and easily accessible. As a matter of fact, in most of our hospitals, the physicians that are on our hospital staffs have to sign an agreement that they will function, while in that facility, in conformity with the Ethical Directives.

If we didn't have it, I don't know what we'd be using for an articulation of Catholic principles for our pluralistic medical and nursing staffs. I'm sorry I wasn't clear enough, but I don't think all the Bishops have realized the value put on that document and the use to which the *Ethical Directives* has been put in this country.

BISHOP: Some of the reasoning behind the mergers and the thrust for getting together and combining some of our institutions has been the overall desire for debedding in many areas because of the DRG's and things like that. With the age crisis coming in, it seems to some of us that there may be, really, a change in this whole question. We may end up in the next five years needing many, many more beds than we have needed before. Is that something that we should consider as we do the planning? Is that something which can affect the future of mergers and consolidations in Catholic hospitals?

SISTER MARGARET JOHN: The interesting thing is that we are currently overbedded in acute care but we are seriously underbedded in long term care. In most of our hospitals on any given day, you probably have twenty to thirty to forty patients in what we call an alternate level of care. They are patients who do not need acute care. They should be in long term care facilities but there are no facilities to send them to. That has an economic impact because the hospitals are reimbursed at a much lower level for those beds.

We need long term care beds desparately and we will undoubtedly need more AIDS beds. However, there is controversy going on right now whether we want to have more deinstitutionalized care for AIDS patients with more hospice care and less institutional care.

If we would just take care of our long term care needs in a more responsible fashion, we would probably have need for those excess hospital beds. Also, with people living longer, and the number of chronic diseases that we have, we will need many more beds for those chronically ill patients as well the MS and ALS patients, for example, are on the increase and require a great deal of nursing care. We will have those patients for a longer time. And there are other chronic diseases that will present the same kind of need.

In planning we tend to look at the immediate crisis and our planning agencies are not very sympathetic beyond the present year's budget. In New York City, for example, they are now suffering dramatically from a lack of beds. They are really draining off the resources from the whole State of New York to support the uncompensated care that is occurring in the New York City hospitals because of the AIDS crisis. So the AIDS situation and the increased elderly population are certainly impacting delivery and financing of care but we have not gotten hold of it, yet.

BISHOP: Sister Margaret John, in our Diocese, we have the unusual situation of the number of our Catholic hospitals increasing by three-fold in the last two or three years, from one until three. I guess that's bucking the trend.

What actually happened, two religious congregations bought two separate hospitals, one in a rural area, which is experiencing considerable difficulty in a very poor area, the other, a psychiatric care hospital, again a small hospital, specializing in psychiatric care and in drug treatment.

In both instances, I think those acquisitions have been successful and I think a great witness to the religious communities as well as to the larger Church. Is there any kind of a trend of that happening countrywide, that you know of?

SISTER MARGARET JOHN: Yes, there is a trend, Bishop. Perhaps I shouldn't say a trend, but there are sufficient examples to indicate that there might be a trend developing.

The Church has acquired a good many hospitals, some are publicly owned facilities because, with the tax base eroding, many of the municipalities and counties do not want to be involved with health care. In Washington, several hospitals have been acquired by Catholic systems. Pennsylvania is trying to close their acute hospitals. Even though several years ago the public health facilities were transferred from the government to other sponsors including some religious congregations, one hesitates to take on hospitals because they're losers. The trend is emerging.

Some of us project that perhaps, in the future, we may have, just the way we started in this country, a lot of Catholic hospitals and denominational hospitals and very few public and no for-profit hospitals.

The for-profits are now withdrawing from hospital work. The for-profit companies were the darlings of Wall Street in the retrospective payment period, when you were reimbursed for costs. Now, when you have a specific cost for every diagnosis, the for-profits are withdrawing from the hospitals. Some think that, over the next five–ten years, we may be the remaining hospitals, because it will only to be a matter of service and charity, not economic advantage that will keep sponsors in health care unless health policy changes dramatically.

Right now health care is a commercial enterprise, which I think is contrary to its whole nature, but it has been growing since the late seventies and the early eighties. I think as the tax base erodes, as the costs go up, people will not want to have hospitals as their responsibilities in towns, cities, counties and states.

I don't think the for-profit hospitals will continue much longer. They are concentrating generally now in rehab and psychiatric care, and drug dependency but they're not in the difficult, costly medical-surgical areas.

BISHOP: Our concern for all health care workers is that they become another Christ because of their role as priest, prophet and king by virtue of their baptism. Can we not extend this program of pastoral education to doctors, nurses and all other health care of as Catholic doctors and Catholic nurses.

FATHER NIKLAS: My experience is not very successful in dealing with doctors and inviting them to come to meetings for ethics or Church theological teachings. Some of them have gone to Catholic universities and medical schools and they feel they know enough theology. Another point is that most doctors are very conservative theologically and politically. They tend not to want changes in the Church teaching or developments to occur.

It was mentioned earlier that the residents are being forced by the regulatory agencies to have ethics classes. That has helped me in my hospital so that I can provide ethics programs for them. But, ironically, it's not the Church or priests or anybody who is influential, but a state organization or a national organization that's demanding that ethics be taught!

Some hospitals do have retreats for their employees or they have days of recollection. Those are means to try and achieve the goals that you speak of.

BISHOP: Do you have any comments concerning cooperative programs between hospitals, affiliation type programs? Do they, more or less inevitably, lead to mergers? Or is there a lot of cooperation going on that's quite successful and continues to be quite successful while still having independent hospitals remain independent?

SISTER MARGARET JOHN: I really don't know how to answer that. I do know, though, that when you have a major employer in an area, you're going to have more pressure for collaboration. That can be very healthy because I believe, as Catholic hospitals, we have a dual role of service and witness. When we meet with other groups and we share our perspectives, that's a very positive force.

The regulatory agencies are going to force health care agencies and providers to work more together. There's absolutely no question. We're going to have that. The key would be, do we want to be proactive or just reactive?

One of the important things is to get the medical staffs to understand what it is that makes us Catholic. That's where I see a real lack. I think many of the physicians don't see much difference in the hospitals. And maybe that's valid.

214

But if we want to retain our Catholic identity, it's important that we have Catholic integrity. And then there will not be a possibility of *informal* mergers and consolidations taking place. None of the mergers I studied were initiated by the sponsors. They were all initiated by someone else, physicians, administrators or major employer. What we really need, as sponsors and as stewards of these facilities, is to be active in our planning processes and know where we want to go. The best deterrent to an unhealthy situation is a very good planning process and a planning process which is based on mission. When you visit your hospitals, it would be good just to check and see if your long range plan is mission-oriented or finance-oriented, or is it a blend of the two?

The mission is foremost, we're there for ecunumerical efferent, efficacious service, but we're there for Christian witness as well. The universal need would be good education as to why we exist and then, secondly, a very strong planning process which is mission oriented and proactive.

BISHOP: What you have said about Catholic hospitals and the difficult situation they find themselves in, especially financial reasons, apply also to other denomination of hospitals and to the secular hospital, in general?

SISTER MARGARET JOHN: Yes, it does. It hurts all of us. It's because of the reimbursement system primarily, that we're in trouble right now, but it also is the advent of high technology and everyone wants the latest and best.

It may affect the Catholic hospitals more because we are frequently located in areas with a high charity case component and, therefore, it could be more devastating to us. Also, because by our ethical stance, we do not, as Monsignor Cassidy pointed out, perhaps, have a full range of services in the obstetrical/gynecological areas we may not receive some contracts in managed care.

But I would say there is also a financial crisis. In New York State, I think we have very few hospitals that have a black bottom line. In Connecticut, things are hard. In Massachusetts, we don't even have a budget for next year, so the hospitals don't know what they're going to get. Mass. has also just cut back the uncompensated care pool in that state.

Texas has had 19 hospitals close in the past year. We, in our system of 43 hospitals, have just closed two hospitals. Because of their location and the fact that they have so much free or discounted care they cannot continue. This is a very sad commentary but as the saying goes, "No margin; no mission."

BISHOP: How important do you consider this element of for-profit or non-profit as far as being the criterion for Catholic identity?

SISTER MARGARET JOHN: I think there's nothing Catholic about being not-for-profit or for-profit. As a matter of fact, the Trappists have their jelly, and the Christian Brothers their wines, and they have been for-profit for a long time.

I think our hospitals, though, as hospitals, better remain not-for-profit. We're getting into some trouble because of some of the for-profit activity. There are, right now, 22 states that have legislation directed toward removing the tax exempt status of not-for-profit hospitals because of their activities and competition with other businesses.

In Tennessee there have been several rather celebrated cases about taxing hospitals. In Pennslyvania, we have a situation where one Catholic hospital has promised services in lieu of taxes while another Catholic not-for-profit hospital has litigated and has retained its tax-exempt status. So the not-for-profit question is coming up more frequently. We must be sure that we are acting as not-for-profits, which doesn't mean you can't make a profit, but that you have a different philosophical base and the manner in which the revenues are used is quite different.

BISHOP: Where you don't have the direct ownership by a Catholic group, if you have some lay board that might have some Catholic participants do you think that to establish Catholic identity at this institution, you can secure that by a contract that regulates the type of governance and the kind of ethical and moral principles that are going to be involved in the operation of that institution?

SISTER MARGARET JOHN: If you want a personal opinion, my answer is no. I believe that we have the strong Catholic hospitals that we have today because of the ongoing commitment of women religious in this country.

They have given a lot to those institutions. We have now marvelous leaders among the women and have had charismatic leaders from way back. The value has been the continuity and the stability

216

the religious congregations have provided in terms of mission. That has made our hospitals what they are.

Now, I know there are some diocesan hospitals, but the same continuity exists because you Bishops usually stay for a pretty long time in a certain area and you have core people who do the same thing as religious congregations have. Church organizations have a character which is not totally subject to the personality of the chief executive officer.

My personal bias is that, without that historical continuity of mission, you set up a situation where you have private individual leadership. I also think that it's very hard to monitor Church identity. The lay sponsorship models appear to be extremely difficult to monitor in terms of advancing the Church mission in a positive, proactive manner.

There are two lay sponsorship models in place now, one in New York and one in Tennessee. They have lay people responsible to the Bishop. The Bishop really has the last word on their Catholicity. I don't know how they are going to work. Father O'Rourke as a canon lawyer, I think, has confidence in them. I don't have the same level of confidence because I think that you need a strong corporate culture and this is more readily achieved through a corporate reality like a congregation or a diocese.

So we have two difficulties in the totally lay model. First, a corporate culture and corporate vision may be missing; secondly, church compliance will be very difficult unless we have a marvelous formation program for all of our lay leaders. And I do not see that happening to the degree and depth required.

I do see it happening in some places but I've sat with too many Boards and physician groups all over this country who are genuinely surprised when you mention things about the basic Catholic moral and social teachings. And that's our fault. We have not done a good job and at this point we have several major survival problems that we need to concentrate on. We, ourselves, sisters and diocesan sponsors need a lot of education but trustee education in Catholic identity is just beginning.

I think the best model is a collaborative model which brings the laity and the religious together so that we have continuity, stability as well as loved representation. That's the vision of Vatican II, as well, at this point in history, I don't think we have sufficient

217

Christian formation and Apostolic formation to have effective models that do not include a bonded tie-in to Church. Maybe someone wants to argue that and feel free. It's a personal opinion from my own perspective and is not universally shared but it grows out of my national experiences with a great many Church institutions and sponsors as well as with other Christian and non-demonstrational institutions.

PART THREE

PREBORN AND ANENCEPHALIC INFANTS

Chapter 14

TISSUE AND ORGAN DONATION BY ABORTED PREBORN AND ANENCEPHALIC INFANTS: MEDICAL ASPECTS OF HUMAN FETAL TRANSPLANTATION

Christopher M. DeGiorgio, M.D.

Introduction

For the last 10 years investigators in Scandinavia, the United States, and Mexico have been experimenting with fetal tissue for animal and human transplantation.[1,2,3] From initial work in Parkinson's disease, research has expanded into using tissue for diabetes, bone, blood, endocrine, and other disorders. Use of human fetal tissue has generated significant controversy, which has been compounded by mixed and preliminary claims in the lay press and medical literature.[3,4,5,12] Further complicating the medical issues are the ethical dilemmas which have not been fully addressed, and the fact that abortion has made fetal tissue in high supply. There exists a host of incurable diseases for which human fetal tissue may have an application, generating significant interest in and demand for human fetal tissue.

Parkinson's Disease as a Prototype

The most intense research to date has focused as Parkinson's disease. Parkinson's disease is a progressive nervous system disease, characterized by tremor, rigidity, immobility and dementia; 60,000 new cases are reported yearly.[6,7] Parkinson's disease is caused by a loss of neurons in the area of the brain called the substantia nigra. These neurons normally secrete a substance called dopamine. Current medical therapy uses drugs which contain dopamine precursers or drugs which stimulate the release of dopamine by the remaining neurons. Medical therapy may control the symptoms of rigidity, tremor, or slowing for several years, but after prolonged treatment, medical therapy often becomes ineffective or results in untoward side effects.

Initial efforts by researchers in Mexico and Sweden to transplant dopamine secreting cells from the patients own adrenal gland were hailed with initial enthusiasm.[8,9] Attempts to confirm these results have largely failed in the United States. However, fetal tissue, especially neurons from the substantia nigra, have been shown in animal models to survive longer, produce more substantial neural connections and result in longer and more sustained neurologic improvement.[10,11] Most work has been performed in rodents; it was only in May, 1986 that the first fetal substantia nigra transplants were reported in monkeys.[2] Since that time, only a handful of substantia nigra transplants in humans has been attempted, and it is too early to adequately assess the success or failure of these few transplants.[3,12] Preliminary reports of fetal tissue transplantation into two humans by the Mexican group has already met with severe criticism from a scientific standpoint,[3,4,5] and Lindvall's group in Sweden has reported no success in two patients who received human fetal substantia nigra.[12]

Why Fetal Tissue

Fetal tissue is in high supply. It is estimated that of the 1.3 million abortions performed yearly in the United States up to 90,000 may produce tissue suitable for Parkinson's disease transplantation alone.[6] Various diseases may need young (less than 11 weeks) fetal tissue (e.g. Parkinson's Disease); other diseases may require tissue from older fetuses. Therefore, it is conceivable that fetal tissue may be useful at a wide spectrum of gestational ages for a wide variety of diseases, making all aborted fetuses potential donors. In the case of Parkinson's disease, fetal substantia nigra is well suited because the neurons are more viable, have not yet sprouted significant connections, are not well differentiated and may generate a less intense immune response than neurons from adult tissue.[10,11] Exact mechanisms why fetal tissue is more viable have not been fully delineated.

Spontaneous Versus Induced Abortion

The question arises whether fetal tissue from induced abortions is more viable, and a better source for transplantation than fetal tissue from spontaneous abortions. This question has not been fully addressed. Investigators such as Madrazo have reported initial success using tissue from a spontaneous abortion.[3] Fetuses from spontaneous abortions may be exposed to varying degrees of hypoxia, or a lack of oxygen, depending on the interval between death and retrieval of the fetus. Fetuses from spontaneous abortions may also have chromosomal abnormalities in approximately 20 percent, and may be infected with a variety of organisms, possibly causing the spontaneous abortion.[15] Such infections could be transmitted to the recipient, and could lead to disastrous consequences. Both the mother and fetal tissue should be tested for infectious agents prior to transplantation. There is also a risk that fetal tissue from *induced* abortions could be infected, (e.g. with the AIDS virus), and suitable means of screening such tissue would be necessary before transplantation. Therefore, the risk of infection is not unique to spontaneous abortions, and if adequate safeguards are used, should not preclude their use. Furthermore, fetal tissue has been obtained from spontaneous abortions for years, providing a source for tissue culture and other experimental purposes, and it is likely that some fetal tissue could be used for transplantation purposes.

The Method of Abortion

Abortions are usually performed using suction curettage, which may traumatize the tissue and makes fetal tissue (especially from small areas such as the substantia nigra) difficult to dissect. In contrast, tissue from monkeys has been obtained from hysterotomy, i.e., surgically removing the fetus from the uterus.[2] It is not clear whether the two techniques yield equally viable tissue. Substantia nigra from human fetuses obtained by suction curettage has been successfully transplanted into rodents,[10] In Lindvall's recent report of the failure of fetal substantia nigra transplants in two patients, all tissue was obtained from induced abortion, presumably by suction curettage.[12] Future investigators may change or modify the abortion technique in order to best harvest optimal "donor" fetal tissue.[15] Prolonging a pregnancy near or beyond viability solely for optimizing the yield would be a flagrant violation of current federal guidelines governing fetal experimentation.[16] Such an attempt to optimize fetal tissue viability and yield solely for transplantation purposes would also blur the distinction between the abortion procedure and the transplant, and would seriously compromise the ethical integrity of those involved.

Selected Ethical Concerns

Human fetal transplantation from induced abortion raises new, serious, and as yet unresolved ethical concerns. All recognize that the intention of curing currently incurable degenerative and progressive diseases such as Parkinson's, Alzheimer's and diabetes is a noble one. It must also be recognized that to date there is no evidence in animals or humans that these diseases can be controlled in the long-term, let alone cured, by fetal transplantation. However, many are advocating human experimentation before the long-term efficacy and safety of fetal transplantation has been demonstrated in animal models.

The Link to Abortion

The ethical dilemmas may eclipse the technical issues involved. A fundamental problem is the link between fetal transplantation and abortion. The abortion debate is beyond the scope of this article; however, abortion creates a large supply of potential fetal donors, whose tissue is currently being "wasted." Thus, fetal transplantation would not be so vigorously advocated if that tissue was prohibitive in terms of cost, supply, and difficulty of harvesting. Some would argue that, if fetal tissue is available, whether one supports or condemns abortion, it would be wasteful not to use this tissue for benefit of others. These would also argue that sufficient safeguards could be erected to totally insulate the act of abortion from the harvesting and transplantation of fetal tissue. In reality, the two cannot be separated. Firstly, human fetal tissue transplantation creates a need for fetal tissue, and as shown above, the converse is also true: abortion makes fetal transplants a viable option. Secondly, abortion is a difficult and distressing decision for any woman. Would not the knowledge that the fetus could be used to save another life seem sufficient to justify the abortion for the sake of the greater good or for the benefit of humanity? Could society and medicine directly or indirectly coerce woman into having an abortion by simply giving her the hope that her fetus could benefit another, thus mitigating guilt, anxiety, and distress? It is conceivable that human fetal transplantation may actually increase the number of abortions performed yearly. This point has been underscored by James Bopp, and in a recent article by Greely et al. in the New England Journal, his argument could not be refuted. " ...
[I]t is possible, of course, that even with these restrictions, the

225

mere knowledge that a beneficial use may be made of the fetal tissue could influence some women considering abortion."[14]

Another dilemma involves the ethics of transplantation. Organ or tissue transplants may be ethically taken from two classes: live, freely consenting donors, or brain-dead cadaver donors. The ethical criteria for donors applicable to either class cannot be fulfilled by fetal transplantation of tissue from induced abortion. Mahowald et al summarize the three criteria for transplantation from live donors.[17] Transplantation is acceptable if three conditions are met: 1) the donor or donors proxy has provided free and confirmed consent; 2) the burden of the donor (including loss of an organ or tissue risk and possible pain of the procedure) is proportionate to its expected benefit to another or others; 3) other means of obtaining the expected benefit are not available. It is difficult to argue that either criteria one or two could be met by fetal transplantation. The fetus is not asked his opinion, and it is questionable that the same woman contemplating terminating a live fetus could be his/her free proxy. Fulfillment of the third criteria is dependent on whether there are other sources or alternatives of transplantable tissue. We will investigate this in the last section, but alternative sources for fetal tissue do exist, or could be developed in the near future.

A counter argument to circumvent this inability to fulfill basic ethical principals would be "Fetuses are not human beings and therefore not subject to the same rigorous criteria." Again we must recognize why the use of human fetal tissue is being advocated in the first place: precisely because it *is* human. The dignity of the fetus has been underscored in the recent article by the Stanford Bioethics Committee. . . . "A fetus is not simply a mass of tissues; it is at least a potential human life and should be treated with dignity."[14]

Another counter argument would be: "The aborted fetus is not a live donor, but rather a cadaver, and a cadaver can be used for transplantation, regardless of the cause." In answer to this contention, if consent for transplantation is given after the decision to abort but *prior* to the actual abortion, (as has been recommended),[15] the fetal donor is at that time a *living donor* capable of feeling pain. He has not yet met any criteria for determination of brain death, nor is he a cadaver.

Alternatives To Human Tissue From Induced Abortions:

Several alternatives to fetal tissue from induced abortions do exist, or can be developed for use in the near future. Since all fetal transplantation is highly experimental, to reject alternative sources solely because they are experimental would be unsound. If alternative sources of fetal tissue could be developed, the ethical dilemmas could be avoided. Three sources of fetal tissue include:

1) fetal tissue from spontaneous abortions;
2) fetal tissue from other species (rodent, primate);
3) tissue cultures of specific cells; e.g. Neuroblastoma.

Fetal tissue from spontaneous abortions has been used, albeit with questionable results. As mentioned previously, disadvantages include a high rate of infection, chromosomal abnormalities and hypoxia.[15] Some have argued that transplantation of such tissue should not be used, because to transplant infected tissue into a human would be "indefensible".[15] However, all fetal tissue, whether from spontaneous or induced abortions could be potential sources of infection, and would need to be screened for such infections prior to transplant. The viability of tissue from spontaneous abortions should be investigated further, but it is obvious that such tissue would be ethically less problematic than tissue from induced abortions. This assertion has been emphasized in the Stanford Bioethics Committee recommendations.[14] Cross species transplantation has been successfully performed between mice and rats, rabbits and rodents, and even from humans to rats.[10] It is conceivable that because fetal tissue generates a mild immune response, primate or rodent donors could be used. However, the safety and efficacy of rodent transplants into monkeys (primates) would need to be verified before such tissue could be transplanted into humans.

Lastly, a potentially unlimited source of transplantable tissue could be obtained from tissue culture of specific cell types. One example is human neuroblastoma cells. Neuroblastoma cells are cells which have been resected from a brain tumor and cultured in such a way that tumor growth has been arrested. This tissue could be cultured to secrete specific neurotransmitters, such as acetylcholine or dopamine (potentially for the treatment of Alzheimer's disease or Parkinson's disease).

Kordower et al. have reported successful transplantation of human neuroblastoma cells into monkeys, with survival of the graft, and production of the neurotransmitter without development of a tumor. Kordower concludes that . . . "cultured cell lines, such as differentiated neuroblastoma cells, may be a viable and practical source of donor cells for transplantation.[18] Transplantation of tissue from cell cultures has multiple advantages including potentially unlimited supply, and lowers the risk of transmitting infectious agents through proper screening. Futhermore, the specific tissue needed could be selected more easily than allowed by current dissection techniques. Most importantly, the ethical problems associated with using fetuses from spontaneous abortions would be eliminated.

Current Legal Status of Human Fetal Transplantation

In May, 1988, a moratorium on federal funding for research and fetal tissue transplantation from induced abortions was announced. A draft executive order banning federal funds for such transplantation has not yet been signed, pending the Bush Administration's review of the recommendations of an NIH advisory panel. This NIH advisory panel voted 15 to 2 to allow fetal transplantation under certain conditions.[19] Regardless of the draft executive order, transplantation of tissue from induced abortions could conceivably proceed with private or other non-federal funds.

Summary

Human fetal tissue transplantation has the potential for controlling or possibly curing many diseases. Nevertheless, the efficacy and safety of these transplants has yet to be fully demonstrated in animal models, let alone humans. Use of human fetal tissue from induced abortions introduces new and serious ethical and moral dilemmas. Alternatives to such tissue do exist or can be developed

228

which are more acceptable from an ethical and medical prospective. Such alternatives should be aggressively investigated.

The author wishes to thank Alice Sharp for her assistance in the preparation of this manuscript.

References
1. Bjorklund A, Stenevi U: Reconstruction of the nigrostriatal dopamine pathway by intracerebral nigral transplants. Brain Res 1979; 177:555–560.
2. Redmond D E, Roth R H, Elsworth J D et al: Fetal neuronal grafts in monkeys given methyphenyltetrahydropyridine. Lancet 1986; 1125–1127.
3. Madrazo I, Leon V, Torres C. et al: Transplantation of fetal substantia nigra and adrenal medulla to the caudate nucleus in two patients with Parkinson's disease. N Engl J Med 1988; 318:51.
4. Dwork A J, Pezzoli G, Silani V, et al: Transplantation of fetal substantia nigra and adrenal medulla to the caudate nucleus in two patients with Parkinson's disease (letter). N Engl J Med 1988; 319:370–371.
5. Freed C R: Transplantation of fetal substantia nigra and adrenal medulla to the caudate nucleus in two patients with Parkinson's disease (letter). N Engl J Med 1988; 319:370.
6. Fine A F: The Ethics of fetal tissue transplants. Hastings Center Report 1988; 18:5–8.
7. Richardson E P, Beal M F, Martin J B: "Degenerative diseases of the nervous system," Harrison's Principles of Internal Medicine, ed. 11 E. Bramwald, K. Isselbacher, Petersdorf R G et. al eds. (New York: McGraw Hill, 1987).
8. Madrazo I, Drucker-Colin R, Diaz V et al.: Open microsurgical autograft of adrenal medulla to the right caudate nucleus in two patients with intractable Parkinson's disease. N Engl J Med 1987; 316:831–834.
9. Madrazo I, Drucker-Colin R, Leon V, Torres C: Adrenal medulla transplanted to caudate nucleus for treatment of Parkinson's disease: report of 10 cases. Surg Forum 1987: 38:510–511.
10. Brundin P, Nilsson O G, Strecker R E et al.: Behavioral effects of human fetal dopamine neurons grafted in a rat model of Parkinson's disease. Exp Brain Res 1986; 65:235–240.
11. Brundin P, Bjorklund A: Survival, growth and function of dopaminergic neurons grafted to the brain. In Seil F J, Herbert E, Carlson B (eds), Progress in Brain Research Vol 71, Elsevier, 1987, pp. 293–308.
12. Lindvall O, Gustavii B, Astedt B: et al.: Fetal dopamine rich mesencephalic grafts in Parkinson's disease. Lancet 1988; ii:1483–1484.
13. Bopp J: Use of fetal tissue will increase the number of abortions. National Right to Life News. November 17, 1988:4.
14. Greely H T, Hamm T, Johnson R et al: The ethical use of fetal tissue in medicine. N Eng J Med 1989; 320:1093–1096.
15. Annas G J, Elias S: The politics of transplantation of human fetal tissue. N Eng J Med 1989; 320:1079–1082.

229

16. National Commission for the Protection of Human Subjects of Biomedical and Behavorial Research, Report and Recommendations: Research on the fetus. (Washington, 1975).

17. Mahowald M B, Silver J, Ratcheson R A: The ethical options in transplanting fetal tissue. Hastings Center Report 1987; 17:9–15.

18. Kordower J H, Notter M F D, Yen H H, Gash D M: An in vivo and in vitro assessment of differentiated neuroblastoma cells as a source of donor tissue for transplantation. Ann NY Acad Sci 495: 606–622.

19. Consultants of the Advisory Committee to the Directors of the National Institutes of Health Report of the Human Fetal Tissue Transplant Panel. Washington D.C.: National Institutes of Health, 1988.

Chapter 15

ANENCEPHALY: SELECTED MEDICAL ASPECTS*

D. Alan Shewmon, M.D.

Anencephaly is generally defined as the congenital absence of skull, scalp and forebrain (cerebral hemispheres). In most cases, the cause is unknown; whatever the teratogenic factor, it must operate very early in embryogenesis, around the time of closure of the cephalic end of the neural tube (3½ weeks of gestation.)[1]

Animal models and early human fetuses demonstrate that the exposed anterior portion of the neural tube initially proliferates, as though attempting to form a forebrain, resulting in a disorganized mass of primitive glial, neural, and vascular tissue arising from the

---

*Originally appeared as "Anencephaly: Selected Medical Aspects" *Hastings Center Report* October/November, 1988, 11–19. Reprinted with permission from the Hastings Center.

upper end of the brainstem. This stage in the evolution of anencephaly is known as exencephaly. During gestation, this tissue typically degenerates, leaving by term only a remnant of varying amount called the cerebrovasculosa. Although the term "anencephaly" literally means "no brain," the actual amount of nervous system tissue compatible with that diagnosis can vary anywhere from only a few grams up to a normal full-term brain weight.[2] Anencephaly is classically subdivided into two forms: holoanencephaly (complete absence of forebrain and cranium) and mero-anencephaly, in which "the cranium and the brain are present in rudimentary form."[3] Others employ the related terms "holoacrania" and "mecroacrania," referring to the degree of bone absence.

The brainstem in anencephaly can display a spectrum of involvement anywhere from relatively normal to totally absent, with the congenital defect extending all the way into the spinal canal (craniorachischisis). There may also be associated malformations of other organ systems.

Differential Diagnosis

In the great majority of cases, the diagnosis of anencephaly is very obvious, and there is little, if any, chance of mistaking it for another condition. Nevertheless, not all cases are so straightforward. If anencephaly were clearly distinct from all other congenital brain malformations, it should be possible to give an operational definition of it that includes all cases of anencephaly and excludes all cases of everything else, yet such a definition has not been offered by anyone so far.

In their textbook on anencephaly, Lemire and colleagues stated: "An almost incomprehensible array of synonyms and classifications of anencephaly exists in the literature; many include entities now considered to be pathogenetically unrelated to the anencephaly spectrum."[4]

Another expert on congenital neuropathology, Josef Warkany, wrote:

As a congenital malformation that cannot be overlooked, [anencephaly] exemplifies the problems and difficulities of teratologic research in man. The terminology is confusing. I use the terms "anencephaly" for partial or total absence of the brain, "exencephaly" for exposure of the brain... and "pseudencephaly" for massive "area cerebrovasculosa" imitating the shape of the brain that it replaces.[5]

Although "exencephaly" is usually considered to be a mere stage in the evolution of anencephaly, his definition implies that what is exposed may be something more than mere cerebrovasculosa, and that exencephaly is not necessarily restricted to early fetuses.

Clearly, mutually exclusive operational definitions of anencephaly and exencephaly cannot be given, because the two conditions differ only in terms of the amount of exposed tissue, and therefore represent but two overlapping regions of a continuous spectrum. On the other hand, if exencephaly is to be included within the general category of anencephaly, as most authors conceive it, we must either abandon the notion of anencephaly as "brain absence" (even "forebrain absence") or provide mutually exclusive operational definitions for "brain" and "exencephalic tissue." The latter distinction is based on the degree of neural organization present, and is difficult, if not impossible, to determine by gross visual inspection.

This leads directly to the problem of overlap with another spectrum of congenital malformations called "encephaloceles," defined by Warkany as "hernias of the brain protruding through a congenital opening of the skull." He remarks that:

Encephaloceles are closely related to exencephaly and anencephaly. If the protruding brain of an exencephaly deteriorates, anencephaly results. If it is covered by skin or epithelium, and persists, encephaloceles are formed.[6]

A major problem arises, however, if the covering of encephaloceles may, by definition, be merely "epithelium" (a thin membrane composed of surface-lining cells), because the cerebrovasculosa of anencephaly and exencephaly is also typically covered by an epithelial membrane continuous with the skin at the edge of the cranial defect.[7] Rendering the distinction even more obscure, he states: "In experimental teratology exencephalies are encountered frequently. Sometimes they are covered by skin or thin epithelium (Fig. 24–1) corresponding to encephaloceles in man."[8] Although this passage describes his Fig. 24–1 as illustrating an experimental exencephaly, the corresponding figure legend refers to the lesion as an "encephalocele."

Other investigators distinguish the conditions more on the basis of the degree of neural organization than on the thickness of covering. But the cerebrovasculosa in anencephaly/exencephaly may contain rudimentary cerebral ventricles and/or patches of laminated cortex, leading some investigators to reject "the widely accepted view that the area cerebrovasculosa is totally disorganized, and that anencephaly is characterized by absence of the forebrain."[9] Conversely, the tissue in some encephaloceles is so abnormal that it is probably devoid of neurophysiologic function. The parameter "degree of neural organization" is therefore hopelessly vague for the purpose of unambiguously distinguishing anencephaly/exencephaly from encephalocele.

In particular, mero-anencephaly (meroacrania), which involves only a *partial* absence of brain and calvarium, by definition admits of degrees to which both these structures may be present. The least severe forms of mero-anencephaly may involve relatively small skull and scalp defects, thereby forming a continuum with the most extreme forms of microcephaly with encephalocele.

A more explicit acknowledgment of the ambiguity inherent in these terms is provided by Lemire and colleagues in describing the picture of an infant with a partial skull defect, through which a round nubbin of brain tissue protrudes, the diameter of which is about half the length of the face (Fig. 4–12).[10] The figure legend states:

> Lateral view of an infant with meroacrania who lived for several weeks. Since there is no skin covering, the basic lesion is that of anencephaly rather than of encephalocele (which is skin covered)... Because there is a significant protrusion of dysplastic cerebral cortex, it can also be classified as exencephaly.

If the "skin" covering of encephaloceles is understood in Warkany's sense of any sort of surface membrane of unspecified thickness, and if the lesion had happened to be covered by an epithelial membrane, then it could legitimately have been classified as any of the three entities.

These are not the only examples of such diagnostic ambiguity. A Dallas woman told the *American Medical News* "that her child, a daughter, lived fourteen months after being diagnosed—initially by the obstetrician—as having microcephaly with encephalocele, and later by a pediatric neurologist as having anencephaly."[11] This overlap between meroanencephaly and microcephaly with encephalocele is important to acknowledge, because the latter constitutes a continuous spectrum of its own, at the other end of which are encountered quite functional individuals.[12]

Amniotic band syndrome, which encompasses a broad continuum of severity, can mimic anencephaly, as occurred in one large epidemiologic survey.[13] Other investigators would consider amniotic bands not so much a misdiagnosis, as an actual cause of anencephaly, constituting yet another blurred boundary between anencephaly and some other condition.[14]

These examples are not intended to exaggerate the potential for diagnostic confusion surrounding anencephaly: it is still quite true that in the vast majority of cases the diagnosis can be made easily and without risk of error. Nevertheless, the commonly encountered contention that "anencephaly" is so well defined and so distinct from all other congenital brain malformations that misdiagnoses cannot occur and that organ-harvesting policies limited to "anencephalics" cannot possibly extend to other conditions, is simply false.

Prevalence and Prenatal Screening

The prevalence of anencephaly varies widely around the world, ranging in previous decades from as high as 6.7 per 1,000 births in parts of Ireland to as low as 0.29 in Denmark.[15] There is a declining gradient from Europe to the Far East, with intermediate prevalences in the western hemisphere.[16] Ethnic differences also obtain; for blacks and Jews the prevalence rates are some three to seven times lower than for other races. For unknown reasons, the sex ratio is quite skewed toward females, who constitute around

70 percent of anencephalic births.[17] Of great interest is the world-wide steady decline of the prevalence of anencephaly over the past several decades.[18]

In the United States, various studies reported rates of anencephaly ranging from 1.93 per 1,000 births in the early 1950s to 0.45 to 1.39 in the '60s and early '70s.[19] Rates from the late 1970s were lower, between 0.35 and 0.48.[20] The most recent data indicate still lower prevalence rates. In California between 1983 and 1984, just prior to the institution of a statewide prenatal screening program for neural tube defects, it was 0.3.[21] The Birth Defects Monitoring Program database, a nationwide source, gives an average rate of 0.26 between 1984 and 1986, and the Metropolitan Atlanta Congenital Defects Program reports an average rate of 0.35 during the same period, figures believed to be relatively unaffected by prenatal screening.[22] Taking into account all of the above, a reasonable estimate of the natural prevalence rate of anencephaly in the United States in 1988 is around 0.3 per 1,000 births. With some 3.75 million births per year during the latter half of the 1980s,[23] that makes the estimated number of anencephalic infants potentially born yearly in this country to be around 1,125.

This incidence is, of course, drastically reduced in areas with active prenatal screening programs. Either ultrasound or maternal serum alphafetoprotein (MSAFP) measurements will identify nearly all anencephalic fetuses tested during the second trimester. Experience here, as in other countries with well-developed screening programs, indicates that the vast majority of detected anencephalic fetuses are electively aborted.[24]

In California, where mandatory offering of MSAFP screening has been in effect since the spring of 1986, about 50 percent of all pregnancies have actually been screened during the second trimester. About 95 percent of all anencephalics screened have been detected in this way, and around 95 percent of the detected anencephalics have been electively aborted.[25] This does not include those diagnosed by ultrasound alone and electively aborted. It is probably fair to estimate that overall around 50 percent of the anencephalic fetuses in the state are being aborted. An educated guess as to the proportion of pregnancies nationwide that are being prenatally screened might be around 20 percent, and this is likely to increase over the next few years to a realistic maximum of around 50 percent, if the California experience turns out to be representative.[26]

The number of anencephalics aborted would probably diminish somewhat if their use as organ sources were to become widely accepted and routinely practiced, given that a fair amount of the impetus toward this in the last year seems to have come as much from parents of anencephalics as from transplant surgeons. It is the impression of the genetics counselors at the University of California, Los Angeles, however, that this would still have a relatively small impact on the total number of second trimester terminations for the condition. The diagnosis is so emotionally devastating to parents, and so many more months of pregnancy still lie ahead, that the vast majority of women want to get it over with and return to normal life as soon as possible.

Moreover, many obstetricians consider it improper to encourage a woman to carry a second trimester anencephalic fetus to term, given the increased risk of complications to the pregnancy.[27] For these reasons, the possibility of organ donation would be expected to have much more of an impact on parental decisions to terminate pregnancy following a diagnosis in the third trimester than in the second.

Thus, taking 20 percent as a very rough estimate of the nationwide proportion of pregnancies prenatally screened for neural tube defects during the second trimester, and 95 percent as the proportion of detected anencepahlic fetuses that are electively terminated, the theoretically projected 1,125 anencephalic births per year in the U.S. (which is based on trends from earlier years, relatively unaffected by prenatal screening) reduces to 911.

Prenatal diagnosis, although it permits improved obstetrical planning for high-risk cases, is unlikely to lower significantly the high rate of stilbirths associated with anencephaly. These infants' predisposition to stillbirth is probably due to their inability to withstand the pressures on and mechanical distortion of the exposed brain during its passage through the birth canal. Thus, the only effective way to lower the stillbirth rate would be by performing elective cesarean sections prior to the onset of labor, a maternal risk that virtually everyone agrees would be unwarranted in this setting. The proportion of anenecephalics who are stillborn is difficult to determine from the literature, with estimates ranging from around half to as high as 90 percent.[28] A middle figure of around two-thirds is therefore not unreasonable, making the estimated annual number of *live* anencephalic births in the country 304.

Neurologic Functioning

Little has been published concerning the neurologic functioning of anencephalic infants. Given that the structural anomalies of the brainstem can range from severe to relatively mild, it goes without saying that a corresponding spectrum of neurologic dysfunction can occur. Abnormal fetal movements have been observed by means of real-time ultrasound.[29] Apart from absence of the visual cortex, many anencephalic infants would be peripherally blind on the basis of associated maldevelopment of the eyes, with small optic nerves that end blindly without connection to the brain.[30] Similarly, the middle and inner ears may be anomalous.[31] Thus, the pupillary light reflex, vestibulo-ocular and oculocephalic reflexes, and response to sound could all be absent on a peripheral basis, providing an occasion for the potential misdiagnosis of brain death.

Because the neural structures that mediate typical newborn behaviors are located mainly in the brainstem, those anencephalic infants with relatively intact brainstems exhibit many such behaviors, for example, purposeless back-and-forth movements of the extremities, sucking and swallowing, normal orofacial expressions to gustatory stimuli, crying, withdrawal from noxious stimuli, and wake/sleep cycles. The main behavioral difference described between normal newborns and those without cerebral hemispheres, whether due to anencephaly or hydranencephaly (*in utero* destruction of both cerebral hemispheres, with intact skull and scalp), is increased irritabilty and lack of habituation to repeated stimuli,[32] although even these differences are not universally observed among infants lacking forebrains.[33] Some hydranencephalic infants have even demonstrated a capacity for paired associative learning[34] and visual tracking.[35] Of particular interest is the occasional high performance of these infants on measures of state-regulatory behaviors, such as self-quieting and hand-to-mouth facility, and of social behaviors, such as responsiveness to cuddling, consolability, and distinguishing mother from other adults by non-visual cues.[36] Thus, it is hardly surprising that parents of hydranen-cephalic infants often mistake their child for normal during the first month or two of life. Similarly, though on a milder scale, new-borns who have suffered a massive hemispheric stroke, which would produce a profound hemiplegia in an adult, often manifest only a subtle, if any, abnormality in muscle tone or movement.

These behavioral similarities between decerebrate and normal newborns are consistent with current knowledge of developmental neuroanatomy: even though cerebral hemispheres are present in gross structure in normal newborns, they are very immature microscopically compared to the brainstem.[37] In addition, patterns of regional cerebral energy metabolism, revealed by positron emission tomography, also suggest a relative lack of cerebral cortical function in normal human newborns.[38] In an older child or adult, such a metabolic pattern would constitute strong evidence for a persistent vegetative state (PVS). Nevertheless, newborns are able to carry out complex behaviors and sensory discriminations that would never be attributed to PVS patients.[39] Only gradually does the human cortex assume its adult-type primacy in the functional hierarchy of the brain—a developmental process known as "encephalization."

Animal experiments and comparative neuroanatomy also reveal that the brainstem is potentially capable of much more complex integrative activity than is usually attributed to it, including some functions generally considered to be "cortical" even in animals.[40] Both the clinical and experimental evidence strongly suggest that this is also the case with the human brainstem (at least in the newborn). This is not to say that the newborn cortex is physiologically irrelevent or that decerebrate infants mainifest all the complex (and probably cortical) sensory and cognitive abilities that specialized testing can reveal in normal newborns. But neither should one falsely minimize the functional capacity of those anencephalic infants with relatively intact brainstems.

Consciousness in Anencephalics

All this has obvious bearing on the issue of anencephalic consciousness. Whether or not an anencephalic infant, or even a normal infant, is "conscious" or capable of "suffering" is a philosophical question that is empirically unanswerable, if by these terms one means a subjective self-awareness associated with the respective behavioral reaction to environmental stimuli.

It seems established beyond doubt that in the mature human brain, the content of consciousness is processed in the cerebral cortex, while behavioral arousal and receptivity of the cortex is governed by the reticular activating system of the brainstem.[41] Children and adults with bilateral destruction of the cerebral cortex remain in a vegetative state, characterized by wake/sleep cycles, yet without evidence of any content of consciousness or voluntary movement during the periods of alert facial expression.[42]

Based on such considerations, there has been a traditional (usually unspoken) assumption that newborn infants, particularly prematures, because of their relative lack of cortical function, are not "conscious" even though they may be awake, and that their crying following painful stimuli does not necessarily reflect any subjective experience of unpleasantness or pain, any more than the reflex facial grimacing of patients in persistent vegetative state does. A practical consequence is that circumcisions and other types of surgery have traditionally been performed on newborns in the absence of anesthesia or analgesia. Needless to say, if this theory is true, it would apply all the more to infants born without cerebral hemispheres.

For this inference to follow logically from established principles of "adult" neurophysiology, however, a second (usually unspoken) premise must be accepted, namely, that the newborn brain is like a miniature adult brain with respect to the physiology of consciousness, and therefore, a newborn operating from a mere brainstem is equivalent to an adult operating from a mere brainstem. Although this may yet prove to be the case, discoveries in developmental neurobiology over the past several decades indicate that this is an extremely hazardous assumption, because the newborn brain does function quite differently from a "miniature adult brain" in many other (and relevant) ways.

240

The fact that decerebrate newborns behave much more similarly to normal newborns than to decerebrate adults is already an important distinction that cannot be overemphasized. This is no longer the case by around 2 months of age, when decerebrate infants begin to exhibit the rigidity typical of PVS patients. But at the newborn stage, the essential difference between normal and decerebrate infants is in the area of potential for future development, with only subtle differences in actual, present functioning. Also, associative learning and conditioning, which can occur in some decerebrate newborns, have, to my knowledge, never been reported in older PVS patients.

Secondly, it is a great fallacy to assume that the functional deficit associated with congenital absence of a certain part of the brain is the same as that associated with destruction of that part in a fully formed brain. The literature on developmental neuroplasticity is overwhelming on this point.[43] As a general rule in both animals and humans, the earlier the neurologic lesion, the greater the capacity of other parts of the brain to reorganize in a functionally compensatory way.[44]

The most relevant question with respect to neuroplasticity in anencephalic infants is whether subcortical structures are capable of taking over certain "cortical" functions, if the cortical lesion occurs early enough in fetal development. Unfortunately, the evidence on this point is both meager and conflicting. In rats and rabbits, no evidence has been found for such compensation.[45] In higher species, however, it has been clearly shown to occur to a limited extent. For example, cats rendered decorticate neonatally are capable of complex social behaviors and of learning stimulus discrimination coupled to an adaptive motor performance, in contrast to the more severe deficits of adult-lesioned animals.[46] Subcortical assumption of otherwise "cortical" visual and motor functions has also been implicated in other experiments involving neonatally lesioned cats and monkeys.[47]

The point is not, of course, to imply that plasticity can permit a brainstem to substitute for a cerebral cortex; clearly the extent to which it can assume lost cortical function in higher newborn animals and man is very limited. The point is, however, that decerebrate newborns are not merely miniature PVS patients, and that brainstem plasticity might possibly suffice to provide a decerebrate newborn with some primitive form of awareness. Just as we are now beginning to recognize that the brainstem is capable of more complex functioning than was previously realized, and as clinical practice is beginning to take into account the apparent reality of newborn pain,[48] so should we remain open-minded about the possibility that the subjective experiences of anencephalic infants, like their external behaviors, may resemble more those of normal newborns than of older PVS patients. The inherent uncertainties about infant consciousness are an important yet overlooked factual premise for various ethical analyses.

To be sure, anencephalic infants with complete craniorachischisis or severe brainstem maldevelopment cannot experience consciousness or suffering. But these are not the ones of interest as organ sources, because they are almost invariably stillborn. Concerning those with more intact brainstems, it simply begs the question to state categorically that they lack conscious awareness because they lack cerebral hemispheres. Much less is there any logical or physiological basis for the claim of some that an anencephalic infant can neither feel nor experience pain "by definition."[49] For practical purposes, one should presume, at the very least, that anencephalic infants are no less aware or capable of suffering than some laboratory animals with even smaller brains, which everyone seems to feel obliged to treat "humanely."

Life Span and Cause of Death

The life span of an individual anencephalic infant depends on both the severity of dysgenesis of the brainstem and the intensity of medical and nursing care provided. Although it is commonly stated that these infants invariably die within a few days of birth, various large studies and a number of anecdotal reports of longer survivals cast serious doubt on this contention. According to one study of 181 such infants, 42 percent of those born alive survived longer than twenty-four hours, 15 percent survived longer than three days, and 5 percent longer than seven days.[50] The longest survivor died on the fourteenth day. A review of the California Birth Cohort File between 1978 and 1982 revealed that of the 205 liveborn anencephalic infants with birthweight greater than 2,500 grams (and therefore of greatest interest *vis à vis* organs), 47 percent died within one day, an additional 44 percent between one day and one week, 8 percent between one week and one month, and 1 percent around three months of age.[51] There are also documented cases of anencephalic infants living five and a half months,[52] seven months,[53] and fourteen months.[54]

The cause of death in anencephaly has never been systematically studied and remains essentially unknown. It undoubtedly varies from case to case, depending upon the severity of the anomalies of the brain and other organ systems. If the brainstem respiratory and/or vasomotor centers are abnormally developed, then one would expect hypoventilation and/or blood pressure instabilities to set in within a short period of time. Trauma to the exposed brain during the birth process, less severe than to cause stillbirth, could also result in hypoventilation during the first several hours. These are the most likely explanations for the many deaths within the first day.

The infants whose brainstems are intact enough to maintain respiratory drive and regulate blood pressure may succumb over the next few days to endocrine abnormalities. Common findings in anencephaly are absent or hypofunctioning pituitary glands, as well as hypoplastic, poorly functioning adrenal glands.[55] These could result in ultimately fatal electrolyte imbalances and inability to handle various physiological stresses, eventually leading to either hypoventilation or a cardiac arrhythmia as the immediate cause of death.

Although the brain is exposed, infection is rarely, if ever, cited as a cause of death, probably because these infants tend to die before infection can set in. Those who live longer tend to have less extensive cranial defects, which are also more likely to be covered by an epithelial membrane, protecting the brain not only from infection but also from damage by direct contact with air. The cause of death of the rare infants who survive several months or more is probably aspiration, to which they would be highly prone.

From what we know of the anatomy and pathophysiology of anencephaly, therefore, it is unlikely that the primary cause of death of these infants is progressive brainstem destruction or degeneration. The final apnea may result from a developmental lack of chemoreceptormediated respiratory drive, from systemic disorders, or from potentially transient trauma-induced brainstem dysfunction; in any case, it does not necessarily indicate progressive and irreversible structural damage to the brainstem, as occurs in brain death. Theoretically, therefore, artificial ventilation and intensive care should help to preserve the integrity of the brainstem just as much as that of the other organs, and the only accomplishment would be to postpone the moment of death until some systemic complication were to supervene.

Utility of Organs for Transplantation

Anencephalic infants tend to be born prematurely (53 to 58 percent of cases), with a mean gestational age of thirty-three to thirty-six weeks.[56] In addition, most have intrauterine growth retardation, with 33 percent having weight below the mean by greater than two standard deviations.[57] According to various series, 50 to 80 percent have birth weights less than 2,500 grams.[58] It is reasonable to assume, therefore, for purposes of calculation, that around 60 percent of liveborn anencephalics will be too small to provide useful organs for transplantation, reducing the above-estimated yearly 304 liveborn anencephalics to 122 potentially useful ones.

Although there is no hard data on the proportion of brain-dead children whose parents are willing to donate their organs, the experience in UCLA's pediatric intensive care unit approximates 75 percent. In the case of anencephalics, there will be a need either to prolong the infant's dying process (by means of a ventilator and intensive care, while awaiting "brain death") or to remove the organs while the infant is still alive (if the laws change). Neither of these alternatives will be acceptable to some parents, so it is safe to assume that a somewhat lower proportion, say two-thirds at best, will be willing to donate. This brings the annual number of useful, donated anencephalic infants down to eighty-one.

One-third to one-half of anencephalic infants have associated gross malformations of at least one other organ system.[59] Around one-third have urinary tract malformations, most of which are nevertheless compatible with transplantable kidneys. Even though the kidneys tend to be hypoplastic, once transplanted they can grow and function normally.[60] Nevertheless, the overall experience with long-term graft survival from infant kidney donors in general has been poor.[61] Furthermore, the ability to support infants in renal failure by means of chronic peritoneal dialysis has improved enough that pediatric nephrologists prefer to maintain infants this way until several years of age, when the likelihood of a successful transplant is much higher. Typically, the kidneys from infant liver or heart donors go unclaimed, as was the case with the famous baby Gabrielle, Loma Linda University Medical Center's first anencephalic heart donor.

Cardiovascular malformations occur in some 8 to 41 percent of anencephalics, including a 5 to 10 percent rate of "major" malformations.[62] A large proportion of the hearts are hypoplastic, and some may be unsuitable for transplantation merely on the basis of their size. Around one-fourth of anencephalics have gross gastrointestinal anomalies,[63] and their livers tend to contain decreased glycogen (energy stores),[64] which may compromise organ viability during a transplant procedure. Although in one series, the liver weights of anencephalics born at term were near normal (92 percent of controls),[65] in another series, of the infants with birth weight over 2,500 grams, 55 percent had livers smaller than one standard deviation below the mean.[66] Size is much more crucial for liver transplants than for heart, and selection criteria generally require that donor and recipient livers be similar in size (ordinarily judged preoperatively on the basis of body weight).[67] Thus, say around 15 percent of the hearts and 25 percent of the livers will be unusable on the basis of malformation or size, reducing the estimated annual number of usable kidneys, hearts and livers available from anencephalics to zero, sixty-nine, and sixty-one, respectively.

Not every potentially transplantable organ finds its way into a recipient, however. For various reasons, around 25 percent of all organ referrals (all ages combined) are found acceptable by established organ sharing networks.[68] The figure is lower for hearts, usually because an excessive amount of medication is required to maintain the potential donors' blood pressure before referral, disqualifying them under most protocols. At present infants with biliary atresia almost always receive a palliative surgical procedure (Kasai procedure) first and then are placed on the national transplant waiting list at age four or five months.[69] Nevertheless, there are still some at this age who have failed to gain weight and are therefore small enough to be size-compatible with a newborn donor. For both hearts and livers, blood type compatibility between potential donor and recipient is preferred, unless the latter is listed as having less than twenty-four hours to live. If there is no potential recipient in geographic proximity, some parents would be reluctant to allow the body of their child to be flown to a distant city for organ harvesting. In spite of national computerized organ sharing networks, the need for temporal coincidence of potential donors and compatible potential recipients remains a major reason for the nonuse of transplantable organs.

Some of these problems have already been illustrated by the experience with Loma Linda's anencephalic protocol, which went into effect in mid-December 1987. Out of thirteen anencephalic infants donated as of August 9, 1988 (including the first case, referred from Canada prior to the formal establishment of their protocol), only three were declared "brain dead" within the specified seven-day limit, and from those only a single vital organ, a heart, made its way into another child.[70]

Based on the meager experience so far, it is difficult to estimate the proportion of organs that would actually be used from potentially suitable and donated anencephalic infants, if similar protocols were to become widespread or laws changed to relax the requirement that anencephalic "donors" be dead. Even if the latter were to come about, it is highly doubtful that any more than 25 and 15 percent of otherwise suitable hearts and livers, respectively, would ever be used, reducing the yearly number of used anencephalic kidneys, hearts, and livers to zero, seventeen, and nine, respectively, at most.

Finally, the proportion of infant recipients actually benefitted is not entirely clear, as there has been so little experience to date with transplantation in such a young age group. Few institutions perform heart transplantation in newborns. To date, of the seventeen heart transplants in infants under six months of age performed by Dr. Leonard Bailey at Loma Linda, thirteen are alive, with follow-up periods ranging from a few days to two-and-a-half years.[71] The eventual proportion of long-term survivors will undoubtedly be somewhat less than 13/17, with the current state of the art. Dr. Constantine Mavroudis, at the University of Louisville, has performed seven heart transplants in infants, six of whom were newborns. Four of the seven are alive at eight months to two years of follow-up.[72] Based on the experience at these two centers, a 50 percent long-term survival is optimistically reasonable. Liver transplantation in newborns is in a much more preliminary stage of development. Even some of the most active liver transplant teams in the country, for example at UCLA and the University of Pittsburgh, usually reject offers of newborn livers on account of the high incidence of complications, preferring instead those from somewhat older infants.[73]

If we use estimates of 50 and 20 percent long-term survival for recipients of newborn hearts and livers, respectively, the yearly number of patients in the country actually benefitting from anencephalic kidneys, hearts, and livers optimistically projects to zero, nine, and two, respectively.

It is interesting to try to project these figures into the near future, say ten years from now. Based on present trends, there will probably be around 4,000,000 births annually. The natural anencephaly prevalence rate of 0.3 per 1,000 births will probably have fallen by, say, 3 percent per year, which over 10 years will bring the rate to 0.22. Prenatal screening will have become more widespread, resulting in, say, termination of 50 percent of anencephalic fetuses nationwide. Let us assume that the proportion of stillbirths, the mean gestational age, organ malformation rate, and the proportion of parents willing to donate, remain about the same. For the sake of argument, let us suppose that the use of neonatal kidney donors were to become standard (with, say, 15 percent of kidneys unusable). The logistics of matching donors and recipients will have improved somewhat, so that, say, 25 percent of otherwise suitable kidneys, hearts, and livers would be used (a high estimate of the current salvage rate across all ages). The outcomes of neonatal transplantation will also have improved, so let us assume that the proportion of long-term survivors receiving neonatal kidneys, hearts, and livers will be optimistically 75, 75 and 50 percent, respectively. Combining all these figures, and assuming two kidney recipients for each anencephalic "donor," the annual number of infants in the country who will benefit from anencephalic organs ten years from now projects to at most twenty-five, twelve, and seven, for kidneys, hearts, and livers, respectively.

Such present and future projections ought to be borne in mind in discussions of the impact of anencephalic organ harvesting upon the many hundreds of children who die each year from congenital kidney, heart, and liver disease, before we expend great effort in modifying diagnostic criteria for brain death, changing statutory definitions of death, or relaxing fundamental principles of transplantation ethics in order to obtain anencephalic organs.

NOTES

1. Ronald J. Lemire, "Neural Tube Defects," *Journal of the American Medical Association* 259:4 (January 22/29, 1988), 558–62.

2. Michael Melnick and Ntinos C. Myrianthopoulos, "Studies in Neural Tube Defects II. Pathologic Findings in a Prospectively Collected Series of Anencephalics," *American Journal of Medical Genetics* 26:4 (April 1987), 797–810.

3. Josef Warkany, *Congenital Malformations* (Chicago: Year Book Medical Publishers, 1971), 195.

4. Ronald J. Lemire, J. Bruce Beckwith, and Josef Warkany, *Anencephaly* (New York: Raven Press, 1978), 5.

5. Warkany, *Congenital Malformations,* 189 (note 3).

6. Warkany, *Congenital Malformations,* 211 (note 3).

7. Warkany, *Congenital Malformations,* 192 (note 3); Jeanne E. Bell and Robert J. L. Green, "Studies on the Area Cerebrovasculosa of Anencephalic Fetuses," *Journal of Pathology* 137:4 (August 1982), 315–28.

8. Warkany, *Congenital Malformations,* 212 (note 3).

9. Bell and Green, "Studies on the Area Cerebrovasculosa" at 315 (note 7); see also Toshihiko Terao *et al.,* "Neurological Control of Fetal Heart Rate in 20 Case of Anencephalic Fetuses," *American Journal of Obstetrics and Gynecology* 149:2 (May 15, 1984), 201–208.

10. Ronald J. Lemire *et al., Normal and Abnormal Development of the Human Nervous System* (Hagerstown, MD: Harper & Row, 1975), 62.

11. Diane M. Gianelli, "Anencephalic Heart Donor Creates New Ethics Debate," *American Medical News* (November 6, 1987), 3, 47–49, at 49.

12. Pictures of cephalic lesions further exemplifying this diagnostic ambiguity are found in Warkany, *Congenital Malformations,* Fig. 22–11 at 198, 24–4 at 213 (note 3); Yvonne Brackbill, "The Role of the Cortex in Orienting: Orienting Reflex in an Anencephalic Human Infant," *Developmental Psychology* 5:2 (September 1971), 195–201; J. M. Nielsen and R. P. Sedgwick, "Instincts and Emotions in an Anencephalic Monster," *Journal of Nervous and Mental Disease* 110:4 (October 1949), 387–94.

13. Patricia A. Baird and Adele D. Sadovnick, "Survival in Infants with Anencephaly," *Clinical Pediatrics* 23:5 (May 1984), 268–71.

14. H. Urich and M. Kaarsoo Herrick, "The Amniotic Band Syndrome as a Cause of Anencephaly. Report of a Case." *Acta Neuropathologica* (Berlin) 67:3–4 (August 1985), 190–94.

15. J. Mark Elwood and J. Harold Elwood, *Epidemiology of Anencephalus and Spina Bifida* (Oxford: Oxford University Press, 1980), 87-90; J. Haase *et al,* "A Cohort Study of Neural Tube Defects (NTD) in Denmark Covering the First Seven Years of Life," *Child's Nervous System* 3 (1987), 117–20.

16. Ntinos C. Myrianthopoulos and Michael Melnick, "Studies in Neural Tube Defects I. Epidemiologic and Etiologic Aspects," *American Journal of Medical Genetics* 26 (1987), 783–96.

17. Mary J. Seller, "Neural Tube Defects and Sex Ratios," *American Journal of Medical Genetics* 26:3 (March 1987), 699–707; Elwood and Elwood, *Epidemiology* 130–38 (note 15).

18. Lechaim Naggan, "The Recent Decline in Prevalence of Anencephaly and Spina Bifida," *American Journal of Epidemiology* 89:2 (February 1969), 154–60; Ian Leck, "Spina Bifida and Anencephaly: Fewer Patients, More Problems," *British Medical Journal* 286 (May 28, 1983), 1679–80; David H. Stone, "The Declining Prevalence of Anencephalus and Spina Bifida: Its Nature, Causes and Implications," *Developmental Medicine and Child Neurology* 29:4 (August 1987), 541–49; Elwood and Elwood, *Epidemiology,* 107–19 (note 15).

19. Elwood and Elwood, *Epidemiology,* 89 (note 15); Myrainthopoulos and Melnick, "Studies, I" (note 16); Roberta H. Raven *et al.,* "Geographic Distribution of Anencephaly in the United States," *Neurology* 33:9 (September 1983), 1243–46.

20. Sherman C. Stein *et al.,* "Is Myelomeningocele a Disappearing Disease?" *Pediatrics* 69:5 (May 1982), 511–14; Gayle C. Windham and Larry D. Edmonds, "Current Trends in the Incidence of Neural Tube Defects," *Pediatrics* 70:3 (September 1982), 333–37. (Prevalence rates for each sex are shown separately on their graphs; the total prevalence rate of 0.48 cited here was provided through the courtesy of Mr. Edmonds.)

21. Personal communication, Linda Lustig, M.S., Chief, Neural Tube Defect Section, Genetic Disease Branch, California Department of Health Services, Berkeley, CA.

22. Data made available through the courtesy of Larry D. Edmonds, M.S.P.H., Birth Defects Branch, Centers for Disease Control, U.S. Department of Health and Human Services, Atlanta, GA.

23. U.S. Bureau of the Census, *Statistical Abstract of the United States: 1988* 108th edition (Washington, DC: U.S. Government Printing Office, 1987), Tables 81 and 83 at 59–60.

24. See, for example, H. Thom *et al.,* "The Impact of Maternal Serum Alpha Fetoprotein Screening on Open Neural Tube Defect Births in North-East Scotland," *Prenatal Diagnosis* 5:1 (January 1985), 15–19.

25. Personal communications, Linda Dobbs, R.N., Southern California Regional Coordinator for the AFP Screening Program, UCLA Medical Center, Los Angeles, CA, and Linda Lustig (note 21).

26. Personal communication, Linda Dobbs (note 25).

27. Jack A. Pritchard, Paul C. MacDonald, and Norman F. Gant, *Williams Obstetrics* (New York: Appleton-Century-Crofts, 1985), 17the ed. 462, 802–803.

28. Elwood and Elwood, *Epidemiology,* 58, 75–76, 84, 109 (note 15); Windham and Edmonds, "Current Trends" (note 20).

29. G. H. A. Visser *et al.,* "Abnormal Motor Behavior in Anencephalic Fetuses," *Early Human Development* 12:2 (November 1985), 173–82.

30. Lemire, Beckwith, and Warkany, *Anencephaly,* 52–53 (note 4).

31. I. Friedmann, J. L. W. Wright, and P. D. Phelps, "Temporal Bone Studies in Anencephaly," *The Journal of Laryngology and Otology* 94:8 (August 1980), 929–44.

32. Brackbill, "The Role of the Cortex" (note 12); Patricia L. Francis, Patricia A. Self, and Mary Anne McCaffree, "Behavioral Assessment of a Hydranencephalic Neonate," *Child Development* 55:1 (February 1984), 262–66. (Judging from the authors' description, this infant probably suffered from maximal hydrocephalus rather than hydranencephaly.)

33. Gary G. Berntson *et al.,* "The Decerebrate Human: Associative Learning," *Experimental Neurology* 81:1 (July 1983), 77–88; Frances K. Graham *et al.,* "Precocious Cardiac Orienting in a Human Anencephalic Infant," *Science* 199 (Jan. 20, 1978), 322–24.

34. David S. Tuber *et al.,* "Associative Learning in Premature Hydranencephalic and Normal Twins," *Science* 210 (November 28, 1980), 1035–37; Thomas Deiker and Ralph D. Bruno, "Sensory Reinforcement of Eyeblink Rate in a Decorticate Human," *American Journal of Mental Deficiency* 80:6 (May 1976), 665–67; Berntson *et al.,* "The Decerebrate Human: Associative Learning" (note 33).

35. Glen P. Aylward, Anthony Lazzara, and John Meyer, "Behavioral and Neurological Characteristics of a Hydranencephalic Infant," *Developmental Medicine and Child Neurology* 20:2 (April 1978), 211–17. (One cannot entirely exclude the possibility, however, that the visual tracking reported in this case was mediated by a shrunken remnant of occipital lobe.)

36. Julius Hoffman and Leopold Liss, " 'Hydranencephaly.' A Case Report with Autopsy Findings in a 7-Year-Old Girl," *Acta Paediatrica Scandinavica* 58:3 (May 1969), 297–300; James H. Halsey, Jr., Norman Allen, and Harrie R. Chamberlin, "Chronic Decerebrate State in Infancy. Neurologic Observations in Long Surviving Cases of Hydranencephaly," *Archives of Neurology* 19:3 (September 1968), 339–46; Francis *et al.,* "Behavioral Assessment of a Hydranencephalic Neonate" (note 32); Nielsen and Sedgwick, "Instincts and Emotions" (note 12).

37. Lemire *et al., Normal and Abnormal Development,* 40–52, 231–39, 260–65 (note 10).

38. Harry T. Chugani, Michael E. Phelps, and John C. Mazziotta, "Positron Emission Tomography Study of Human Brain Functional Development." *Annals of Neurology* 22:4 (October 1987), 487–97.

39. Marshall M. Haith and Joseph J. Campos (volume editors), "Infancy and Developmental Psychobiology," in Paul H. Mussen, ed., *Handbook of Child Psychology* 4th edition, Vol. II (New York: John Wiley & Sons, 1983).

40. Robert J. Noman *et al.,* "Classical Eyeblink Conditioning in the Bilaterally Hemispherectomized Cat," *Experimental Neurology* 44:3 (September 1974), 363–80; Ann M. Travis and Clinton N. Woolsey, "Motor Performance of Monkeys After Bilateral Partial and Total Cerebral Decortications," *American Journal of Physical Medicine* 35:5 (October 1956), 273–310; Stanley Finger and Donald G. Stein, *Brain Damage and Recovery. Research and Clinical Perspectives* (New York: Academic Press, 1982), 245–50; David A. Hovda, Richard L. Sutton, and Dennis M. Feeney, "Amphetamine-Induced Recovery of Visual Cliff Performance After Bilateral Visual Cortex Ablation in Cat: Measurements of Depth Perception Thresholds," *Behavioral Neuroscience* (1988), in press; Dennis M. Feeney and David A. Hovda, "Reinstatement of Binocular Depth Perception by Amphetamine and Visual Experience After Visual Cortex Ablation," *Brain Research* 342:2 (September 9, 1985), 352–56.

41. Fred Plum and Jerome B. Posner, *The Diagnosis of Stupor and Coma* 3rd Edition (Philadelphia: F. A. Davis, 1980), 1–30.

42. Ronald E. Cranford, "The Persistent Vegetative State: The Medical Reality (Getting the Facts Straight)," *Hastings Center Report* 18:1 (February/March 1988), 27–32.

43. See, for example, Hans Flohr and Wolfgang Precht, eds., *Lesion-Induced Neuronal Plasticity in Sensorimotor Systems.* (Berlin: Springer-Verlag, 1981); Carl W. Cotman, ed., *Synaptic Plasticity* (New York: Guilford Press, 1985); Jaime R. Villablanca, J. Wesley Burgess, and Charles E. Olmstead, "Recovery of Function After Neonatal or Adult Hemispherectomy in Cats: I. Time Course, Movement, Posture and Sensorimotor Tests," *Behavioural Brain Research* 19:3 (March 1986), 205–26, and sequels II and III in 20 (1986), 1–18, 217–30; Finger and Stein, "Brain Damage and Recovery," 63–81, 103–52, 287–302 (note 40).

44. See, for example, M. A. Jeeves, "Age Related Effects of Agenesis and Partial Sectioning of the Neocortical Commissures," in *Functional Recovery from Brain Damage,* Marius W. van Hof and Gesine Mohn, eds. (Amsterdam: Elsevier/North-Holland, 1981), 31–52;

Sid Gilman, James R. Bloedel, and Richard Lechtenberg, *Disorders of the Cerebellum* (Philadelphia: F. A. Davis, 1981), 263.

45. Brian Kolb, Ian Q. Whishaw, and Derek van der Kooy, "Brain Development in the Neonatally Decorticated Rat," *Brain Research* 397:2 (November 12, 1986), 315–26; P. M. Stuurman, M. W. Van Hof, and J. Hobbelen, "Behavioural Effects of Early and Late Unilateral Ablation of the Occipital Lobe in the Rabbit," in van Hof and Mohn, *Functional Recovery,* 121–29 (note 44).

46. L. M. Bjursten, K. Norrsell, and U. Norrsell, "Behavioural Repertory of Cats without Cerebral Cortex from Infancy," *Experimental* Brain Research 25:2 (May 28, 1976), 115–30.

47. David A. Hovda, Jaime R. Villablanca, and B. L. Shook, "Sparing of the Visual Field Is Associated with Less Metabolic Depression in the Superior Colliculus of Neonatal versus Adult Hemispherectomized Cats," *Society for Neuroscience Abstracts* 13 (1987), 1692; Patricia S. Goldman and Thelma W. Galkin, "Prenatal Removal of Frontal Association Cortex in the Fetal Rhesus Monkey: Anatomical and Functional Consequences in Postnatal Life," *Brain Research* 152:3 (September 8, 1978), 451–58.

48. K. J. S. Anand and P. R. Hickey, "Pain and its Effects in the Human Neonate and Fetus," *New England Journal of Medicine* 317:21 (November 19, 1987), 1321–29.

49. John C. Fletcher, John A. Robertson, and Michael R. Harrison, "Primates and Anencephalics as Sources for Pediatric Organ Transplants. Medical, Legal, and Ethical Issues," *Fetal Therapy* 1:2–3 (1986), 150–64, at 155.

50. Baird and Sadovnick, "Survival in Infants with Anencephaly" (note 13).

51. Jeffrey Pomerance and Barry S. Schifrin, "Anencephaly and the 'Baby Doe' Regulations," *Pediatric Research* 21:4 (Part 2, April 1987), 373A; Jeffrey Pomerance *et al.,* "Anencephalic Infants: Life Expectancy and Organ Donation," *Journal of Perinatology* (in press).

52. Brackbill, "The Role of the Cortex in Orienting" (note 12).

53. Personal experience, Warwick J. Peacock, MD, Associate Professor of Pediatric Neurosurgery, UCLA Medical Center, Los Angeles, CA.

54. Gianelli, "Anencephalic Heart Donor Creates New Ethics Debate," at 49, col. 4 (note 11).

55. L. Pajor, A. Németh, and T. Illés, "Functional Morphology of the Adrenal Cortex in Newborns. I Morphometric Study," *Acta Morphologica Hungarica* 34:1–2 (1986), 31–37; L. Cavallo *et al.,* "Endocrine Function in Four Anencephalic Infants," *Hormone Research* 15 (1981), 159–66; Bruce R. Carr *et al.,* "Regulation of Steroid Secretion by Adrenal Tissue of a Human Anencephalic Fetus," *Journal of Clinical Endocrinology and Metabolism* 50:5 (1980), 870–73.

56. Elwood and Elwood, *Epidemiology,* 55–56 (note 15); A. Giroud, "Anencephaly," in *Handbook of Clinical Neurology,* Vol. 30, P. J. Vinken and G. W. Bruyn, eds. (Amsterdam: North-Holland, 1977), 173–208 at 176.

57. George Cassady, "Anencephaly. A 6 Year Study of 367 Cases," *American Journal of Obstetrics and Gynecology* 103:8 (April 15, 1969), 1154–59.

58. Cassady, "Anencephaly" (note 57); Pomerance *et al.,* "Anencephalic Infants" (note 51).

59. Melnick and Myrianthopoulos, "Studies, II" (note 2); Lemire, Beckwith, and Warkany, *Anencephaly,* 66–84 (note 4).

60. P. Kinnaert *et al.,* "Transplantation of Both Kidneys of an Anencephalic Newborn to a 23-Year-Old Patient," *European Urology* 7:6 (1981), 373–76.

61. Robert B. Ettenger and Richard N. Fine, "Renal Transplantation," in *Pediatric Nephrology,* Malcolm A. Holliday, T. Martin Barratt, and Robert L. Vernier, eds. (Baltimore: Williams & Wilkins, 1987), 2nd ed., 828–46; Caliann T. Lum, Steven J. Wassner, and Donald

E. Martin, "Current Thinking in Transplantation in Infants and Children," *Pediatric Clinics of North America* 32:5 (October 1985), 1203–30.

62. Melnick and Myrianthopoulos, "Studies, II" (note 2); Lemire, Beckwith, and Warkany, *Anencephaly,* 73–74 (note 4).

63. Melnick and Myrianthopoulos, "Studies, II" (note 2); Lemire, Beckwith, and Warkany, *Anencephaly,* 79–80 (note 4).

64. Richard L. Naeye and William A. Blanc, "Organ and Body Growth in Anencephaly: A Quantitative, Morphological Study," *Archives of Pathology* 91: (February 1971), 140–47.

65. Naeye and Blanc, "Organ and Body Growth" (note 64).

66. Extrapolated from Lemire, Beckwith, and Warkany, *Anencephaly,* Fig. 306 at 80 (note 4).

67. Lum, Wassner, and Martin, "Current Thinking in Transplantation" (note 61); Carlos O. Esquivel *et al.,* "Liver Transplantation Before 1 Year of Age," *Journal of Pediatrics* 110:4 (April 1987), 545–48.

68. Personal communication, Barabara L. Schulman, R.N., Transplant Coordinator, Regional Organ Procurement Agency of Southern California, UCLA Medical Center, Los Angeles, CA.

69. John R. Lilly, Roberta J. Hall, and R. Peter Altman, "Liver Transplantation and Kasai Operation in the First Year of Life: Therapeutic Dilemma in Biliary Atresia," *Journal of Pediatrics* 110:4 (April 1987), 561–62.

70. Robert Steinbrook, "Center Modifies Baby-Organ Harvesting," *Los Angeles Times,* April 16, 1988, Part I, 20; personal communication, Stephen Ashwal, MD, Division of Pediatric Neurology, Loma Linda University Medical Center, Loma Linda, CA.

71. Personal communication, Anita Rockwell, assistant director of community relations, Loma Linda University Medical Center, Loma Linda, CA.

72. Constantine Mavroudis *et al.,* "Infant Orthotopic Cardiac Transplantation," *Journal of Cardiovascular Surgery* (in press).

73. Esquivel *et al.,* "Liver Transplantation" (note 67); Lum, Wassner, and Martin, "Current Thinking in Transplantation" (note 61).

Chapter 16

ETHICAL ASPECTS OF TISSUE AND ORGAN "DONATION" BY PREBORN AND ANENCEPHALIC INFANTS

Janet E. Smith, Ph.D.

Introduction

There has been much interest in the popular media about the possible usefulness of organs from anencephalic babies. Proposals have recently been made to place these babies on respirators immediately upon their birth, in order to keep their organs fresh for implantation when they die. The prospect of having a source of organs such as kidneys or hearts for ailing infants or of helping victims of Alzheimer's and Parkinson's has excited many. But in the professional world of medical research, this excitement has been tempered in recent months. As Dr. Alan Shewmon has persuasively argued, there are truly very few anencephalic babies that are likely to be suitable as sources for organ sources, certainly as long as so many are aborted.[1] Indeed, Loma Linda, the research facility that performed a successful heart transplant from an anencephalic baby, has stopped doing organ transplants from anencephalic babies since it has found the practice "medically unfeasible".[2] Nevertheless, although the use of organs from anencephalic infants may not be the boon it initially seemed to be, the arguments used to justify such use must be carefully examined; they raise ethical problems in their own right and quite readily lend themselves to justifying the harvesting of organs from other infants with birth defects, and from the comatose and dying.

While abortion reduces the availability of anencephalic babies, it provides an immense supply of fetal tissue possibly useful for many medical treatments; researchers speak of such tissue a "precious resource" that can be used to alleviate maladies from Parkinson's to hearing loss. Although some researchers are expressing more and more doubt about the ultimate usefulness of tissue from unborn babies,[3] the research community as a whole seems eager to have access to this tissue.[4]

Some of the crucial ethical questions that must be faced are these; 1) Is the human dignity of anencephalic infants being fully respected or are they being treated merely as instruments and means for the well-being of others?; 2) Are these infants truly dead when the organs are removed or are we tampering with definitions of death to facilitate removal of organs?; and 3) in regard to the use of tissue from aborted babies, we must ask, does this practice involve complicity with abortion? Before we get to these specific questions it may be useful to state the principles governing organ transplantation in general.

Principles Governing Organ Transplantation

Moralists have articulated four basic principles that ought to govern the practice of organ donation.[5] They are these:

1. The recipient has a serious need that cannot be fulfilled in any other way.

2. The functional integrity of the donor as a human person must not be impaired, even though anatomical integrity may suffer.
3. The burden to the donor must be proportionate to the expected benefit to the recipient.
4. The donor or the donor's proxy must give free and informed consent.

Let us first note that the first principle—that the recipient have a serious need that cannot be met in any other way, is easily met in the situations for which organs from anencephalic infants are sought. Other infants do need these organs but there are few infants available for organ transplants. Yet, the practice of using organs from anencephalic babies seems to have manifest coflicts with the other principles; these conflicts will become clear as we discuss the morality of organ transplantation in general and the specific problems associated with taking organs from anencephalic infants.

The practice of organ donation and transplantation is now so common that few question why it is moral for one to donate his or her organs to another. It was not so long ago that this question was hotly debated and that many, if not most, moral theologians were opposed to the practice. Many thought that since organ donation requires a sort of mutilation of the body of the donor, it would be immoral to subject one's self to such mutilation. This position was, of course, not altogether without merit. But a crucial distinction was made between what has been called anatomical integrity and functional integrity.[6] That is, since we have some organs such as a second kidney that we do not need in order to function, it is morally permissible to sacrifice our anatomical integrity as long as we maintain our functional integrity. That is, it would not be morally right for us to donate an organ that we needed to function in order to assist another—thus we insure functional integrity—but we can give to others organs that we do not need for survival, although we may have to sacrifice anatomical integrity. After death, of course, it would be permissible to donate healthy organs to another for one is not endangering one's own life, and one may be able to do enormous good for another.

Nature of the Body

As the above distinction suggests, it is important to remember that our bodies are not our property—they are not ours to do with as we will. We may give away our property quite freely and even whimsically and on occasion others may even have rights to our property. But our bodies are not ours in this sense. Rather our bodies *are* us in several important senses. The Catholic Church holds that the human person is not a soul housed in a body, but that the human person is a unity of body and soul. Our body, then, is not something we inhabit, it is not just a set of parts that our soul unifies; rather, it, in some meaningful sense, in union with the soul, *is* us. The importance of this point here is twofold. First, we must note that as with the abortion debate where many wish to argue that unborn babies are not fully human, so, too, do many wish to argue that anencephalic babies are not fully human. This point will be addressed more fully momentarily, but here we must ask if these babies are not human, what are they? They have living human bodies—what more do they need to qualify as human beings? Is it possible for something that is not human to have a human body?

That fact that the body is a part of the human essence also entails that what we do to our bodies is a matter of great ethical concern for these are actions done to human persons. We may, for instance, freely tamper with the parts of our cars, replace these parts at will and even demolish the car when it becomes appropriate, but our bodies are not to be subject to such treatment. Our bodies share in the dignity of the human person and must thus be treated in accord with that dignity.

Organ Donation: Act of Charity, not Justice

There are a few moralists who argue that individuals have an obligation to donate their organs,[7] but much more common—and defensible—is the view that we are not duty bound to donate our organs to others.[8] Others have no rights to our organs, but we can make gifts of them. This is one of the reasons behind prohibitions for selling organs—charity is the motive of the donation and charity is negated by a sale. Donation of organs is justifiable, then, not under the principle of justice but under the principle of charity. In fact, there are even limits to this gift giving. That is, as was mentioned above, it would be wrong to donate an organ that one needed for one's self. One may be able to assist a famous research scientist by donating one's heart to him so that he might be kept alive, but if one needed to commit suicide in order to do so, this would be a misuse of the gift of life that God has given one. Human beings, then, are not a set of parts, to be divvied up and to be given to those who most need them; human beings, with their bodies, have an inherent worth and identity that puts severe restrictions on the use of them.

The advocates of using organs from anencephalic babies generally hold views at odds with the principles stated above. They generally assume 1) that these babies are not fully human and therefore that it is permissible to treat them differently from other human beings and 2) that these babies will have greater worth if they, who have no chance of a long life, make a life-saving gift to those who do have a prospect of a normal life. Let us examine these assumptions.

Humanity of Anencephalic Babies

The literature on the use of organs from anencephalic infants constantly betrays the view that advocates of organ transplants do not view such infants as fully human. An article written by doctors from Loma Linda speaks of anencephalic infants' "marginality as human beings."[9] Many advocates of the use of organs from anencephalic infants argue that anencephalic babies are not human and others claim they are not persons. The argument in both cases is essentially the same: these babies are denied membership in the human species or in the class of human persons because they do not have sufficient brain tissue to have, either actually or potentially, such specific human abilities as thinking and having self-awareness. The dangers of using such standards to determine who qualifies for human rights are well-known—for one quickly finds out that many who are disqualified, such as any who do not exhibit signs of consciousness; for instance the comatose and those in a persistent vegetative state. Many, of course, do not shrink from disqualifying these individuals as human—and recommending that they, too, be harvested for organs[10]—but neither the philosophic

257

community or society at large are ready yet to accept such refinements on the definition of who qualifies to be treated as human. Personhood is a condition susceptible to many different definitions—under some definitions preborns and newborns and the comatose may qualify, under some they do not. What is not clear is why one must meet some definition of personhood to qualify for human rights. Why is it not sufficient simply to insist that any who are living human beings have human rights? And those are easy to identify: any creatures who have human parents should count as human beings and be entitled to be treated as such.

Anencephalic babies are born of human parents; they may not have a full brain but they can live for awhile on their own without artificial support systems; they can cry, and nurse, and make the bodily movements characteristic of newborns. Yet, some have even gone so far as to suggest that some animals have more rights than anencephalic babies since they display signs of greater intelligence.[11] But, again, it is the nature of one's being, not one's intelligence that confers rights on one. Certainly some dogs and cats may be more mannerly and loving than some humans but having these characteristics does not qualify them for a change in species or a change in rights. Those who are genetically human are those who have human rights—the absence of eyes, ears, legs, and even parts of the brain do not change one's genetic make-up, do not detract from one's humanity. The ultimate irony, of course, is that it is precisely because anencephalic babies are genetically human that makes their organs so desireable for transplant and makes it so tempting for some to want to treat them as less than human in order to have access to their organs.

The defining of anencephalic infants as less than fully human leads to some very disturbing proposals. One is the proposal that it would be morally permissible to take organs from these babies while they are still alive.[12] In other words, though they would hesitate to speak so bluntly, some find permissible the killing of these infants in order to benefit other infants. We find such an admission in a report by a committee of doctors and ethicists from Michigan; they argue for removal of the organs from these infants when they are still alive—a true advocacy of vivisection—since they do not consider them the same as other infants: "infants born with the top half of their brains missing are so very different from other living infants—and their future so radically limited—that it is permissible, with the fully informed and freely given consent of the parents, to remove their organs for transplantation." This report speaks of these infants as being "in a class that is entirely *sui generis,* and one for which special rules and laws should apply."[13] The special rules and laws are ones that define them as not fully human and allow the removal of their organs when they are not truly dead.[14] Indeed the most blatant effort to secure the means to treat anencephalic babies different from other human beings is the proposal to make an exception to the "brain death" criteria accepted by physicians and the law and to declare anencephalic babies "dead" at birth.[15] Laws have been proposed in both California and New Jersey to this effect. It has been proposed to define "brain absent" as "brain dead." Yet these infants are neither "brain dead" nor "brain absent": certain portions of their brains are absent but they have an intact brain stem that enables them to breathe spontaneously and occasionally to live quite some time after birth.[16] The proposal to declare them dead upon birth is an obvious attempt to use definitions not to describe reality but to advance a certain agenda—here the agenda of obtaining useful organs for transplantation.[17] The dangers of strategically changing the definition of death to facilitate some desired goal are clear—we could start redefining all sorts of other diseased, handicapped, or retarded humans as "dead" and thus make ready use of them for our purposes.

The argument for removing vital organs from anencephalic babies when they are still alive definitely violates principles two and three for moral transplantation of organs. That is, removing vital organs violates the functional integrity of the donor and the donor suffers a disproportionate burden—that is, his or her death—to benefit another.

Human Worth

Let us address the second assumption: that these babies have little or no worth beyond what they can contribute to another through the donation of their organs. First, it is crucial to establish the principle that human beings do not derive their worth from what they contribute to the rest of society. Of course, most every one would prefer to make some grand contribution to society but we must remember that each and every human being has inestimable worth simply by virtue of his or her humanity. Christians teach that humans are made in the image and likeness of God and thus share in God's infinite worth. We have this worth whether or not we enter into any human relationships, whether we live for ten years or ten minutes. Those not particularly comfortable with the Christian definition of man as a creature made in the image of God are often drawn to Kant's dictum that it is never right to use a human being as a means to an end. Whatever the justification for the principle, Western civilization has endeavored to protect each and every human life as valuable in its own right. It is important to establish this principle, for many want to argue that anencephalic infants can be said to have a worthy life if—and it seems *only* if—they are sources for organs for other needy infants. Such a claim completely ignores the inherent value and worth they have simply through being human.

The proposal to put anencephalic babies on respirators upon birth provides another piece of evidence that these babies are not fully valued in their own right for this treatment is not initiated to benefit these infants; rather it is initiated to keep their organs fresh for transplantation. And it is likely that the procedure causes them some discomfort, for which reason the Loma Linda protocol required cessation of such treatment after seven days; it seems that the babies are thought to have suffered long enough by that time. But, from the moment of their birth there is more than a little suggestion that they are being treated like a set of parts for someone else's use.

Consent

The fourth criterion listed above for legitimate organ transplantation is that the organ donor or the donor's proxy must give free and informed consent. This principle seems to have two justifications. One is that the donor must be assured that his or her interests are being honored and that he or she is not being plundered for the sake of the well-being of another; fair treatment is best ensured by having the donor or someone with the donor's best interest in mind give consent. And, as was stated above, organ donation is a matter of charity and not justice; thus, we must have reason to believe that the organ donor would have wanted his or her organs to be donated before their organs are used. Clearly an anencephalic baby is not able to give such consent. Thus, one would naturally turn to the parents. But the parents in this instance are as likely as anyone else to be tempted to undervalue the humanity of the baby. Let us consider that approximately 95% of anencephalic babies diagnosed as such during pregnancy are aborted. Even mothers who do not abort make remarks such as "if transplantation were not possible, I would have aborted the baby." Thus, it would be the rare instance where the baby was not being treated merely as a means to an end. Could such a baby be said to have a proxy who is acting in his or her best interests?

Assessing the legitimacy of proposed treatment for anencephalic infants, then, requires that several basic criteria be determinative of this assessment. 1) First and foremost all treatment must be predicated on the full humanity of the child; 2) The child should in no way be thought of or used merely as a means to the good of another. The dignity and worth of the child must be fully respected. Nothing should be done to the infant that is not fully in accord with its human dignity no matter what good might be obtained for another. 3) Parties making decisions about the infant should unquestionably have the interests of the child in mind.

But, let us grant that it is at least theoretically possible to envision a situation where a couple gave birth to an anencephalic baby and where they and their doctors exhibited full respect for the infant and cherished it for however brief an existence it might have. Would there be anything wrong with their giving permission for the donation of organs from this baby? I have found a report of one such instance that I believe meets the requirements for moral treatment of an anencephalic infant. This is the story of a baby named Hope born in Knoxville.[18] Hope's mother learned during her pregnancy that she was going to have an anencephalic baby. Because of her and her husband's strong Christian commitment and their respect for life, they rejected the suggestion that they might "terminate the pregnancy." It was only after she had made the decision not to abort, that Kay, the mother, learned about the possibility of donating some of her baby's organs. She was not enthusiastic about having Loma Linda take her baby since they would place her on a respirator and Kay did not want her baby uncomfortable if she didn't need to be. But when they got Loma Linda to agree to use a respirator only if it were needed for Hope's well being, they sent Hope off to Loma Linda. Kay immediately regretted having sent her off alone and found a charity to send her and her husband to be with Hope. There, unlike the parents of other anencephalic infants, they were daily by her bedside, caring for her; they saw her open her blue eyes and saw her smile. They expected her to die within seven days, but she lived. Her parents went home and left Hope in California, but again found themselves missing her dreadfully when they came home. Loma Linda flew Hope back to Knoxville in their private jet. Hope lived for fifty nine days under the loving care of her family. Kay tells how Hope brought her and her stepdaughter closer together; she said "I think she [my stepdaughter] saw that if I could love a baby with no brain then I sure as heck could love her, as sweet and dear as she is. In the end, Hope really made a family out of us." After her death, Hope's parents donated her cornea and her heart valves and donated her body for research. Since she was not on a respirator when she died her other organs were not in a condition suitable for transplantation. Although the plans for donation of Hope's liver to another baby did not work, had they worked, Hope's story shows that it is possible for transplantation of organs from anencephalic babies to be done in a moral fashion—for Hope was accorded the full respect due a human being. Her parents truly loved her and acted in her best interests.

We must note, though, that few anencephalic babies are loved like Hope was. And, apart from the fact that this is, unfortunately, the rarest of occurrences and thus not a good basis for the making of policy or law, it is also true that there is at least one great technical difficulty in the way of being true to the principles for organ transplantation and this is the difficulty of determining with certainty that death has occurred.

Brain Death

As Dr. Shewmon has shown, the criteria used to determine brain death in adults does not work well for anencephalic infants.[19]

Doctors generally find such criteria unreliable for infants under a week old. Infants rarely die because their brains have stopped functioning. Moreover, their brains are more resilient than adult brains and it is not easy to determine when all brain activity has irreversibly stopped functioning. It is disturbing to read reports that the doctors at Loma Linda who performed a heart transplant from an anencephalic baby declared the baby dead after only three minutes of respiratory failure and then also administered an anesthetic to the baby since they wanted to ensure that it experience no pain.[20] But a dead body feels no pain, and if they were certain that the baby was dead, there was no need for an anesthetic.

Thus we can add one more requirement to the list given above for moral criteria for use of organs from anencephalic babies: 4) There must be no "fudging" on the determination of death. No organs should be taken from a child who has not been declared dead with certainty.

Finally, let us address one of the most common justifications for the use of organs from anencephalic babies. Many argue that such donation will help console the parents of these babies; that they will sense that some good has come out of their tragedy. But if such consolation is impossible without the dehumanization of their baby, it would hardly seem to be appropriate consolation. As Shewmon and others have argued, the fact that few such transplants have worked may lead to further grief for the parents.[21] They may even come to suffer from doubts about their eagerness to bring good out of tragedy; they may worry that they had some part in their baby's death. But as Shewmon and others have pointed out, it is possible for them to make the cornea and other nonvital organs available for transplantation and experience some consolation in this way, as did the parents of baby Hope.

Use of Fetal Tissue from Aborted Babies

The use of fetal tissue from aborted babies is an issue closely related to the issue of organ transplantation from anencephalic babies. Some argue that it would be immoral to let them go to further waste by tossing out their remains—rather some good could come of their lives—however brief they may have been—by using their bodily parts to help others. But to others it seems patently exploitative to take the organs or tissues of aborted babies to help others. They have already paid a big price—the price of their lives—to help out someone else—usually their mothers. Who has shown these babies any of the love or respect they deserve as human beings? Futhermore, our using them to help others may amount to a kind of cooperation in the death that they had. Our refusal to harvest them for organs and tissue may be the last remnant of respect we can pay them.

With the increased number of abortions and thus the increased amount of fetal tissue and with the considerable (if unrealistic optimism) about the possible therapeutic use of such tissue, plans for great experimentation in this area have burgeoned. Because of the inevitable use of federal funds in such projects, a special committee was set up by the National Institute of Health to investigate the morality of this practice. As is well known, last November seventeen of the twenty-one members of the committee voted to permit this practice. Two dissenters were Father James Burtchaell from Notre Dame, and James Bopp, chief legal counsel for the National Right to Life Committee.[22] In their work and that of others we find several fundamental objections to this practice. Certainly there is the same tendency to view these babies as less than fully human as there was with anencephalic babies. But the most forceful objections here have to do with the difficulty in determining a suitable agent to give consent for donation of organs or tissue from an aborted baby. And there is also the very troubling question of complicity with abortion and the prospect of women or clinics trafficking in human tissue.

Informed Consent

The fourth principle listed above for moral donation of organs is that the donor or his or her proxy must give free and informed consent. Again, a proxy is permitted when someone can be found—usually next of kin—who can be said to have the best interests of the donor in mind. But the donor we are talking about here is an aborted fetus and the most natural and suitable proxy is his or her mother, who decided to kill this very baby. It's hard to fathom that the mother, in this instance, could be said to have the baby's best interest in mind. Others, such as the father, grandparents, doctors, or state could possibly be construed as likely candidates to be a protective proxy, but unless they have all vigorously opposed the abortion it would be hard to see any of them as proper proxies.

Complicity in abortion

There is a lot of tissue available from aborted fetuses and it does seem that their mothers would likely give permission for this tissue to be used. Isn't it possible that even those opposed to abortion may morally use the remains of aborted babies? Wouldn't it be a humanitarian thing to do? Couldn't one remain free from any association with abortion?

First, let us note that direct cooperation in abortion is not an unrealistic possibility. It is possible that the best tissue to be gained is from late term abortion, from abortions that are done through hysterotomy—a procedure very like a caesarian section. Since most women get abortions through the suction D and C, in the first trimester, there would likely be some attempt to talk these women into having later term abortions. These abortions are more dangerous for the health of the woman, are done on fetuses capable of experiencing more pain, and on fetuses more likely to survive an abortion. Ethicists are troubled by these factors but some are willing to allow them in their eagerness to have fetal tissue available for medical treatment.[23]

Analogies with medical experiments done by doctors in Nazi Germany seem inevitable and right. These doctors could claim that they had nothing to do with the decisions to kill the Jews and that it would be foolish to pass up such a golden opportunity to make medical discoveries. At least some good could come from these deaths. And, of course, experimentation was done on live subjects for the reason that their death was imminent. The parallels of this situation with the use of aborted babies—and anencephalic babies, too—are obvious. The fears of those who imagine research scientists sitting in abortion clinics directing how abortions are done have been confirmed as valid by a recent event. A doctor recently, in defiance of a national moratorium on research using aborted fetal tissue, took fetal brain tissue from an aborted baby to implant in a patient with Parkinson's disease. He reports that he spend one day a week for three weeks in an abortion clinic in order to find suitable tissue.[24] How does he differ from the doctors of Nazi Germany who eagerly used victims of the Nazis for research purposes?

Trafficking and Other Bizarre Occurrences

Comparing current medical practices with Nazi Germany would seem to be the most damning kind of evidence one could give against a project. And in no way is such a comparison with the past a product of exaggeration or scare tactics. Future possibilities almost certainly to follow the permission to use fetal tissue from aborted babies are even more horrifying and suggest the medical doings of Nazi Germany are relatively tame compared to what we have on the horizon. Consider that shortly after the possibilities of the use of fetal tissue become known more popularly, a woman requested that she be fertilized with sperm from her father, a sufferer of Alzheimer's. She intended then to abort the baby and use its brain tissue to assist her father.[25] And consider the views of one ethicist who has argued that since women are the "point of origin" of fetuses and thus fetal tissue, they should be able to profit from the sale of their aborted fetuses.[26]

Another danger of the beneficial use of such tissue or rather, the desire to find a beneficial use for such tissue, threatens to supplant the search for morally acceptable means for treating the various condition fetal tissue may help treat. There is some evidence that this has already happened.[27]

Whether or not the expectations for the usefulness of such organs or tissue are realistic, it is important to fight these practices for, as we have seen, the justifications made for them strike at the root of the principles governing moral use of human organs and tissues. By reducing these helpless human beings to mere sources of parts for others, by redefining who is human and who is not, by creating industries dependent upon the aborting of millions of babies, these practices contribute to the increasing dehumanization of those on the edges of life and ultimately to a general devaluation of the worth of all human life.

Acknowledgement: I would like to thank Mark Recznik from the Human Life Center, Steubenville, Ohio; Richard Doerflinger of the NCCB pro-life office; and David Andrusko of *National Right to Life* for providing research assistance for this project.

NOTES

1. D. Alan Shewmon, "Anencephaly: Selected Medical Aspects," *Hastings Center Report* (October/November 1988), 11–18.

2. Louis Sahagun, "Harvesting of Baby Organs Not Feasible" *Los Angeles Times* part 1 (August 24, 1988); and see "Anencephalic Organ Donor Program Suspended; Loma Linda Report Expected to Detail Findings" *JAMA* 260:12 (Sept 23/30) 1988, 1671–2.

3. See particularly Peter McCullagh, *The Fetus as Transplant Donor: Scientific, Social and Ethical Perspectives,* (New York: John Wiley & Sons, 1987) and Leslie Bond, "Whether Fetal Tissue Transplants Works, 'A Very Big If," Bioethicist Caplan Says," *National Right to Life News* (August 11, 1988), 11.

4. James W. Walters and Stephen Ashwal, "Organ Prolongation in Anencephalic Infants: Ethical and Medical Issues," *Hastings Center Report* (Oct./Nov. 1988), 19–27.

5. See Benedict M. Ashley, O.P., and Kevin D. O'Rourke, O.P., *Health Care Ethics: A Theological Analysis,* (St. Louis, MO.; The Catholic Health Association of the United States, 1982, 2nd ed.) 309–312.

6. Ibid.

7. See, for instance, Richard McCormick, "Proxy Consent in the Experimentation Situation," *Love and Society: Essays in the Ethics of Paul Ramsey,* edited by James T. Johnson and David H. Smith (Missoula, Montana; Scholars Press, 1974), 209–227.

8. For an explanation of the principle of charity, see Paul Ramsey, *The Patient as Person* (New Haven; Yale University Press, 1970).

9. James W. Walters and Stephen Ashwal, "Organ Prolongation in Anencephalic Infants: Ethical and Medical Issues," *Hastings Center Report* (Oct./Nov. 1988), 21.

10. See, for instance, Ronald E. Cranford, M.D., and David Randolph Smith, J.D., "Consciousness: The Most Critical Moral (Constitutional) Standard for Human Personhood," *American Journal of Law and Medicine,* 13: 2&3 (1987) 234–248.

11. See, for instance, Mary Anne Warren, "Can the Fetus be an Organ Farm," *Hastings Center Report* (October 1978) 23–24; "It is clear that if we are to make a reasoned judgment about the moral status of fetuses, and of nonhuman animals, alien life, forms, intelligent machines, and other problematic entities, we must develop a criterion for the possession of moral rights that is species-neutral. That is, it will not do to make 'genetic humanity' (mere genetic affiliation to the human species) either a necessary or a sufficient condition for the possession of full moral rights. To make it necessary is to beg the question against all nonhuman entities, even those which may prove to have intellects and sensibilities comparable or superior to our own... " (23).

12. See, for instance, Mary B. Mahowald, Jerry Silver, and Robert Ratcheson, "The Ethical Options in Transplanting Fetal Tissue," *Hastings Center Report* (Feb. 1987) 9–15.

267

13. The Ethics and Social Impact Committee, Transplant Policy Center, Ann Arbor, MI., "Anencephalic Infants as Sources of Transplantable Organs," *Hastings Center Report* (Oct./Nov. 1988) 28.

14. See Mahowald, et al. Ibid.

15. For a report on this proposal see Alexander Morgan Capron, "Anencephalic Donors: Separate the Dead from the Dying," *Hasting Center Report* (February, 1987) 5–9.

16. For a review of such arguments, see D. Alan Shewmon, "Caution in the Definition and Diagnosis of Infant Brain Death," op. cit. Chapter Four in *Medical Ethics: A Guide for Health Professionals* edited by Monagle, T. F., and Thomasma, D. C. (Aspen, Rockville, MD; 1988).

17. For an argument that calls for creating a category of "nonviable" fetuses and infants and that thus makes them available as organ sources, see Mary B. Mahowald, et. al., op. cit.

18. See "A Legacy of Hope" a Special Report in *The Knoxville New-Sentinel* (Sunday, July 3, 1988).

19. D. Alan Shewmon, "Commentary on Guidelines for the Determination of Brain Death in Children" *Annals of Neurology* 24:6 (December 1988) 789–791 and "Caution in the Definition and Diagnosis of Infant Brain Death," op. cit. See also, Norman Fost, "Organs from Anencephalic Infants: An Idea Whose Time Has Not Yet Come" *Hastings Center Report* (Oct./Nov., 1988) 6.

20. Fost questions whether the Loma Linda criteria for death are valid (Ibid, p. 7). The information about the length of respiratory failure and the use of anesthetic was found in Richard Doerflinger, "Guest Opinion," *Catholic Standard* (December 24, 1987) 13.

21. Shewmon, et al., 28.

22. Their dissenting report has been published in *National Right to Life News* 16:1–2 (January 22, 1989) pp. 14–15. See also, James Tunstead Burtchaell, "University Policy on Experimental Use of Aborted Fetal Tissue," *IRB: A Review of Human Subjects Research* 10:4 (July/August 1988) 7–11.

23. See Mahowald et al., op. cit., 13.

24. Leslie Bond, "First U.S. Fetal Brain Tissue Transplant Performed," *National Right to Life News* 15:22 (Dec. 5, 1988) 1.

25. Temar Lewin, "Medical Use of Fetal Tissue Spurs New Abortion Debate," *The New York Times* (August 16, 1987), 1.

26. Ibid, 7.

27. See Leslie Bond, "Adrenal Autografts: Dashed Hopes Lead to Premature Dismissal, Says Gash" *National Right to Life News* 16:1–2 (January 22, 1989) 7.

Chapter 17

PASTORAL CONCERNS
PREBORN AND ANENCEPHALIC
INFANTS

BISHOP: Would you be able to tell me, how many anencephalic infants would be at Loma Linda waiting to have their organs harvested?

DR. SHEWMON: Actually, Loma Linda called a moratorium on their protocol several months ago becaue they found that the practice of placing these infants on ventilators, waiting for them to become "brain dead" was not working, that the infants were not dying. And so after six such infants, they suspended their program. Of the six, not a single organ was obtained from any of them. So it proved to be a failure from a practical point of view. And that's why some of these other places, like the one in Michigan that Janet mentioned, are talking about removing the organs from live anencephalic infants rather than waiting for them to die.

But your question allows me to elaborate a little bit, if I may, on the issue of brain death in the anencephalic infant. One of the catch phrases that have been used to describe these infants is "brain absent". And, in fact, that phrase was the basis for Senator Milton Marks in California to introduce a bill that would have defined an anencephalic infant as *ipso facto* "dead" according to the law, because, according to Senator Marks and not a few other people, there is no difference between being "brain dead" and being "brain absent." As I tried to show in the slides, these infants are not really "brain absent," but rather "cerebral hemisphere absent." The brain stem is the part of the brain that controls blood pressure and respiration and, in infants, the sucking reflex and other vital functions. That part of the brain is present and functioning in most of these anencephalic infants. And so they're not really "brain absent;" they're just "cerebral hemisphere absent." Therefore, they're not equivalent to being brain dead because an adult or a child with a functioning brain stem but nonfunctioning cerebral hemispheres is not dead.

I see from the program that Dr. Plum talked to you the other day about the persistent vegetative state. These infants have been likened by many people to patients in a persistent vegetative state rather than patients who are brain dead. Now, as a pediatric neurologist, I would even take exception to that analogy, because if you look at the neurologic functioning of perfectly normal newborn infants, what do they do? They move around in a very stereotyped way, their arms and legs go back and forth, but they don't have any purposeful movement. They suck, they sleep, they wake, they cry, and that's more or less all they do. They have intact brain stem functions but they don't have much of a functioning cerebral cortex. In fact, the cerebral cortex in a newborn infant is just beginning to function, and over the next number of years, up to adolescence, there is a continuum of development of the cerebral cortex. If you do a scan of the brain that looks at the energy metabolism (a measure of the functioning of the various parts of the brain) in the newborn human infant, most of the cerebral hemispheres have very little energy metabolism and are not functioning very much at all. So almost all of the behavior of normal human newborns comes from the brain stem.

Why aren't normal human newborns like patients in a persistent vegetative state? The answer is that during development—postnatal development—other centers of the brain develop and

270

start to inhibit the brain stem. The cerebral cortex begins to inhibit brain stem reflexes like sucking and so forth. Finally, the cerebral cortex takes over.

There's a process called encephalization that goes on during the first year of life. During the newborn period and the first weeks and months after birth, the cerebral hemispheres are not inhibiting the brain stem, and neither are the parts of the brain between the cortex and the brain stem, which are also not yet fully developed. So the brain stem has these functions. Also, many of the connections between the brain and the spinal cord have not developed yet either. In a persistent vegetative patient, there is spasticity and lack of spontaneous movement, because the brain stem-spinal cord connections *have* developed but are unopposed by influences from the cortex, thereby resulting in an imbalance of muscle tone called spasticity. Because the brain stem-spinal cord connections are not developed yet in the newborn period, normal newborns are not spastic and motionless like persistent vegetative patients.

The point of all this is that an anencephalic infant is behaviorally very much like a normal newborn infant, because at least those anencephalics who have functioning brain stems, wake, sleep, cry, move around, suck, and behave in ways quite similar to normal newborns. They're not at all similar behaviorally to adults in a persistent vegetative state. Therefore, they are neither brain dead nor are they in a persistent vegetative state. I think this is important to understand, in light of what Janet was saying with regard to the humanity.

If we're going to say that the anencephalic isn't human because it doesn't have cognition, well then, you'd probably have to argue that the normal human newborn isn't human either, because it doesn't have cognition. The difference is in the potential for development of that capability rather than the actuality.

What they were trying to do at Loma Linda was place these infants on ventilators and hope that the brain would become destroyed somehow, so that the infant could then be declared brain dead while on the ventilator and the organs used according to existing standards. But there's really no reason why the brain stem would become destroyed. And placing the infant on the ventilator would theoretically only serve to protect the brain stem from damage, just as much as it protects all the other organs from damage.

Theoretically, you wouldn't expect them to become brain dead. Actually, I and a number of other physicians predicted this, way back at the beginning of Loma Linda's protocol, and now the experience has borne it out. Because that approach just didn't work, they called a moratorium on it.

BISHOP: I have two questions for Dr. Shewmon and one for Dr. De Giorgio. We often in the newspapers see mention of spina bifida. Does that have anything at all to do with anencephaly? In many of the cases they start to raise questions about whether to remove feeding from the children.

The second question that I had was: you mentioned that the worst type of anencephaly is going to be stillborn. The next type up, it seemed to me you said will die probably the first day. The other types that you mentioned after that weren't quite as severe as that, or the type that you said wasn't fully anencephalic, i.e. part of the brain outside with some kind of a casing on it. How long will they live? Is it a matter of weeks? Or could they go on for many years?

And the question for Dr. DeGiorgio: I'm a little confused. You had said that the reason that the tissue of children like this is desirable is that, in the case of adults, because of brain death, the tissue wouldn't be suitable. But it would seem to me we couldn't approve of going ahead with the use of an infant tissue either unless there was brain death. Why would infant tissue be any more useful than that of an adult?

DR. SHEWMON: Well, in answer to the first question, recall the first slide that I showed of the neural tube. If the bottom opening in that neural tube doesn't close, then you get spina bifida or meningomyelocele. So it is a condition very closely related to anencephaly: it's just at the opposite end of the nervous system.

In terms of life span, the less severe the lesion, the longer they are likely to live. That's a very good question that you raised, because one of the claims of advocates of using anencephalics is that they will inevitably die within a day or within a few days at most. And that's actually not true. The most severe ones will. And if you look at the statistics of it, about 44% or so of the live-born anencephalics will die within the first day. But 5–8% will still be alive after a week. And in one series, 1% were still alive after around three months. So the life span is very limited, but there is certainly no foregone conclusion that these infants will die within a day or a few days.

BISHOP: None of them are going to last ten or fifteen years?

DR. SHEWMON: No. The record, as far as I know is 14 months. And that's very unusual.

DR. DeGIORGIO: To clarify your question, anencephalics or brain dead individuals may be suitable for organ transplantation of kidneys, lungs, pancreas and heart. They would not be good donors for brain tissue because the brain has been so severely injured. For Parkinson's disease, or brain tissue transplantation anencephalics and brain dead patients would not be good donors, whereas for heart disease, they would.

BISHOP: The reason I asked that question was the implication at Loma Linda that they had been using children who were not brain dead, at least that was the plan, apparently, to use them when according to the ordinary definition they were not dead.

DR. DeGIORGIO: I think that the problem which we alluded to was that anencephaly is a special situation; they do not meet brain death criteria. Loma Linda was trying to use the guidelines under the Uniform Anatomical Gift Act, which requires brain death for organ donation. They were trying to wait for the anencephalic to become brain dead when, in reality, logically, it really isn't to begin with brain dead and isn't likely to become brain dead in spite of their protocol. But they were trying to fit them into the brain dead category.

BISHOP: This might be related to what the other Bishop is getting at. Is there some special property in the fetal brain tissue if the fetus has been aborted, that allows it to be used for a longer time or to be usable for a longer time?

DR. DeGIORGIO: Well, for example with brain death, the tissue has sustained an irreversible injury (anoxia) to the tissue that makes it really nonviable. Whereas, fetal tissue, coming from a spontaneous abortion or an induced abortion, is collected early enough after the abortion. It may not have undergone the cell-injuring effects of the lack of oxygen and, therefore, may be much more viable for transplantation.

BISHOP: If the product of the abortion did not have those effects in the brain, would it be certainly dead?

DR. DeGIORGIO: Well, for example, the most common procedure performed is a suction curettage, where the baby is basically disintegrated. So the baby would be so disintegrated that he would indeed be dead. But there are spontaneous abortions where there may still be transient brain function for a few minutes afterwards, for a few minutes, such a child might not be brain dead. But with the effects of the lack of oxygen and the lack of blood flow, within just a few minutes the infant would certainly be dead within a few minutes.

BISHOP: Would that kind of tissue be more desirable for treatment of Parkinson's or something?

DR. DeGIORGIO: The fresher the tissue, i.e., the shorter the interval after the spontaneous or procured abortion, the more viable the tissue would be. Actually, they have tried to transplant tissue that was a few hours old. Some of it took; some of it didn't. But the earlier the tissue is taken after the abortion, the more viable it is.

DR. SHEWMON: The whole anencephalic infant debate has brought out into the open a very interesting phenomenon. Many of the people who have been using the term "brain death"—people in the transplant field, neurologists, ethicists, and surgeons, especially—have had a notion of brain death that really, in the final analysis, does not regard the brain-dead person as truly dead. What I mean to say is that they have taken the term "brain death" to mean death of an organ, the brain. And I've had person after person, including physicians, say to me something to the effect that, "Well, we know that even though the brain is dead, the person isn't really dead yet." They seem to imply that "brain death" was merely invented to facilitate organ transplantation.

Now, if you asked the people on the President's Commission and the people who introduced brain death legislation, which is in just about every state now, they wouldn't say that. They would say, "No, what we mean by 'brain death' is just another way of diagnosing one and the same state of death that has traditionally been diagnosed by the cessation of heartbeat." So, for example, the President's Commission criteria regard this as simply a different way of diagnosing death. But there's a unitary notion of death.

But the whole anencephalic issue has brought out into the open that there are an awful lot of people who don't look at it that

way and who consider a brain-dead body as simply a deeply comatose patient who is still alive. And somehow, they regard that state
as justifying the removal of vital organs like the heart. I think it's
important for everybody to understand what we mean when we
use the term "brain dead." In fact, I think it's a term that probably
ought not to be used any more, because it is so confusing to people. There are surgeons who remove hearts from patients thinking
that the donors are deeply comatose and alive, not dead. I think
that such people are just playing games with words when they talk
about brain death, and that those surgeons who look at it that way
are subjectively guilty of murder, even though objectively, they
may not be.

So I think a better term to use would be "neurologic criteria
for diagnosing death." It's a little bit more cumbersome, but it gets
away from this idea that there are two kinds of death: cardiac death
and brain death. I think for any kind of an organ transplantation to
be moral, everybody involved has to be sincerely convinced that the
patient is "dead dead," and not just deeply comatose.

BISHOP: What I am going to say does not necessarily require
an answer but it is merely an observation. A section of the bioethics of the International Federation of Catholic Universities met for
two years, from December, 1987 to June, 1988, to study the question of anencephaly. And it came out, not in a public document,
with the following conclusions, which seem to me is not congruent
with some of the things said here. The conclusion is premised on a
key question, that is, whether an established anencephalic is a person or not.

And it says:

In cases of established anencephaly, the following considerations apply:

1. We do not claim to know or to study here the full essential requirements for being a person. That remains
   an important and still open ethical and legal question.
   But the enjoyment of moral protections provided to
   those thought to be persons demands a minimal biological substrate as a basis for future development.
2. In the absence of biological conditions for the possibility of any capacity for future relationships or self-

consciousness, there is either no human person or no longer a human person.

3. Therefore, those who advise or choose to terminate a preganancy in which anencephaly has been clearly established cannot be said to be acting in a way that is morally wrong unless on other grounds.

4. Furthermore, the use of anencephalics after delivery as the source of organ or tissue retrieval is not a violation of personal dignity. Therefore, if such retrieval is considered morally wrong, it must be on other grounds.

I was disturbed by this morning's session, because this is not for me a merely academic discussion. I am working in a remote area and I had a case presented to me on this. And more or less, I based my decision on this statement emanating from the Federation of Catholic Universities with its medical faculties.

DR. SMITH: Well, I think I agree with you. I think they do violate some of the principles that we have articulated here. The question of personhood is a very complicated philosophical issue. And then it gets to be a practically complicated issue when you suggest that rights are rooted in personhood as opposed simply to humanity.

It is not clear to me why one wants to say that only persons have moral rights whereas humans may not have moral rights. The burden of proof in argumentation is on those who think that somehow personhood confers rights whereas humanity does not. And then it seems to me that there are many other questions involved. Again, whose definition of personhood do we accept? What degree of relationship, what degree of cognition, what degree of self awareness and consciousness constitutes personhood? We are all people with varying degrees of consciousness, for instance, so at what point do you say, well, here we have a person? Different people have different levels of consciousness. But humanity is something that is easily discernible. It is a matter of genetic makeup. The degrees of cognitive awareness, consciousness, etc., on the other hand, are very subjective.

Then, take it another step further. How do you determine who, in fact, has those qualities? Who, in fact, qualifies as a person? It seems to me that the benefit of the doubt always has to be that if there are signs of humanity we assume there is also evidence of personhood. The pro-life movement has dealt with this for years, that if you have any suspicion that a creature may be a person it seems to me you must treat this entity as a person.

And, again, going back to kind of a simplistic but compelling argument. I spoke of the woman named Kay who has an anencephalic baby named Hope. She certainly entered into a personal relationshop with this baby. Who would want to say that the baby did not enter into a personal relationship with her? I don't think she was relating to her baby as she would relate to her cat or her dog. She knew she was relating to another human being and I think she would say she was relating to a human person. It's curious to me that those guidelines can suggest that these babies are not capable of human relationships. Because we've seen them enter into human relationships. So, I think the problems with those criteria are profound.

DR. DeGEORGIO: Perhaps Dr. Shewmon could comment on this but, whether or not there's personhood or humanity, the other issue is whether there's a soul. And, if I'm not mistaken, the Church might give conditional baptism to an infant who might have anencephaly or some other severe developmental anomaly.

Did you want to address the issue of soul?

DR. SHEWMON: Yes. Well, I understand the thinking behind the argument that anencephalic infants are not persons because of the lack of potential for future intellectual activity and volitional activity. I'm very concerned that such recommendations have been made, because they apply not only to anencephalic infants but also to every infant with a severe congenital brain malformation. It applies to persisitently vegetative patients. It applies to a whole host of patients who are severely mentally disabled. And even if, in a classroom of philosophy, we wanted to argue from a purely theoretical point of view that all of these types of patients are not human beings any more, to apply that in practice, I think, is extraordinarily risky, because we have to be at least open to the idea that these are persons. And if there is any possiblity that they are persons, then, as Janet said, we need to treat them as such, or else we run the risk of committing direct abortions or homicide or whatever. So the bottom line for me is, even though I understand the arguments and I can recognize that, okay, maybe there is a theoretical possiblity that these are not human beings, to turn that into a practical policy of allowing the removal of organs from such patients is very frightening.

BISHOP: I would like to make three comments just very briefly. As a reaction to the panelists, the mentioning of conditional baptism. Well, to my knowledge of theology, of moral theology, the administration of conditional baptism is not a cogent argument to state the presence of the soul.

It is merely a caution, a safe approach to the problem. Therefore, it cannot be used as an argument of presence of personhood, in the case of person implying soul. Second, the document was requested; the conclusion was not published or requested by the European Bishops. Third, as an answer to Dr. Shewmon, there is a nota bene in the document which says, "The above considerations are not intended to apply to those human beings who will have or who have or who have had the biological capacity for human self awareness and human relationships. But they may raise the questions whether those who have genuinely and irretrievably lost such a capacity might be judged, under certain conditions, to have died."

In the light of this final remark, as a layman in this very complicated field, I am disturbed by what seems to me an illogical proposition. On the one hand, we said that the concept of personhood does not belong to biological science. It belongs to metaphysics and ontology. On the other hand, we find scientists making a decision that, in this case, is biologically verifiable, personhood is assumed. I find that a little disturbing and illogical.

DR. DeGIORGIO: I certainly don't know, and I don't even suggest I might even know, whether these are persons or not. They certainly are human beings. And I wouldn't know whether they had a soul or not. I think that the issue of conditional baptism reflects uncertainty as to their moral status. I was just trying to say that perhaps there is a degree of uncertainty, moral uncertainty, in this issue. And perhaps, we shouldn't necessarily communicate that there is certainty.

DR. SHEWMON: Yes, I would just reiterate that. I agree that I don't think, just from the purely biological considerations, we can conclude whether there is or is not a person or a soul. But I do think that we have to be open to the possibility that this is a person and is a human being, simply because it is the product of conception of human beings and looks like a deformed human being. And therefore, to give it the benefit of the doubt of humanity is, I think, the safer course of action: to treat it as a human being.

BISHOP: I want to thank my brother bishop for raising the question, not because I'm pleased with that report he gave. I find it a little bit disturbing. But it does, I think, highlight something of a weakness. I address my question to Dr. Smith. The whole question of the *humanum,* rather than speaking of personhood, as you speak of the *humanum,* I got the impression that you put the weight of the answer very simply on whether this comes from two human parents. And I'm wondering if that's adequate enough. And I'm wondering if maybe you're either simplifying too much or putting too much weight on that, because referring to the classical pastoral manuals, there was reference to that whole category of monsters. It sounds like a horrible word today, but that was the classical word used. And in sacramental practice, yes, it was conditional. With newborns, it was not conditional upon whether the minister was conscious or willing; it was conditional upon whether it was human. So there was a doubt there. Now, by way of the conclusions, I would not dispute the conclusions. I think in the order of pastoral caution, we simply cannot take any chances. I'm not disputing the conclusions, but I'm wondering if, perhaps, there might be a bit of an overkill there if we're suggesting that there is no doubt that this is human and therefore one who is fully "personal." I think we can draw the same conclusions without having that forceful sort of absolute premise.

DR. SMITH: I don't particularly want to move away from my claim that the offspring of human parents is a human being. But, obviously, these are metaphysical questions. Good ethics are rooted in good metaphysics and good metaphysics is hard to come by. I don't know that you'll get it from me. I'd like to give you a sketch of the kind of problems I think we're addressing here. You've brought up the word "soul" several times which, perhaps, is very much to the point. Just a little review. The classical tradition has taught that anything that is living has a soul. Carrots have souls, tomatoes have souls, dogs have souls, cats have souls. They don't have immortal souls but they have souls. There are sensate souls, vegetative souls, and rational souls. A human being has one soul which has vegetative, sensate and rational capacities. Now, when you have something that is genetically born of human parents and genetically human, now what kind of a soul does it have? Again, when you make those divisions, sensate, vegetative and rational, are you really saying that there are certain parts of a soul or is this one soul that has all these capacities? Could you say that a certain infant has a vegetative, sensate soul but not a rational soul if, in fact, it is genetically human? Or are you simply saying that it doesn't have the material or the organs—say a brain—by which to manifest the rational soul—that it's there but it simply cannot operate? There are certain organs that people might be born without, such as the eye. Does it really mean that this individual has no potential to see? It seems there are different grades of potentiality. A stone or rock has virtually no potential to see. But a human being, even without an eye, by the nature of its very being, has some potential, in a meaningful sense, to see. He has more potential, obviously, if he has an eye, even if he has a defective eye, than if he has no eye. But he, by his nature, has the potential to have an eye, and thus has the potential to see. But there are different grades of potentiality.

So it seems to me that all those questions enter into this very complicated question of personhood, the nature of the soul and the nature of human life. But I really don't feel challenged at this point to back away from the statement that any creature born of human parents is human and deserves to be granted with the full panoply of human rights.

BISHOP: I never heard of the International Federation of Universities. I was wondering if Archbishop Lagasti or somebody from Pope John XXIII Center could tell us who they are, what they do and what the make-up of it is? It's completely new to me.

BISHOP: First, regarding the International Federation of Catholic Universities. This is an adjunct, a UNESCO affiliate, and is under the Holy See. The present president is the President of the University of Leger. It is composed of all Catholic universities over the world, and about ten years ago it established a section of all the members with a faculty of medicine. Five years ago, an international study group was formed under the umbrella of U.N., precisely to study the questions about bioethics. It is a group composed of the Secretary General and people who are experts in bioethics. At least, that is what I understand. And they have been studying about abortion, etc., but always with the idea of not coming out in publication, although it came out in one book recently, in order to permit the meeting of theologians, philosophers and specialists, scientist, in the area.

The last topic they discussed was anencephaly. They met in Milano, then in Germany, and the last one was in Vienna where they finalized these conclusions for some discussion. Again, I would like to repeat, the conclusions were not meant to be publicized but merely to guide, to give an answer to those who have asked for guidance. Who are the persons involved in these studies? It depends on the field. But it is always a meeting of theologians and scientists. And the scientists and theologians need not be Catholic.

BISHOP: This is really a matter of curiosity more than anything else. But in the donation of such organs as heart, liver, kidney of an anencephalic infant, which obviously is very, very young, very small, how old can the recipients be or must they be? Infants, too? How many months? How does that work?

DR. SHEWMON: Maybe I could answer that. The recipients of the hearts and livers must be newborn infants. In fact, for a liver transplant, the size of the donor liver and size of the recipient liver must be very similar, within about 20% of each other for the transplant to work at all.

Obviously, the small, newborn heart would not be able to pump blood through an adult or an older child, and so the recipients of those hearts would also be newborn infants.

In terms of kidneys, there have been reports of newborn kidneys being transplanted into adults—specifically, anencephalic kidneys being transplanted into adult humans. Those kidneys can grow in the recipient, and eventually two infant kidneys can fulfill the function of one adult kidney. The infant kidneys will grow and fulfill the renal function in the adult. But the reason that that isn't done, right now, anyway, is because the success of transplanting infant kidneys, newborn kidneys especially, is not nearly as good as the success of transplanting kidneys of older donors, because the vessels are so small that the surgical connections tend to clot off and then the organ is lost. So most of the centers that transplant kidneys into children, and UCLA is one of those, will not even accept donor organs from infants less than three years of age, because of this problem of clotting of the vessels. And they prefer to keep the recipients on hemodialysis or peritoneal dialysis until they are old enough to receive an older donor organ.

BISHOP: Well, perhaps my question did have a moral dimension after all, because I was wondering about the technology of this, and if it has to do with, say the heart, there is the whole danger of perhaps hastening death. You know, it seems to me to be so complex to get the two together that I'd be kind of worried about any overt actions that might be taking place to help this, to foster this, if that exchange had to be almost instantaneous. My question, simply, again, was: how old does the infant have to be to be a recipient? Could it be some months or does it have to be just newly born?

DR. SHEWMON: No, it could be some months old, but the recipients of infant heart transplants typically are of two types. One is what's called hypoplastic left heart syndrome. And those infants die within a few days inevitably. There is an operation that is used on some of those infants called the Norwood procedure which does not have a very good long-term success rate. And that's the best we have to offer. So a heart transplant is really the best thing for those infants if it could be done from a truly dead donor.

BISHOP: Dr. Shewmon, please. I'm getting very uneasy about the application of EEG and the use of it as a determining factor in life and death. I asked Dr. Plum about this and he said that, in his estimation, this could not be used by itself alone to determine death and that he did not agree with a lot of things that were being done. And so, it seems to me that we have allowed to be written into law a determination of death which is not really absolute. He stated that when brain death occurs, it is not really absolute. And I think that we can all agree with that, as long as we know what we're talking about. But technically, I was very curious to know, when you apply an EEG, what part of the brain does it test? And, in your estimation, Dr. Shewmon, how absolute is death when one is brain dead?

DR. SHEWMON: A very good question. The EEG measures the electrical activity of the brain cells that are within about a centimeter from the skull. So most of the brain is not measured by the EEG. And it's quite possible to have a completely flat EEG with a perfectly normal brain stem. So Dr. Plum was quite right that a flat

EEG, in and of itself, in no way diagnoses brain death. Now, one thing that you said isn't quite factually correct; EEG criteria are not enshrined in law. What the laws state is that death must be diagnosed according to acceptable medical standards. I don't know of any law that specifies that death can be diagnosed by a flat EEG. And there are no medical standards that would accept a flat EEG as diagnostic of brain death. So, anybody who would claim to diagnose brain death merely on the basis of a flat EEG doesn't know what he's talking about.

What else is involved in diagnosis? There has to be a known cause for complete brain destruction. So this is usually, in the case of organ donors, head trauma from a car accident or whatever. Brain destruction can also result from, say, a brain tumor that keeps expanding, and finally the whole brain just herniates through the bottom of the skull into the spinal canal. Cardiac arrest with severe anoxia to the brain can result in massive brain swelling and lack of blood flow getting to the brain, and that can destroy the whole brain.

So we need to know what is the cause of the brain death and, in knowing that cause, we have some basis to infer that this is, indeed, irreversible destruction of the brain. And that's how we know that there is irreversible lack of function. We also need to have evidence of lack of all neurological functions. That's why the clinical examination is very important. There has to be lack of the pupillary reflex, lack of all the brain stem reflexes as well as lack of all cerebral cortical function. The EEG can be helpful in confirming a diagnosis of brain death, but in and of itself, taken in isolation, cannot constitute a diagnosis of brain death.

DR. DeGIORGIO: Like Dr. Shewmon said, the EEG is used to confirm the diagnosis of brain death made clinically: respirations, cranial nerve reflexes, pupillary reflexes must all be absent, and then an EEG is performed to confirm brain death. The reason for that is that there are times when a patient fulfills the clinical criteria for brain death, that is, absent respiration, absent pupillary response, etc., and then the EEG shows brain activity. That does occur, of course, quite frequently in my hospital because of barbiturate or other drug overdose or an incomplete hypoxic injury.

And so actually, the EEG can be very, very helpful in identifying patients who are not brain dead. But if the clinical criteria are met, the patient does not have respirations, and you have a clear cut cause of the brain death itself, then the EEG is a very reliable confirmatory procedure. But in terms of routine practice, it is not used as the sole determinant of brain death. It's used to confirm brain death and it also can be very helpful in identifying patients who are incorrectly diagnosed as being brain dead.

BISHOP: Doesn't the problem become more acute for us, then, when we're talking about these kinds of patients who are on mechanical respirators, etc.? Because we're sustaining these functions, they have them. And therefore, doctors use the brain death test because it's the last one that's left.

DR. DeGIORGIO: Well, the only function that is being sustained by the mechanical ventilator is respiration. So it's not going to give you other brain stem reflexes or other neurological functions. And in a patient on a ventilator, who you suspect is brain dead, you test for absence of spontaneous respiration by overoxygenating him and then stopping the ventilator for a while, usually five minutes or so, to see whether he has any spontaneous respiration when the carbon dioxide builds up enough in the blood to cause a respiratory drive. So, you're right—that does confound the diagnosis of brain death, but there are still ways of diagnosing it, getting around that problem.

BISHOP: Yes, from the obstetrics point of view, Dr. Shewmon, we know that in the prenatal care of an anencephalic infant, the mother usually suffers from a hydramnios. Normally, we induce preterm deliveries for this condition as well as in women who had a previous cesarean section. What about the mothers of these anencephalics preterm? If they have acute hydramnios, they have to be hospitalized for several weeks for medical treatment so you can have the baby go to term. You can have a delivery with the mature infant and then it is possible to donate the organs. Is this possible? What is your experience in this field.

DR. SHEWMON: Well, not being an obstetrician, I have very little experience personally. But it is true that hydramnios, which means excess amniotic fluid, is a very common complication of anencephaly. And, as far as I know, the treatment of that would be to treat hydramnios just the same way you would with any other case of hydramnios, namely, doing amniocentesis and drawing off the excess amniotic fluid as often as that needs to be done. And when the infant reaches a viable age—it doesn't have to be to term, but at least a viable age—labor could be induced or a section could be done.

I would think that the treatment of the hydramnios would have to be undertaken without a view toward possible future organ donation, because first of all, it's very unlikely that the organs would ever be donated anyway. And so I think you would have to treat the hydramnios completely independently of possible organ donation or of the fact that the fetus happens to be anencephalic.

DR. DeGIORGIO: One final comment. We've been focusing on the eithics of anencephaly but we haven't really talked about the ethical issues involved in fetal transplantation. And I just want to summarize that this is an area that has tremendous ethical implications. For example, what are the ethics of using fetal tissue from spontaneous abortions? We haven't addressed that issue. Also, what are the ethics of prolonging a pregnancy in order to procure ideal fetal tissue for future transplantation? Who should control where the parts go? And this is a very highly contested issue. If a woman decides to have an abortion, does she then have the right to determine where the fetal parts should go, if they could be used for transplantation purposes. If she doesn't have the right to control it, who does? Who then takes responsibility for the fetal tissue? You know, issues of property rights and the like are ethical implications of fetal tissue. Also, lastly, is the procedure by which fetal tissue will be obtained going to be changed solely to optimize the fetal tissue? For example, in most fetal experimentations, the fetus is obtained by hysterotomy rather than suction curettage. For example, with a monkey or a rat, they try to extract the fetus without chopping it up like they typically do in human first trimester abortions. What would happen, for example, if the physician decided, well, if we chop up the fetus it won't be very useful; so we're going to have to modify the abortion technique in order to procure a better fetus for transplantation purposes. These are some of the ethical dilemmas that would occur if fetal transplantation were to be allowed.

PART FOUR

THE HEALTH OF THE CLERGY

Chapter 18

PROMOTING THE HEALTH AND WELL-BEING OF OUR PRIESTS

The Reverend David E. Brinkmoeller, M.A.

Thanks to the Pope John Center and to each of you for giving me the opportunity to be with you this afternoon. I was originally asked for suggestions regarding who could give this presentation. I suggested several bishops. I suggested several experts. I did not suggest myself!

The planning committee, however, honored me with the invitation. Although I initially hesitated, I eventually accepted. I accepted because I care deeply about the subject. And I know that bishops typically care deeply about the health and well-being of priests. In spite of my own limitations, I welcome the opportunity to be here this afternoon, because I know that we are talking together about mutual concerns, and that all of us want to do our best for priests.

Last week I attended a workshop on the state of Catholic preaching. In many ways it was a wonderful program. But, as you might suspect, priests and bishops were battered again. How can you have continuing education of priests, it was said, unless you've first had education. There's such a drive for lay preaching, it was said, because you can't get any worse than the homilies currently being given. The speakers were intelligent people, who love the Church and long for its growth. They probably love the priesthood, many of them being priests themselves. But their generalizations and their lack of nouance were inaccurate and hurtful.

Surely we priests are oh-so-human. We are limited, wounded, short-sighted, of less than consumate talent. But I've never met a priest who knelt before his ordaining bishop without a holy dream, without some profound hope to serve humankind, to serve God. These are the men whose health and well-being you will be discussing today.

This is a wonderful time in which to be a priest. It is a difficult time, for sure, and a challenging time, but also a time of great opportunity. For this world deeply needs the Gospel.

Much talk these days is given to the question of morale among priests. The talk has yielded description of legitimate concerns, and has led many dioceses to give due priority to a carefully designed ministry to priests. This is not the time, however, for priests and bishops to circle the wagons in solipsistic groaning. For we are a blessed body—a challenged, if wounded, body—and we have enviable opportunities before us. These opportunities, as those of the past, may at times feel more like Good Friday than Easter Sunday. But these opportunities make this a wonderful time in which to be a priest.

I am asked today to address the topic of "Promotion of the Health and Well-Being of Priests." In doing so, I have divided this presentation into 3 sections, the first providing a foundational comment about the topic, the second addressing several concerns about the health of priests, and the third providing comments about 7 additional factors—beyond physical health—which impinge upon the well-being of priests.

Before getting to these three sections, however, I want to say that in all of this paper I am operating upon the assumption that the priest himself must see that he has primary responsibility for his own health and well-being. He must have primary responsibility for his own spiritual life. He must have primary responsibility for his own happiness. This primary responsibility does not belong to the bishop, does not belong to the Personnel Board, does not belong to the Parish Council, although all of these can make important contributions to the priests' well-being.

I. The Heart of Well-Being:
Well Chosen Beliefs

I recently attended a stress management workshop. When you feel stress, the instructor of this workshop said, do these exercises (neck roll, stiff arm rotation, etc.), have a sense of humor, don't feel guilty(!), prioritize your time, eat healthy food. He was a funny man. He teased participants and made us laugh. He said sometimes insightful things. By the time the workshop ended, however, I decided that much of the program had missed the point; I was, thereby, full of stress!

My stress was not that he said wrong things. It was that he made no reference to choosing beliefs about life and love and God as an important part of stress management. It was that he made no reference to the ability to love and be loved. This, for me is the foundation for our discussion about the health and well-being of priests.

Tending to our health and well-being is not to deny the pain. It requires more than a regular whistling of the currently popular tune, "Don't worry, be happy!"

Life's hurts really hurt. Some of life's confusions are impossibly confusing. The unfulfilled longings in us are truly empty. This is true for all of us.

But we believe that life is worth living, even if it is at times disillusioning, and that love is worth giving, even if at times we get burned in our love, and that God is All in all, even if God sometimes seems so elusive. I am not arguing here against stress management techniques and stress management workshops; they have their place. I am arguing for depth, a depth which knows the Cross, and knows the Light.

So, I believe that this is at the heart of well-being: well chosen beliefs, beliefs chosen in response to the priceless grace of God.

II. Promoting the Physical Health of Priests

To raise the question of health is to confront the possibility of a certain amount of free floating defensiveness. Perhaps we all count among our acquaintances a beguiling if nasty health fascist— someone who quietly makes us feel guilty for not eating oat bran 21 meals per week, someone who eminates a certain disdain for all of us who have not jogged our 6 miles yet today. Perhaps, however, we can discuss health in a non-fascist manner.

It is clearly inaccurate to say that physically ill people are spiritually ill. Sometimes, of course, the contrary is much truer. It is quite accurate to say that one's physical health has important influence upon one's spiritual health and one's ministerial effectiveness. If I do not have enough discipline to get physical exercise, for example, I am likely to have less energy and even to be more prone to depression. If I fail to eat the right foods or the right amount of food, if I fail to get enough sleep, I can expect an adverse impact upon my ability to be present to others and to be present to God, upon my enthusiasm, motivation, energy, and spirit. Discipline is a key factor in matters of health, as in matters of prayers.

In discussing the health of priests, I will first draw comments from the study, "The Health of American Catholic Priests," then describe efforts made in 3 dioceses to promote the health of priests, and finally make some comment about the specific challenges of alcoholism and drug abuse.

A. "The Health of American Catholic Priests" (1985)

Based upon the very positive feedback it received from its 1981 publication, "The Priest and Stress," the Bishop's Committee on Priestly Life and Ministry commissioned Father Joseph Fichter, S.J., to conduct a study on the health of priests. This study along with some reflections by the Priestly Life and Ministry Committee, was published in 1985 under the title "The Health of American Catholic Priests."

The study consisted of self-administered questionnaires mailed to all priests, active and retired, diocesan and religious, in 21 diocese in various areas of the United States.

Things are not as bad as some suspect.

Throughout his report of this study, Father Fichter seems anxious to counter the impression of some that priests are in poor health. He quotes statistics such as these in making his case:[1]

83.6% declare their health to be "excellent" or "good;" 55.7% did not even have one day of illness in the past year.

"The great majority of American Catholic priests," he concludes, "are healthy, happy, hardworking professionals in the service of God and his people."[2] "We can find no cause for alarm in either the overall state of health or in any specific area of ill health."[3] Finally, "instead of being told that bad health is a critical issue," he says, "(priests) ought to get credit and recognition from church leaders."[4]

Similarly, Father Fichter found reason for optimism about the mental stability of priests, observing that "Less than one out of ten (8.2%) said that he could not manage emotional or behavioral problems."[5]

A portion of the study was based on five health habits that have been found to be significantly related to a person's state of health. The beneficial health habits are identified as follows:

(1) sufficient sleep of seven or eight hours;
(2) control of body weight;
(3) adequate exercise;
(4) avoidance of cigarette smoking;
(5) limited alcohol consumption.

Although the statistics indicate that several individual priests have reason for great concern regarding one or the other of those habits, priests' responses about their own activities in regard to these habits are in general similar to those of others. One statistic about each of these categories. Regarding sleep, over 70% of priests get at least 7 hours of sleep per night. Four out of ten priests admit that they are overweight. Two thirds (65.2%) have had fairly frequent exercise. 33.5% of priests once smoked cigarettes but have quit; almost 25% still smoke cigarettes. Almost 20% of priests indicate that they have at least two or three drinks every day, 37% indicate that they rarely or never have a drink.[6] Father Fichter quotes an interesting observation from a similar study in noting that "moderate alcohol consumption" is associated with the most favorable health scores, more so even than complete abstention."[7]

Regarding mortality rates, priests live longer than other American men. Similarly priests live longer than men in professional services, including lawyers and doctors. All of this is consistent with other demographic studies, which indicate that clergy are a population of "low risk" for illness.[8] As we know, however, we all will get our turn; the three main causes of priests' deaths are heart diseases, cancer, and stroke.[9]

In receiving the study, the Priestly Life and Ministry Committee drew attention to several items, two of which I mention here:

(1) The first 25 years of priesthood and especially the first 10 years, contain the greatest amount of stress, strain, worry.[10] All of us can offer opinions about why this study indicates this fact, but it is worth emphasizing that it seems to be a fact, one validated by other studies. A state of serenity, on the other hand, clearly emerges from the statistics about older clergy.

(2) While the study reveals that the vast majority of priests are physically healthy, 39.8% report "severe personal, behavioral, or mental problems" during the past 12 months.[11] This statistic, of course, only reemphasizes what we already know, that we must give careful attention to the support systems available for priests and to the methods we employ in helping priests in crisis. Much money and much personal wisdom is required of us in this regard.

B. Strategies Used by Dioceses: 3 Samples

The 1985 study about the health of priests showed a close association between the physical fitness and mental health of the priest. We must honor this body of ours. Physically fit clergy were "the least tense and nervous, the least worried about things. The healthiest.... are more than twice as likely (46.6% to 21.2%) to report that they are 'very happy' in the service of God and the Church."[12]

Perhaps as a response to this reality, many dioceses encourage priests to have a regular physical exam; some even require such an exam for priests over the age of 40. Many provide the financial resources for this through either health insurance or diocesan subsidy, some including provision for copayment by the individual priests. Several have enlisted the help of a local Catholic hospital. The 1985 study indicates that 77% of priests report having had a physical within the past 2 years. But no information is provided about how extensive or how limited the exams were.

1) The first sample diocese takes a simple and straightforward approach: it has encouraged regular physicals for several years. The diocese indicates that priests make extensive use of the physicals. The results of the physical are given only to the priest, with no report given to the diocese.

In addition to the annual physical, the diocese on its Annual Personnel Report asks priests voluntarily to list the date of their last physical and to comment on the condition of their health, and tries to follow through on any information gained.

2) A second sample is provided by a large Archdiocese, which has developed and funded an extensive program of preventative medicine for priests. The program is under the direction of the Department of Community and Preventative Medicine at a local medical college. The first phase includes an extensive physical exam. The second phase includes programs and counseling on nutrition, smoking cessation, stress control, cholesterol control, etc. A recent clergy bulletin included a blurb for "Cold Turkey Smoking Cessation Program."

I asked the staff person for this program if she noticed any particular needs among the priests. She mentioned three:

1) "Certainly nutrition: priests, she said, eat a lot of rich food, cook with a lot of butter. Cholesterol is a major concern, closely related to cardiovascular problems. We have been able to help many priests to lower their cholesterol."
2) High Blood Pressure—"a common problem for priests, very closely related to stress control."
3) Lack of Exercise—"Even if they start to take walks, they can help themselves."

3) A third sample is provided by a diocese which annually makes available what it describes as a "health risk appraisal," whereby priests monitor their exercise, nutrition, sleep patterns, muscle flexibility, and stress retention. All who participate also have the opportunity for a full physical exam and a psychological assessment. When the data from the test has been compiled, priests are invited to come in groups of 20 to an overnight "feedback" session, at which they are helped to understand the data from the test(s), and to receive more educational background on physical and emotional health, so that each will be in a position to take better responsibility for his own health. And all of this is done with a view of integrating these concerns into the spirituality of the priest.

The leadership of this diocese argues enthusiastically for such a program for priests, and points to the regular participation of priests as a sign of priests' appreciation. "The most precious resource available to a local church is its people," says the priest coordinator of the program, expressing the belief that it's better (even cheaper) to catch things in their early stages (or to prevent them) than to deal with the full blossomed problem. Of the 87 priests who took the physical exam this year, 3, by using the treadmill test, discovered for the first time that they had heart trouble; 2, by the flexible sigmoidoscopy, discovered that they had lumps within them. He points to several examples of doctors who do not know how to give good physical exams and of at least one doctor who was hesitant to speak candidly to a priest patient about the results of a physical exam as evidence of the value of the diocese providing the opportunity for a thorough and carefully planned physical beyond what a priest might get at his doctor's office.

3) Chemical Dependency/Alcoholism

The estimate has been made that 5.6% of priests are alcoholic, active or recovering. All of us know about the pain and confusion associated with this illness—for the priest, for his parishioners and coworkers, and sometimes for his bishop. A diocesan bishop can be grateful indeed if his diocese has clear and fair policies in the matter of chemical dependency, and if he has associates with the ability to recognize the dependency and to lead the dependent priest toward recovery. Similarly, the diocese can be grateful for having a bishop who is compassionate and firm in this regard.

In recent years several dioceses have developed boards, composed of priests and others who understand chemical dependency, to assist priests to recognize their dependency and to find treatment. [In 1977 the Priestly Life and Ministry Committee, under the chairmanship of Bishop Raymond Gallagher, in a study about alcoholism among priests, recommended such boards for dioceses.] These boards are united by the belief that chemically dependent people live in pervasive denial, that they surround themselves with enablers to assist in the denial, but that skillfully compassionate and articulate intervention can break the chain of denial and can lead a person to choose a new path of sobriety. Experience seems to be showing that these boards of priest peers provide a wonderful service for the health of priests.

One last comment about these boards. In some areas there is pressure upon these boards to expand their area of competence, to be ready to intervene in other situations of poor physical or emotional health beyond chemical dependency. My own thought is that this should be done only with caution, and that it may be asking the board to perform beyond its available time or skills. Perhaps another peer group might be developed to respond to the physical or emotional health needs of priests beyond chemical dependency.

In all of this, of course, care must be taken to avoid any impression of diocesan vigilantism, or any intrusion upon the fundamental reality that the priest is responsible for his own life and for his own choices about life. For this reason, it seems to me, these programs must be developed in careful dialogue with the priests of the diocese, perhaps through the presbyterial council, and should be regularly evaluated by them.

III. Promoting the Well-Being of Priests

In the last section of this paper, I will comment on 7 concerns, all of which seem to be closely connected with the well-being of priests. Each of these concerns is an example of a hopeful trend in today's priesthood. In regard to each of these we need to continue the search for improved responses. That priests and bishops are, in fact, searching is a sign of great hope.

1) Spirituality

I believe that the time is ripe for a critical examination of the spirituality of diocesan priests. Spirituality is at the heart of any well-being experienced by priests, is the integrating factor in our lives.

As the Priestly Life and Ministry Committee anticipates the 20th anniversary of its very first publication, *The Spirituality of the American Priesthood,* it is considering the possibility of working anew on this concern, hoping to articulate a spirituality for priesthood that makes sense to priests, and that is grounded in our own experiences in pastoral ministry rather than in someone else's projections of what should be in our experiences. We would be looking for an articulation by priests of what leads them to deeper love, deeper freedom, deeper wisdom.

I suspect that such a process would yield a spirituality which, for a parish priest, is intertwined with his ministry in the parish, a spirituality which:

- helps him to see the Mysterion in the baby to be baptized, the shut-in to be visited, and the assembly gathered around the Sunday altar. (We are ordained as signs of God's presence, of the Church's presence; we need a spirituality which reflects this).
- frees him to be able to be present to the individuals and to the parish. (Most of you know that the ability to listen and be present is fundamental to almost all of the ministry we do.)

- builds community, especially through the Eucharist.
- leads toward mission, making us, in the words of the Eucharistic Prayer, "an everlasting gift to you."

Two other concerns about spirituality

1) A major concern in regard to the spirituality of priests and to our well-being is our psychosexual development—a concern made all the more pressing by the publicity given to pedophilia cases and to priests with AIDS. In this regard I join you in asking God's blessing upon Fr. Groeschel's session this afternoon. Priests are looking for help in the continuing development of our sexual maturity. We are looking for help in understanding how to live celibacy and why to live celibacy. We are looking for help in understanding how to develop deepening human relationships while remaining faithful to our commitment to celibacy. We need the help of good theologians, psychologists, anthropologists. We need opportunities to discuss these concerns with one another, with our bishops, with the wider Catholic community.

2) Long experience shows that annual retreats are important for the spiritual wellness of priests. I believe that care must be made that retreats for priests are planned to meet the important purpose for which they exist. I believe that, although gatherings whereby priests get to know one another and develop fraternity in the diocese are worthwhile gatherings, they are not retreats. Similarly most priests I know do not have their need for annual retreat met by the single diocesan retreat for all priests. Retreats must go for depth, a depth which different priests find in different ways. I am particularly struck at how many priests have had significant conversion moments in the midst of a private, directed retreat. Finally, I believe that a diocese which provides a variety of good resources and finances for priests' retreats has the right, even the duty, to expect priests to partake of an annual retreat. A great amount of care

can be shown for priests by asking them—in the right way—about their annual retreat.

2) Identity

A second major concern regarding the well-being of today's priests is the question of the identity of the priest. We are ordained *in persona Christi, caput ecclesiae.* The famous passage from *Lumen Gentium,* number 10, provides a key in this discussion: "Although they differ from one another in essence and not only in degree, the common priesthood of the faithful and the ministerial or hierarchial priesthood are nonetheless interrelated." Both halves of this statement are important: difference, interrelatedness. Cardinal Baum recently made this same point in his address about priestly formation. "Our seminarians," he said, "need to know the theology of the common priesthood and the theology of the ordained priesthood, understanding the relationship between them, their mutuality and their differences."[13] Much work needs to be done by today's theological community to help us to understand this difference and this interrelatedness. Much reflection needs to be done by priests in discovering the practical implications of this difference and this interrelatedness. The topic would make for a wonderful conversation among a presbyterate at a diocesan convocation.

3) Collaboration

The discussion about the theological identity of the priest leads logically to what is among the most hopeful developments in today's church—that of the increasing collaboration between priests and others in the mission of the Church. Without a developing sense of his identity as a person and his identity as a priest, the priest himself will be threatened by living and working in mutuality with others; he will be inclined either toward defensiveness, authoritarianism and rigidity, or toward a wishy-washy abdication of his role of leadership.

The lessons we are currently learning about collaboration are filled not only with hope, but also with pain and confusion. Some are tempted to short-circuit the learning because of the pain and confusion, and thereby retreat from the learning. A recent study published by a mid-western diocese indicates that seasoned pastors "shared that their ministry often began by espousing the collaborative model, but that, over time, the mechanics of the implementation eroded."[14] Based upon this, one approach is to say that collaboration has been tried and found not to work. Another approach is to keep learning. I am arguing here that the well-being of most priests—and the well-being of most men and women in ministry—will increase as we learn the skills and attitudes and theology of collaboration. And we will learn it as we see it modeled, however faultingly in the ministry of our bishops.

4) Structural Concerns Affecting Priests

Priests, like bishops, need an opportunity to express divergent perspectives on the realities of church life, diocesan life, parish life. We need a forum where both our hopes and disappointments about the Church can be expressed and understood, and whereby we can develop commitment to mutually-shared goals. All the complications and challenges brought on by the declining number of priests provide but one example of the need for such a forum.

Great progress has been made in this regard, but we have a long way to go. Diocesan synods, convocations of priests, presbyterial councils and diocesan pastoral councils have been examples and have been the source for continuing learning. The central services of some dioceses have even tried to involve priests in the planning and development of diocesan programs! Both priests and bishops are grateful when any such efforts help us all to work together.

A couple of years ago, a recently installed Archbishop was confronted by reporters, who wanted to know how he had dealt with the low morale of priests that had existed in his Archdiocese. He said, "very few priests really talked to me about morale. You've got to remember that the morning after the installation I talked to the Priests' Council and gave them a whole load of projects to take off with. . . . Any process by which you help people to take ownership of their faith life and the life of the Church automatically tends to build morale."

In this regard, some specific concern seems to be developing about the experience of presbyteral councils. A perception is developing among priests in many parts of our country that their concerns are no longer addressed at the presbyteral council. They sometimes say that the agenda is frequently that of the bishop and not also that of themselves, that the Council members are increasingly saying "what the bishop wants to hear" more than what priests themselves believe, that priests no longer attempt to nominate and elect their best priests to council positions, and that these best priests frequently decline nomination.

I do not know how objective this perception is, and I know that it is not universally true, but I recognize it as an increasingly frequent perception. Indications are that both priests and bishops are still learning how to implement the new Code's prescription that presbyteral councils be both consultative and representative. The value of a forum where bishop and priests can speak candidly about the life of the diocese is obvious. The effectiveness of such a forum requires a skill which can be learned and a trust which can be developed on the part of the council members, on the part of the bishop, and on the part of the presbyterate as a whole. Such a forum, however, when effective, will do more than 10 stress management workshops for the well-being of the presbyterate and for the mission of the Church.

Some priests and some presbyterates have given up on presbyteral councils. They would benefit greatly if their bishop would challenge them about this, would tell them of his absolute need for their assistance and wisdom, of his willingness to continue to struggle to learn how to develop structures which enable priests to speak their biggest dreams and to work not just as individuals but as a presbyterate to build the Church.

5) Affirmation/Accountability

An oft raised question of the recent past goes something like this: "Now that we don't make Monsignors anymore, what can be done to affirm priests?" It is an important question, one to which many here would offer differing responses.

My own bias in this regard is described in part by a vote taken recently by the priests of the Archdiocese of Miami, where they were asked if they wanted the custom of naming Monsignors to be reinaugurated. The vote was against naming Monsignors, by a rate of 4 to 1. If I had been asked to vote, I would have voted with the majority, in the belief that there are much more effective, less divisive ways to affirm and support priests. Several of these ways are described in two recent resources: "Reflections on the Morale of Priests" by the Priestly Life and Ministry Committee, and "Companionpiece to 'A Shepherd's Care'" by the National Organization for the Continuing Education of Roman Catholic Clergy.

If I were to select one way of affirmation which I believe is an important way for our future, I would name the process of accountability for priests. Common wisdom says that priests do not want accountability. But I think that this is changing, that styles of accountability are developing which can be affirming and helpful for priests. We priests are increasingly tiring of going it alone, of being the long ranger. We want to do a good job and welcome feedback about how we come across.[15] I do not think that priests welcome additional opportunities to be bashed, or additional opportunities to be controlled by bishop or chancery, but that we welcome feedback on our work, especially when the feedback is rooted in respect. An increasing body of evidence is developing from several dioceses that the struggle to provide accountability is a worthwhile struggle.

6) Leisure

In his wonderful document, *Ecclesiam Suam,* Pope Paul VI made the stunningly insightful statement that "leisure is the mother of friendliness and of prayer." It is a statement that many priests (and bishops) need to hear.

Yesterday, I heard someone say to a group of priests, "If you are too busy for prayer you are too busy."

One bishop, in thinking about the increasing expectations parishioners are putting upon priests and the increasing expectations priests are putting upon themselves, put the question this way: "What can we do to help priests to be satisfied with a reasonable day's work?" I recently received a letter from one priest doing a doctoral dissertation on priests and stress; although he indicates that his research is not yet completed, he says that one preliminary statistic is striking: that the average priest in his survey works 65 hours per week.

This is not to imply, of course, that all priests are on the verge of burn out! Some, in fact, suffer more from being under challenged rather than over challenged. The 1985 study found that many priests get enough rest, regularly take a day off, and regularly get vacation. But many don't. And, because of this, I see cause for all of us in leadership positions to invoke the wise words of Pope Paul that "leisure is the mother of friendliness and of prayer." In this regard I note, finally, the report from several priests that they experience a specific obstacle to finding leisure by living in the same building where they work. Current indication is that we can expect continuing conversation about this issue for some time to come.

7) Continuing Formation

Few things can affect the well-being of priests as deeply as having a sense of being competent, informed, aware. Effective continuing formation programs for priests are valuable for priests and for those served by priests.

Three quick comments about formation:

1) The real purpose of continuing formation programs is conversion, metanioa. And people—priests included—only make conversion when they are internally motivated. Whereas some priests are quite motivated toward ongoing growth, others are not. High quality programs provide motivation; good guidelines and policies of participation (including financial resources) can help the motivation; being inspired by leaders who themselves are continually learning provides motivation; caring confrontation can sometimes lead to motivation. We still have much to learn about motivation.

2) Conversion happens not when we are told by some outside "expert" what we are to think. Rather, conversion happens when we think critically about our beliefs and behaviors and have good resources to deepen our critical thinking. Much as this conference is designed as a "consultation" at which intelligent and professional people meet with each other and with some experts, so also formation events for priests can be "consultations" at which the best methods of adult education are employed—consultations at which the key question is "how can my life and ministry improve?" rather than "did the speakers give a good speech?"

3) Three kinds of continuing formation programs, beyond retreats and especially directed retreats, occur to me as meriting special attention:

a) So-called support groups—especially groups where people can tell the truth to one another about their life and ministry;

b) Transition programs—transitions from seminary to ordained ministry, transition to the first or other pastorate, transition to retirement from administrative responsibility. Most people are especially hungry to learn when they are beginning something new;

c) Sabbaticals—some argue that the decreasing number of ordained priests means that sabbaticals should be discontinued. I argue that the decreasing number of priests makes sabbaticals more necessary.

And so, bishops, I thank you for your having welcomed me to be with you this afternoon. You have allowed me to state my beliefs about some of the great challenges currently facing the priesthood, challenges which are great opportunities as well. We know that, with God's grace, our future is blessed and our well-being is guaranteed. And we know that for priests and for all God's people life is, in fact, worth living, that love is, in fact, worth giving, and that God is, in truth, all in all. And, if God is for us, who can be against us!

NOTES

1. The Health of American Catholic Priests: A Report and Study, Bishops' Committee on Priestly Life and Ministry, 1985, p. 28.

2. The Health of American Catholic Priests: A Report and Study, Bishops' Committee on Priestly Life and Ministry, 1985, p. 43.

3. The Health of American Catholic Priests: A Report and Study, Bishops' Committee on Priestly Life and Ministry, 1985, p. 79.

4. "Clergy Health and Wellness," published in *Continuing Formation of Priests: New Perspectives* by The National Organization of Continuing Education of Roman Catholic Clergy, Fall, 1986, p. 31.

5. "Clergy Health and Wellness," published in *Continuing Formation of Priests: New Perspectives* by The National Organization of Continuing Education of Roman Catholic Clergy, Fall, 1986, p. 33.

6. The Health of American Catholic Priests: A Report and Study, Bishops' Committee on Priestly Life and Ministry, 1985, pp. 36–37, 80, 96–97.

7. The Health of American Catholic Priests: A Report and Study, Bishops' Committee on Priestly Life and Ministry, 1985, p. 56.

8. The Health of American Catholic Priests: A Report and Study, Bishops' Committee on Priestly Life and Ministry, 1985, p. 22.

9. The Health of American Catholic Priests: A Report and Study, Bishops' Committee on Priestly Life and Ministry, 1985, p. 77.

10. The Health of American Catholic Priests: A Report and Study, Bishops' Committee on Priestly Life and Ministry, 1985, p. 4. 81.

11. The Health of American Catholic Priests: A Report and Study, Bishops' Committee on Priestly Life and Ministry, 1985, p. 4, 40.

12. The Health of American Catholic Priests: A Report and Study, Bishops' Committee on Priestly Life and Ministry, 1985, p. 81.

13. William Cardinal Baum, "An Address on The Priesthood," published by The Pontifical College Josephinum, October 17, 1988, p. 15.

14. Gerald T. Broccolo, et al. *Coordinating Parish Ministries,* Department of Personnel Services, Archdiocese of Chicago, 1987, p. 23.

15. Cf, for example, "How the Catholic Priest Cognitively Perceives Sources of Stress During the First Twenty-Five Years After Ordination: A Report to the Bishops' Committee on Priestly Life and Ministry," an unpublished but copywrited report by Richard J. Kalb, S.J., Fordham University, New York, New York, June 17, 1987.

Chapter 19

THE PSYCHOSEXUAL DEVELOPMENT AND MATURITY OF THE CLERGY

The Reverend Benedict J. Groeschel, C.F.R., Ph. D.

When I was first asked to give this presentation I was immediately conscious of the limited time accorded to cover such a vast and, regretfully important topic. It would take several hours to simply review all the important literature on homosexuality and pedophilia and even longer time to describe different therapeutic models and their reported results. Because I have worked as a psychologist with clergy and religious for more than fifteen years I am aware that this audience is primarily interested in practical suggestions. Most, if not all, of this distinguished audience are most interested in the following questions I believe.

Note: I will use the word cleric *throughout to include clergy sem-*

inarians, brothers and most of my remarks will apply to males.
Female homosexuality is a different topic and I have had rela-
tively little experience with the cases of women afflicted by it.

1) Is there any way to accurately predict that a clerical
   candidate will be troubled by homosexual or pedophile behavior in the future?
2) Is there a greater incidence of homosexuality and pedophilia now than there was in the past and if so, why?
3) Once it has been established that a cleric has been involved in homosexual activity or in pedophilia and has
   been sent for assistance, what is the probability of recurrence?
4) Is there anything a superior can do with a sincerely
   contrite cleric in these circumstances to insure that
   there will not be a recurrence?

These four questions are really eight questions because pedophilia is a very different phenomenon from homosexuality. And in
fact there are several different patterns of behavior in each category which are quite distinct. There is also a very important category called pseudo-homosexuality.

Because of the limits of time I am going to assume that you are
all informed of certain commonly known facts about notorious
cases of pedophilia and about treatment programs around the
country which have been established for assisting clerics with
these problems. My omission of these facts is simply an assumption
of your awareness so that we do not have to stop and "reinvent the
wheel."

I also assume that you are aware of the well known positions
of different individuals and groups who more or less disagree with
the teaching of the majesterium on questions of morality.

Before we begin with our questions there are a few definitions
necessary for our discussions. These definitions will be general and
pragmatic. For more precise definitions I suggest you read the *Ho-*
mosexual Person by Fr. John Harvey, OSFS, (Ignatius Press, 1987)
and especially the article in that book by Fr. Jeffrey Keefe, OFM,
Conv.

Homosexuality broadly means a sexual attraction toward a
person of the same sex. However I follow the generally accepted

view in the psychoanalytic world that most people with homosexual attractions are, in fact, heterosexuals who have become fixated in their early development, either in early childhood or early adolescence. They are, in fact, underdeveloped heterosexuals. A truly homosexual person, a syntonic homosexual, is a rare person. He is a person whose body does not match his psyche. Few of these people ever actually enter into the clergy because of the severity of their conflicts. Many, and I think most, so-called homosexuals, (*The Psychoanalytic Theory of Neurosis:* Norton: 1945, and Charles Bocaridies, *Homosexuality:* Aronson, 1978) are men who suffered from an inadequate separation from their mothers at the end of infancy and are subject to only partially repressed but powerful instinctual drives. (cf. Otto Fenishel.) These drives are expressed in a narcissistic attachment to a model of themselves, particularly an attractive male model. Other so-called homosexuals are men who have ambivalently identified with their fathers and other male figures and are conflicted in their sexual identity. They are attracted by the male body but repelled by some masculine behavior and associations. It is important to keep these definitions in mind. If you wish to read about these two types from a more religious point of view I would suggest you read *Crisis in Masculinity* by Leanne Payne, about men who are still over attached to their mothers, and *Homosexuality: A New Christian Ethic* by Elizabeth Moberly about men who have had ambivalent relationships with father figures, (See brief bibliography attached). Both of these books are helpful to give out to troubled persons. Actually I never classify either of these types as a truly homosexual person.

There is also a third kind of person: the man who seems to be well identified with his own gender, is neither dependent on his mother nor ambivalent, but nevertheless is drawn to brief anonymous contacts with other men, so-called "quick sex." Often these are the people who become involved with the police. Dr. Patrick Carnes has written and worked extensively on this problem. (See bibliography). Members of all three categories have been helped substantially by groups like Sexaholics Anonymous and by Courage.

Pedophilia presents a far more primitive drive with its origins in early life. Not much has been written about pedophilia in a popular style unfortunately. It represents, again according to the psychoanalytic theory, a partially repressed oedipal attraction arising from the very basic and instinctual dependency on the mother figure. This primitive attraction is not completely subject to the control of the ego. Strictly speaking a pedophile sees himself in the attractive child and treats the child "tenderly," or in some case where there is a sadistic transformation, "cruelly."

A man attracted to post pubescent boys, called ephebophile, is more like an adult homosexual and is probably better understood by the theories related to homosexuality. Usually he seeks his own lost youth. (For a good review of pedophilia see Chapter 9 in *The Homosexual Person.*)

We proceed now with our questions. Please recall that my goal is to give some very practical answers based on my own experience and not a review of the research.

I. Is There an Accurate Way to Predict That a Clerical Candidate Will be Troubled by Homosexual Tendencies?

The answer to this question was once thought to be found in a process by which everyone was excluded from the ranks of the clergy who was thought to have homosexual inclinations. This answer was generally accepted when homosexuality was a rare and limited phenomena. There is no doubt in my mind that ever growing numbers of people are confused in their sexual identification. The decline of family life and growing number of one parent families will increase these numbers. The question of admissions to religious life is now a more complex one. In evaluating a candidate with some homosexual inclinations we must address the following issues.

1) How sound is the person's overall mental health, especially in terms of control. Does he generally behave in a mature way? And how passive agressive is he? Is he a loser or disaster prone?
2) Does he lead a chaste moral life with relative ease? Persons in late adolescence or early adult life are subject to high levels of hormonal activity and this time is a real test.

3) Is he solidly convinced that the moral teaching of the church on sexuality and is he equally well founded in his faith on which these teachings are based? It is my observation that a loss of a sense of orthodoxy and convictions about faith has lead many clerics to practically reject the teaching of the church on sexuality and then difficulties ensue. This is particularly true when seminarians are given conflicting messages about morality.

If the answer to any of these questions is *no* I believe that serious difficulties are inevitable. Even if the answers are all in the affirmative there can still be trouble, especially if a person does not strengthen his own convictions by prayer, meditation and the reverent use of the sacraments. I have heard many times from young priests that their seminary experience left much to be desired in areas of theological commitment and moral conviction.

If a person has serious pedophile tendencies, even if these have never been acted out beyond deliberate phantasies with auto-erotic behavior, I believe that this person is a serious risk. Pedophilia represents such an instinctual regression that even if repression is therapeutically reduced, the personality changes may be so profound that chaste celibacy is impossible. The case of the person with attraction to teenagers, which has never been acted out, is not as clear cut as the pedophile. The person's overall adjustment and commitment to the teachings of the church and to the spiritual life must be carefully evaluated over a long period of time.

II. Is There More Homosexuality and Pedophilia Now, and Why?

Socaraides makes the point well that the level of homosexual behavior in societies is related to its social acceptance. Many children are "in the middle" or ambivalent as regards sexual identity and it is a function of society by positive teaching, modeling behavior, moral precepts and even taboos, to push children toward a heterosexual adjustment. The media in our country is largely controlled by people with confused sexual identities and deviant morality, and the effects of this on large numbers of adolescents can be seen. Deprived and disturbed adolescents seem to be largely polymorphously sexual and their number is growing. A youngster in Covenant House was recently reported to have said "everybody in this place is gay." Pop psychology with its emphasis on self expression and self indulgence has destroyed the foundations of morality in vast numbers of undergraduates (Presidential Address to American Psychological Association, 1975 by Professor Donald Campbell. Cited in Vitz, *Psychology as Religion* Eerdmans 1977.)

What is appalling is that the religious denominations in the United States have either gone along with the tide or have only weakly resisted it. While I have the greatest sympathy with persons suffering from homosexual proclivities and have seen numbers of these lead devout and chaste lives and others overcome their deviant tendencies, I have no sympathy for any program of any denomination which tacitly or explicitly encourages homosexual behavior. Compassion can bring a person a long way and acceptance of the individual is essential for treatment of personality disorders, but approval of what is destructive is wrong. Should religious groups ever encourage people to be intoxicated, reckless or self destructive? No. Should they encourage sexual deviancy? No.

The question of why the sudden incidence of pedophilia among the clergy is an interesting one. In a more repressive moral climate, such as existed up to the late 1960's, many marginal pedophiles managed to control their impulses. The same was true of clergy with strong sexual needs, either heterosexual or homosexual. As the cultural revolution collided with Post Vatican II changes in what appeared to be a rather euphoric moment, the message was given to all, "don't be repressed, let yourself go; you will be all right." The next message, originally proclaimed by the heterosexual majority was "Sex is for fun. Try it, you will like it." Those mental health professionals and moralists who gave that message neglected to ask what the impact of this message would be outside the ambience of normal heterosexuality. The same change in values and socio-moral functions that caused many priests and religious to get married and many ministers and rabbis to get divorced caused the homosexual community to assert its voice. This included even pedophiles who participated for some years in the Gay Rights demonstrations around the country, with little or no protest from the rest of the so-called gay scene. The wind had been sown, now the whirlwind is being reaped. My suspicion is that things will get worse, except in the single case of pedophilia because of scandal and legal ramifications. Already in a number of dioceses and orders there appears to be a tacit acceptance of the homosexual lifestyle. When this becomes a subculture with gay humor and all the other signs of this phenomena, the possibility of recruiting heterosexual candidates is dramatically reduced. According to some of my friends in the "main stream Protestant Churches" this is exactly what is happening and when one has a celibate clergy, the dangers are all the greater.

III AND IV.

Once it has been established that a cleric has been involved in homosexual activities or in pedophilia and has been sent for assistance, what is the probability of recurrence?

Is there anything a superior can do with a sincerely contrite cleric in these circumstances to assure that there will not be a recurrence?

We will consider these two questions at the same time because they are so closely related. Let's consider the case of the homosexual first. The therapeutic reduction of sexual identity confusion has been debated for years. However, Bieber, a psychiatrist with many years of experience with male homosexuals reported that two thirds of his clients had either adopted a well developed heterosexual identity or had begun lives free of compulsive sexual activity of a homosexual sort. (*Homosexuality, A Psycho-analytic Study of Male Homosexuals,* by I. Bieber, et al Vantage Books: 1965.) Where moral convictions and spiritual motives are present a good deal of success is reported in the therapeutic treatment of homosexuals. (cf. Harvey). The vast majority of cases church officials would be aware of involve persons suffering with compulsive activity. In this case there is an irresistible drive for pleasure, accompanied by self destructive elements. Homosexuality and pedophilia are particularly prone to compulsivity. In such cases the person actually may regret what he is doing while he is doing it and punishes himself afterwards in many ways.

I would like to interject here an analogy that may be helpful for a person unfamiliar with psychoanalytic theory. I am attempting a metaphorical explanation of the understanding of Otto Fenichel in *The Psychoanalytic Theory of Neurosis,* Norton: 1945, cf. p. 333. The infant child is the focus of absolutely imperative drives for pleasure and fulfillment. The baby, in fact, would be a very dangerous person if he had a fully developed mature human body. The baby fortunately is limited by his size and physique. As the infant passes into very early childhood the beginnings of ego develop, one of the functions of ego, according to the psychoanalytic theory is to put a repressive cover on the untamed and unlimited pleasure demands of the infant. Remember that these demands have mostly been directed toward the infant's mother or mother figure. In simple words, the baby is in some way totally in love with his mother. As repression takes place at the end of infancy the normal boy will transfer this powerful affection now in a filtered form to identification with his father. However, for some people their cover of repression is not complete. If the repressive cover is seriously incomplete an infantile personality or a serious character disorder, like a psychopath will emerge. However, in the case of homosexuality it is the view of Fenishel and others that, as it were, a corner of this regressive cover is deficient and a part of the primitive desire of the infant emerges. If I may use the analogy of a cauldron full of burning coals and flames covered by a fire door except in one corner. From that corner emerge bright and living flames. From the fire door itself only emerges heat.

Our difficulty in comprehending serious compulsive behavior including things like compulsive homosexuality and pedophilia is that you and I tend to evaluate the impulse to do immoral and disordered acts from the heat generated by the fire door. We may have impulses to do this or that thing which our moral conscience forbids, as for instance, in the case of heterosexual desires. Many homosexual people however are not dealing with the heat from the fire door. They are dealing with the open flame of infantile desire escaping from an unclosed corner of the fire door. This is why a person with a normal sexual outlook finds it very difficult to understand or have compassion on those who commit sexual crimes.

My impression is that by far the best therapy for compulsives is the program designed by the founders of Alcoholics Anonymous. Compulsives have many things in common and this includes sexual compulsives. A comprehensive change in the person's entire lifestyle with a complete dedication to the spiritual life and conversion accompanied by counseling or therapy is the best treatment by far. The assistance and support of a group of recovering compulsives is to my way of thinking essential. I have worked individually and in group with clergy suffering from sexual additions for about two decades. I still can find no substitute for the group and its processes. The self-respect of the individual is restored, the defense of denial is confronted and helpful steps are suggested. Since the pedophile is dealing with the most powerful of repressed and archaic impulses the support of a professionally directed group is all the more necessary. The pedophile like the narcotics addict is dealing with something more elemental and more destructive to self and to others than alcoholism and compulsive gambling. It seems to me that for a cleric who has been involved in pedophilia, and has had extended residential treatment specifically designed for this problem, it is necessary that there be:

1) close supervision and vigilance
2) A therapeutic support group
3) On-going psychotherapy or counseling with an informed and experienced professional.

While aging may reduce normal sexual desire, and even homosexual impulses, it does not appear to reduce pedophile tendencies.

At this time a responsible ordinary is expected to be an expert on many things. This is often impossible for a busy administrator and spiritual leader. A bishop is expected to understand the sexual problems which may arise in his diocese. It has been suggested that every diocese have a procedure to deal with the legal and ethical ramifications of pedophilia and a team to implement this procedure. I suggest that every diocese and province also have a team to deal with the human side of sexual problems. There should be at least one priest or religious with a degree of sophistication in the behavioral sciences and a team of professionals including psychiatrists and/or psychologists. An ancillary group of recovering sexual addicts is most desirable. This model has been often used effectively in the case of alcoholics. It should be also noted that a well trained and experienced spiritual director is essential. A behavioral approach which ignores the spiritual dimension is a waste of time and a countersign to the message of the Gospel and the church. A compassionate attitude on the part of the bishop is essential, but without these other elements compassion can be disastrous. I have never known an active alcoholic, compulsive homosexual or pedophile who did not lie to himself and to everybody else. Because of misdirected compassion especially on the part of some popular religious spiritual writers, homosexual behavior has been suddenly accepted among the clergy at certain times and in certain places. A pedophile will latch onto this as an approval of his own driven needs. I consider writers who reinforce homosexual behavior no better than liquor advertisements which entice people to drink. I put most "gay rights" movements in the same category as New Year's Eve revelers and barflies. They all encourage compulsions no matter how well intentioned they are. None of these compassionate people will show up in court to offer to pay the fines either for drunken driving or for pedophilia.

Perhaps it is most important to put the discussion of this problem into a broader context. It used to be a truism in history that widespread homosexuality and pedophilia were symptoms of a declining society. There are always many other signs of decline as there were in Greece, Rome, and at the end of the Renaissance. Things fall apart together. We are, I believe, in such times. If we are, then the only real solution is a widespread movement of individual and communal reform. We have to say to the person who is the victim of homosexual or pedophile compulsions what we have to say to ourselves every day, namely, that the time has come, and the Kingdom of God is at hand, and we must repent and believe the Good News. (Mark 1:15)

A sexual addict or in fact any other compulsive will only listen to us if he perceives that we recognize ourselves as fellow sinners in need of repentance. None of us will really make any progress until we recognize that we are, in the words of AA, powerless to control ourselves unless we get help from God. Perhaps the serious moral situation which now obtains in the clergy and religious life of many denominations is traceable to the fact that Christians in our culture have forgotten that they are people called to constant daily repentance. The loss of this awareness may be in fact the root of the problem.

References

Very brief list of books helpful for sexual addicts. (Brevity was the goal in preparing this bibliography of works which can be helpful for distribution to those who need to know about the problems described in this paper.)

Benedict J. Groeschel, CFR

Carnes, Philip, *The Sexual Addiction,* Minneapolis, Minn.: CompCare Publications, 1984.

Groeschel, Benedict J., C.F.R., *The Courage To Be Chaste,* Mahwan, N.J.: Paulist Press, 1985.

Harvey, John F., O.S.F.S., *The Homosexual Person,* San Francisco, California: Ignatius Press, 1987.

Harvey, John F., O.S.F.S., *A Spiritual Plan to Redirect One's Life,* Boston, Ma.: Daughters of St. Paul, 1979.

Moberly, Elizabeth R., *A New Christian Ethic,* Greenwood, S.C.: The Attic Press, Inc. 1983.

Payne, Leanne, *The Broken Image,* Westchester, Illinois: Crossway Books, 1981.

Payne, Leanne, *Crisis in Masculinity,* Westchester, Illinois: Crossway Books, 1985.

Chapter 20

PASTORAL CONCERNS CLERGY ISSUES

BISHOP: You mentioned the need, when you're dealing with this compulsive activity which is described as "immensely imperative," for a support group for the person, the need for vigilance on the part of the supervisor, in which case this would be the Bishop, ongoing counselling, which would be life-long, and the fact that age does not diminish this particular compulsion.

Now, all of those factors taken into consideration, what advice, what counsel, what reflection would you share in terms of attempting to minister to that priest, especially as a Bishop attempts to minister to that priest? And particularly in terms of the assignability of that priest?

FATHER GROESCHEL: Bishop, that is a good summary. Beyond that I would also say that first of all it is absolutely imperative that the priest in question lead a vibrant spiritual life. I believe that the priest in question must commit himself to a daily eucharistic holy hour. The focusing of the priest's personal life and attention on the presence of Our Lord so powerfully presented in the Holy

Eucharist, is a great cure for loneliness and the terrible pain of isolation that so many sexual addicts experience.

Now, when it comes to ministering, the Bishop is in a difficult position because he is both the authority who could, if necessary, put this person on a permanent administrative leave, and at the same time, he is a spiritual father. One of the things learned in psychology very early on is that an authority figure cannot easily counsel someone, because the person is limited in his spontaneity. This is why superiors and bishops are not to hear the confessions of those they are responsible for. This is also why I think that the care of a priest in such a case is best delegated to a well informed priest in the diocese who has had some professional training (at least a Masters Degree in Counseling,) and is himself well founded in the spiritual life. It is understood that the priest counsellor observes confidentiality strictly. It's better that someone else knows what's going on, even if the bishop can't know what's going on.

I also think that the bishop has to examine very carefully the extensive report that is provided by one of the therapeutic agencies, like the Paraclete Fathers or St. Luke's or The Institute for Living. I know that a bishop may get a whole big sheaf of material; but out of all of those papers there's usually one page that's absolutely crucial.

One needs to get a professionally trained person to read it. A Bishop here today showed me such a page that a psychiatrist had written in terms easily understood, but the implications were hidden in the words. A bishop needs a trusted psychologist or psychiatrist to work with. I think it is important to have a panel made up of a counselor, spiritual father, a therapist, someone else who is informed on the relationship of the psychological and the canonical and the legal. Also, a most valuable adjunct would be a recovered addict. You know if you have a priest in charge of AA in your diocese and he's doing his job he's priceless. A recovered addict in the sexual area might be harder to come by but even a priest who is a recovering alcoholic who had a fairly broad view of things could substitute by helping a recovered sexual addict, because he'll know what addiction is.

And then you better say your prayers, because recidivism is fairly high. And a good rule of thumb is, the more bizarre the behavior, the more likely recidivism is to occur. Pedophilia is psychologically much more bizarre than hebephelia or adolescent involvement and is much more bizarre than cruising or anonymous homosexual involvement. The more bizarre, the more regressive, the more archaic and the more powerful the compulsion. If you are the administrator of the diocese, you cannot provide vigilance and supervision yourself. No more than any bishop would care to be in charge of the AA group for your priests should you try to be involved with vigilance in the sexual area.

There is also the fact that the law is vindictive in cases of pedophilia. Two decades ago when I was an intern, I worked at a program for a few weeks in the evening, once a week, which was sponsored by the Teamsters Union for people arrested for sexual difficulties. Most were cases with adolescents. Most of the men were on either probation or adjournment pending dismissal. Suddenly, this has become the great big bear of the American public because there are no other sexual crimes left. Nothing else is illegal, you know. Bigamy is quite acceptable. Violent rape and pedophilia are the only two sexual crimes left. I personally think that the media is getting even with us Catholics for our stand on homosexuality and abortion. I don't think there is any question at all that we're being mugged by the media. And they'll probably continue attacking us through scandal.

You may remember that *The National Catholic Reporter* carried several whole issues on clerical pedophilia. I read those issues. There was not a drop of compassion on one page. It was totally absent.

BISHOP: Even when there's not a law suit and you have to send a person away for the proper help and therapy, it becomes known among the clergy. And because of that, it's very difficult, I think, to reassign them anywhere in the diocese. In my opinion, it's usually necessary to tell the fellow, I just cannot assign you here. If you want to continue as a priest, you know, you'll just have to find another diocese or religious community. Sometimes, you want to encourage the person to apply for laicization but if that's something that he chooses not to do, you just can't force that. So some of us have taken the position that, you just have to find yourself some other assignment.

Is that lacking compassion? Usually, the person does not accept that very well. And I don't know if that harms his ultimate recovery. But for an administrator, we cannot put the diocese in jeopardy with another law suit, especially if you've got a couple pending already. And also, to reassign can cause a moral problem with your own priests. Do you have any observations?

FATHER GROESCHEL: Yes, Bishop, obviously, it's a question that many people have had to face. I think the first thing to say is that the Paraclete Fathers, God bless them, have tried to help the men that they have assisted to get reassigned.

I'm sure they won't recommend someone unless there is solid therapeutic evidence that the person is a good risk. The person can never be more than a good risk. There's a crack in the cup. This is true also of a person who is a recovering alcoholic. Any alcoholic will tell you, "I've got 24 hours and I could fall off the wagon tomorrow." But alcoholism is far less of a risk legally and in terms of publicity.

While I've been here today, I spoke to two Bishops who had taken men who had been through a treatment program. In both cases, it was for hebephilia, not for pedophilia. And both of these Bishops reported to me that the man was doing well. In each case, the pastor knows the whole story. I find it hard to imagine these men being pastors themselves. And if you have many one-man parishes, that practically makes it more difficult for you to accept them. But I think what could happen is that a trade-off might occur where there's been publicity and there are two men of different dioceses who are good risks.

You have to be sure you are very carefully covered by legal documents that your lawyer will accept which indicate that you are not negligent. What the diocese gets sued for is not that the priest misbehaved but that there has been negligence.

The other possibility, and I think this is probably what happens more frequently, is an administrative leave when the man is expected to get a job, support himself, but he is not absolutely finished forever. At least it would give the man some hope and the bishop would not have to go through the difficulty of a canonical process.

I think that you are probably aware most of the bishops were told on their *ad liminia* that the Holy See insists on due process in these cases. This means, putting it bluntly, a second chance. You can't dismiss the man against his will without giving him a second chance. You might not be able to afford a second chance. I think it might be time for a little discussion of all of that, to be held within the shadow of the dome of St. Peters. I think the Bishops in this country are hoping to see some other kinds of procedures. But for the present, an indefinite administrative leave with some real concern for the man, is both compassionate and protective to the diocese.

BISHOP: You mentioned putting a priest on administrative leave indefinitely, that could create even a greater problem, I think, for a Bishop, especially if the priest leaves the diocese, is working someplace else, gets in trouble again. He has no supervision and yet you're still responsible for him. And you could be sued or whatever.

FATHER GROESCHEL: Well, Bishop, some places you could be sued and apparently some you couldn't. I think it's absolutely ridiculous to hold a diocese responsible for a man who is on an administrative leave. If he has a car accident, are you responsible? The foundation of the law suit is that by putting him in a clerical role, you are making people more vulnerable to him. But if you've told him that he cannot fulfill a clerical role why in the world would you be responsible? And it may have to be that one of these cases has got to go all the way to the Supreme Court because it is absolutely unjust to hold the church responsible in such a case. It's ludicrous and I think it's an example of vindictive legislation.

The answer to your practical question would be, if the man is cooperative, to at least make arrangements that he can get therapy. The diocese could undertake the cost. One could look for a suitable priest to be the man's spiritual director. A bishop should take some action to see that the Church is not just throwing him to the wolves. I don't know whether you can have him around in the diocese because the obvious place to put him would be a large religious house of very elderly sisters, and there aren't too many of those left. Maybe he could be in charge of the priest's retirement house or some job that is not involved with the care of the faithful.

BISHOP: Father, I would like to ask you a question concerning number three. I was asked by my ordinary recently to look into a case. It's a married man, a case of pedophilia. He released the psychologist who was treating him. And according to the psychologist, this case is described as regressive pedophilia, which explains to me is just an accident, as it were. The man had problems in his married life and, therefore, well, he fell into that temptation. It was a heterosexual affair, in a way, with a minor. According to the opinion of the psychologist, there is very little probability of recurrence in that. I would like your comment on that.

FATHER GROESCHEL: First, a few facts about pedophilia. Many adult pedophiles are homosexual toward children and heterosexual toward adults. It is not unusual to find a man, who may be married and having normal sexual relations with his wife, who will also fall into an occasion of homosexual pedophilia. That's not unusual nor is heterosexual pedophilia. The most common form of pedophilia in the United States is heterosexual incest. The most common forum of pedophilia is the family.

What is operative in the case presented is something that I think is important for everybody to hear about. Pedophilia, alcoholism, drug addictions are not primary psychological diagnosis. The five major primary psychological diagnosis are neurosis, psychosis, character disorder, borderline psychosis and inadequacy. There are only five major categories. Hopefully, we are addressing today a group of reasonably well adjusted neurotics.

In this case, we have to find out what kind of personality we are dealing with. Suppose this man is a character disorder, who has a defect of the superego or the conscience. One Bishop spoke to me recently about such a person. I wouldn't trust him as far as I could spit. I am as concerned about the fact that he has a character disorder as I am that he's a pedophile. Because if he has a character disorder he has either a self-destructive, passive-aggressive character disorder or, worse yet, he's an active antisocial personality.

If you've got one of those, I don't care whether he's heterosexual, or homosexual, get rid of him. Let him go. Just put him in a poor parish and he'll leave.

What one needs to know is what is the primary diagnosis? When we do psychological screening for the seminary, (and I've done a thousand of those over the years) we're not really looking for the so-called normal person. If anybody tells you some kid is normal, don't believe them. We're looking for reasonably well adjusted neurotics. They rarely get into big trouble and when they do they are very repentant. On the other hand, if someone is never honest with himself, and he gets involved with serious sexual misbehavior, this is very serious. Jemez Springs or St. Luke Institute will focus on the primary diagnosis when they make their report. And that's why you've really got to have a professional read that report for you.

FATHER BRINKMOELLER: From my point of view, I have a need to say we're talking about a small portion of the clergy population. I think everybody agrees with that but it's a big impact upon all of us. Some years ago, people used to project onto priests that they have no sexual energy inside of them. Now, we are like movie screens and people are projecting all kinds of sexual disfunctions upon us.

BISHOP: Dave, while I would agree that it's a very small percentage of the population, nonetheless, it takes up an enormous amount of our time and energy and one of the factors, Father Groeschel, which goes into this is, while we speak of it from a psychological point of view in a discussion like this and we can talk about reasonably adjusted people and also fundamental character defects, we also have to be aware, as we are, that the law views this in a completely different way than we would, either as Church or as psychologists. And the law has introduced elements which are— you used the word "vindictive." I think that's a very good description. But the law has introduced elements into this whole debate that preclude some of the solutions that would otherwise be open to us.

I don't know what direction one can give in facing that reality but the fact is that the law, for all intents and purposes, says that once a person is caught in a pedophilic act, that person, for all intents and purposes, is unassignable because of the liability. The response of a Bishop to a priest is one thing. The response of a Bishop to his local church, to which he also bears some responsibility is another thing. And the law certainly circumscribes that.

FATHER GROESCHEL: It makes it immensely difficult at the present time. My suspicion is that there will be fewer and fewer priests who have either been convicted or indicted for pedophilia who will be assignable, just from the public relations point of view. And you know as well as I do, if you were in administration years ago, that this problem occurred occasionally. Now you are limited in keeping a promising man by reason of notoriety.

324

BISHOP: Dealing with these men with the more severe problems, I don't know exactly how far we should extend ourselves, what our liability is. I realize the liability is on our shoulders.

FATHER GROESCHEL: I think my suggestion of a possibility of trade-off between two modest but equal risks is a very good idea. Your Excellency, are you familiar with some priests who have done some good work when they have recovered? I am sure there are a number of people here that are. It's the same thing with AA or Gamblers Anonymous or something like that. Do realize, too, that the man himself, subjectively, will never have an awareness of guilt proportionate to what the law is doing to him. You could have a man who makes one indiscretion in response to a soliciting adolescent, one indiscretion, perhaps when he's had something to drink. Even Jerome Noldin might not accuse him of a formal mortal sin. But he has ruined the rest of his life. You might have another person who's been leading a life of absolutely deliberate sin for years and nobody's going to care because it's behind closed doors and with an adult. There is no parity between the behavior and the punishment here.

Also, I should say this about priests who are arrested for solicitation, (not pedophilia) but the more common thing of somebody being picked up in the rest room of. the interstate highway. Or walking around the streets of an unsavory part of the city. This person possibly made his evening examination of conscience, said night prayers, his novena to St. Jude, and got into bed at ten o'clock. The moon was full. He got out of bed at eleven o'clock. He goes through his pathetic routine. By six-thirty in the morning he has gone to confession. One evening he gets picked up by a state trooper. And he's in the papers. But he never planned to lead a vicious life. Somebody else has a friend and has been leading a double life for years. They are never going to end up in the paper or be in trouble.

Another entirely different point. Don't always assume that a youngster is innocent. I worked for many years at a residential school for delinquent boys. And we had a little fellow who looked like a model for Hummel figures. By the time he was nine years old he had put two Mafiosi safely up the river with long sentences for pedophilia when the D.A. had been trying to get these guys for years and couldn't. Our little Hummel figure he was absolutely psy-

325

chopathic. And don't overlook that possibility. I wouldn't say that the child is morally guilty, but he may be a solicitor.

There's also the very rare case of the "black widow." In my book, *Stumbling Blocks and Stepping Stones*, I discuss the case of a priest who was solicited by a teenager who had no other purpose in mind than to destroy the priest. The priest didn't know him. He came into church. The priest was not, by any means, an active homosexual. He solicited the priest three times with tears before the priest permitted him to touch him and walked out of the church into the police station. This is what is called a black widow.

BISHOP: At this present moment, with regard to liability, we are extremely vulnerable. If a priest is going to be reassigned, that assignment better be very, very restricted. Children better not be involved in the whole thing. I mean, there are things, perhaps, that can be done about bringing men back and into the active ministry.

FATHER GROESCHEL: Obviously, Bishop, great care is necessary because with sexual addiction it's like alcoholism. The crack is in the cup. And any alcoholic will tell you he could go back to drinking.

I would say this, and please be careful if you quote me: you cannot rely on a pedophile, no matter how contrite or rehabilitated, to always tell you the truth. If he has slipped, he will not tell you. That's why a rule would have to be, with vigilance, "one false move and you're dead." Now, one Bishop I know who went to visit a recovering pedophile priest, looked into his room, and the room was filled with pictures of kids all over the walls. And that was it. Basta. Finito. He was through. And the Bishop was absolutely right. I would defend the decision of that Bishop absolutely.

So, your point is well taken and the best practical thing is to put the man on absolute good behavior. He doesn't go near the kids at all.

BISHOP: I would like to move into a slightly different area. Older priests who have had no prior experience of this, no incidence of this. It seems to have emerged, at least one case in my experience, talking with a major religious superior. There had been no incidence at all of this in the gentleman's history in the past. And this superior said he has a concern that as a person gets older, things that have been suppressed and lain dormant for years, the superior put it rather unforgettably—maybe it's a last chance. Would you comment on the dangers in that possibility for us?

FATHER GROESCHEL: There was a very tragic case in New York not too long ago of a retired District Attorney, 80 years of age, and a married man with grandchildren, who approached a small child. It was tragic because this man had no record of anything like that at all. What happened is something that can happen to a lot of elderly people. If there is the beginning of cerebral arteriosclerosis, or the early symptoms of Alzheimer's Disease, the inhibitory functions of the central nervous system do not work as well. Many elderly people will tell you that they are terribly bothered by sexual thoughts. And they think often that this is the Devil. They've never had sexual problems in their lives and in their old age, they are bombarded with these thoughts.

The highest integrating functions of the human being are located at the outer edge cerebral cortex called the neo-cortex. These functions can diminish with age. A person who has been a very quiet, well behaved person may become garrulous, use obscene speech, and become much more uninhibited. Certain kinds of cerebral arteriosclerosis could cause a person to be sexually uninhibited.

If this kind of behavior is observed, the person must be retired against his will to an institutional setting. This does not mean that they have been involved in pedophilia in the past or even had pedophile tendencies.

BISHOP: From someone who works south of the border, many times religious superiors send priests down to work in Latin America and they don't always inform us that they have problems. In these areas, there is very little supervision, very little vigilance, and especially if I don't know the track record, you just wonder how you can help that individual when the surroundings that we live in, there is a breakdown of healthy defense mechanisms that this person might be able to have. What is the obligation of religious superiors, let's say, after these persons might have been in one of these places—Affirmation Houses or out in New Mexico— to inform the Bishop of what the past track record is?

FATHER GROESCHEL: It is an absolute responsibility in justice.

I know we have a number of Canadian Bishops listed for this program. I should say that there are a couple of Bishops in Canada who have very good programs for priests with difficulties. They include therapy and supervision. I don't want to get myself in trouble with the Canadian hierarchy for saying this, there is one particular archdiocese where they have been very helpful and they have an outstanding program. They are not only willing to help a priest in this kind of difficulty but also a priest who has left the priesthood for a long time.

BISHOP: I just want to take up a part of a question that another Bishop raised in our responsibility to address the confusion and the pain and the sadness and whatever in the people, the shock. I feel, as leaders, we have a responsibility to address that constituency. If we go back 25, 30 or 40 years, our people experienced the same kind of shock in relation to a priest alcoholic. That has been somewhat modified and changed. And so there is the same challenge here on our part. And I was just wondering if you had any suggestions or observations that would assist us in trying to address the Church at large in an educative kind of way.

FATHER GROESCHEL: That is a very fine question, Bishop, and I am afraid, with the media and the hype about the whole thing right now, that we probably couldn't do much. My suspicion is that your model is a valid one and that probably, in the next decade, after all the hoopla dies down, an understanding will grow concerning the problems of the pedophile and of the person driven with other sexual problems including different forms of homosexuality. This understanding will probably come along with an unfortunate lowering of the taboos. You know, there are nothern European countries where the taboos on pedophilia are very low. These countries regularly export pedophile pornography. What this does, unfortunately, is get acceptance for the poor sinner but, at the same time, it destroys the inhibitory functions of social taboos. My suspicion is that the world is becoming more psychologically understanding of sexual problems and that someday, another Graham Greene will write a novel about all of this.

BISHOP: I want to thank both you and Father Brinkmoeller for your presentations. I find this exchange very helpful. Perhaps either or both of you might comment. We do spend a great deal of our time dealing with the difficulties that our priests, a small percentage of them, a relatively small percentage of them, have in the area of substance abuse. The majority of our priests, I think, are not recovering alcoholics and do not have a problem with chemical dependency and are not psychosexually maladjusted, at least in a way that requires special therapy.

But I think the majority of our priests are feeling like they are part of a group that's kind of under siege. And I'm just wondering if you would care to comment on what we can do as we go back to the majority of the priests who don't command a great deal of our time and attention, what we can do? My sense is that they're not feeling very good about themselves or what they do. And I'm just wondering if you would have any comments about how we address that in a positive way.

FATHER BRINKMOELLER: I think it's a very complicated question, of course, Archbishop, and all of us know that. I am aware of several places where dioceses have, in fact, tried to pull priests together and tried to develop some kind of a system where they can say to each other what's on their mind, how they are feeling, what are their dreams and what are their fears. Reports back indicate that that makes a difference. Apparently, it makes a significant difference when the Bishop has chosen to listen carefully to that and try to understand it. Several Bishops, I know, have gone out of their way, in the light of all this publicity, to say as loudly and as clearly as they can that priesthood is as wonderful as it is, even as it is so besieged.

The systems of priestly life and diocesan life are very important. They are the practical expression of the developing theology of *communio* in the priesthood. I think that if we can develop that theology and figure out what are the implications of this communio among priests, we would do ourselves a great favor. So that's one level.

On another level is this question of affirmation and how can the whole body of priests be affirmed. And how can individual priests be affirmed. I think that if priests are sitting around waiting for somebody to come pat them on the head every day or every week or every year, that's not a very healthy wait. But everybody needs to be acknowledged by somebody that they respect. Personal comments are significant, both to individuals and to the whole body of priests.

FATHER GROESCHEL: I totally agree with Father Brinkmoeller on that positive moral push. Bad morale does not do much good at all. There is the other side, too. Morale reflects spirit. The laity are very anxious that priests look like people who are working on their own spiritual lives and their relationship with Jesus Christ. If you ask numbers of young people who have left the Catholic Church to join evangelical churches, they will tell you that they did not hear Christ preached in the Church.

So, I think what we need among our priests, not only are the support systems but the beginning of the recognition that we have to get back to a life of personal conversion. Despite all of the bad publicity about the clergy, in an almost fascinating inverse ratio it is true that if you get up and preach about conversion very directly and with fervor, the people will respond better now than they used to in more religious times.

For example, our little reform community gives missions. Not only do the priests in the community preach but the brothers and sisters give witness talks and things like that. The night of our penance service we rarely finish before midnight. It is not unusual for me to arrive on Wednesday of the mission and find people on the sidewalk in tears, waiting to tell me how much they appreciate the example of young priests and young brothers and sisters who are preaching, to use St. Francis's term, with force and fervor, devotion to Jesus Christ and loyalty to His cause.

The first talk I ever gave to the community was in the Ninth Beatitude which says, "How blessed are you when men shall revile you and say all manner of evil things against you for my sake. Be glad and rejoice." Blessed means happy. And in the middle of all of this, there can be the unique kind of satisfaction of being loyal, even in the face of scandal.

I'm waiting for one of these priests in trouble to become a saint. I'm waiting for two saints. One, a priest who got married. One of them, sooner or later, will become a saint. And another one is the priest who has been in serious trouble. The Catholic Church has always had lots of room for saints who had gotten themselves in trouble. After all, wasn't AA founded by people who got themselves in trouble?

BISHOP MAIDA [Chairman of the Board, Pope John Center]: I, too, add my thanks. It's a very difficult topic and we all know what it means to deal with it.

I would like to give you a little canonical update on where we're at because that's very important in our life as we deal with this problem. Father had mentioned coming together under the shadow of the Dome of St. Peter's. Well, I think we are there. What could be possible, so that we wouldn't have to have the formal court procedure to laicize a pedophile in a serious case.

From a practical point of view, we know that it's very difficult to constitute that formal procedure. There are legal risks. There are defenses that the pedophile has. And there's the publicity. There are so many other problems with the formal procedure, although it is possible it is not very practical. An administrative procedure should be available wherein, in certain kinds of cases, the Holy See, on its own, could laicize a pedophile against the will of the pedophile.

I'm convinced the Holy See is prepared to listen and act quickly and I'm sure they will act as soon as we have a proposal on their desk. Bishop Keating, as Chairman of the Canonical Affairs Committee, is preparing various proposals for consideration by the N.C.C.B. with recommendations to the Holy See.

FINALE

TEACHING MORAL THEOLOGY TODAY
BISHOPS' PANEL DISCUSSION

Chapter 21

CENTRAL QUESTION: HOW DO YOU ASSURE A CONSISTENT MORAL THEOLOGY IN YOUR DIOCESE GIVEN THE PLURALISTIC BACKGROUND OF YOUR CLERGY?

The Most Reverend Oscar H. Lipscomb, Ph.D.
The Most Reverend Thomas J. Murphy, S.T.D.
The Most Reverend Francis X. DiLorenzo, S.T.D.

I. Archbishop Lipscomb

Let me tell you a story about the Bishop's communicating with his priests. Because basically, this is a question of communication and of trust and of confidence in trying to reach out to them with a vision of moral doctrinal consistency, authenticity in a very pluralistic picture of teachings.

This is a story about John and Mary, who had been married ten years and about a man in John's office, Joe, who got married to Sally. And Joe and Sally stayed on the high of the honeymoon for a year and a half. And this kind of magic had gone out of John's marriage. (Bishops, you know, are supposed to be married to their people, a fortiori, to their priests.) So John decided he would ask Joe, "How do you do it?" "Well," he said, "Each day I think of something special that Sally likes and I do it for her. The more unexpected it is, the better the outcome. And that has kept our marriage alive and happy." "Gosh," John said, "That could work for me, too."

So he called up the florist and got Mary the flowers that she liked. He called the confectioner's and bought her the special candy that she loved. He could hardly wait to come to get off from work. Five o'clock arrived and he collected both items. He drove home and he didn't go around to the back. He parked on the side and went up to the front door and rang the doorbell, charged with expectancy, hardly able to contain himself at the thrill that would light up Mary's face when she saw these gifts.

She didn't come at once, so he rang again. And finally, here came Mary, with the youngest of their four children on her shoulder, her hair disheveled, her clothes messed up, the house full of the aroma of burnt meat. She took a look at him and she said, "I cannot believe this. One of the children is sick, two of them have misbehaved and I don't know where the fourth is. I have just burnt the dinner. My life is a wreck, and here you come, now, drunk."

We have to make sure that our gestures and our offerings and our preparations are not misunderstood. How pluralistic can we tolerate the kind of pluralism that is about? Well, the presupposition is that our priests are teaching soundly. That's the first thing. If we give them faculties, that's possibly the highest level of trust a Bishop can impart. So in our efforts to communicate with them, we begin by a level of trust and confidence that stands until the contrary can be proven.

But that level of trust is always measured against something over which we have no control. Bishop DiLorenzo put it rather splendidly in a couple of sentences of his: persons with this religious/moral orientation have arrived at the conviction that there are certain moral insights that lay claim on them as persons within the context of the ecclesial community. We have no right to alter that, no right to change those essential larger insights. These are the principles. The significance, importance and depth of these moral insights are seen as objective, eternal and universal. They are seen as unchanging and unchangeable, timeless rather than timely. And this challenge always has to be given to our priests: that there are some things that remain, in a way, untouchable, and around which we must build the moral path that we are supposed to use on our pilgrim way toward the Lord.

I would suggest that one of the best ways to do this—after the question of formation and the granting of faculties, the assumption that there is sound moral teaching—is to insure that new teaching is communicated clearly, quickly, and with a chance for explanation when questions arise. This should be done by the Office of the Bishop in some way. I feel that we have a beautiful chance for this because, from time to time, we have some advance notice, particularly of those things that are likely to cause questions about perennial teaching, challenges to it. This gives us an opportunity to prepare an instruction and a clarification to our priests at the same time that they are receiving through *Time* and *Newsweek* and all the other secular media, other people's interpretation.

If they never hear the clear voice of the teaching of the Church but instead, read and appropriate these other things as the voice of the Church or an·accepted variant, then we have little room to criticize them later, unless we have come out strongly and clearly and indicated that no, this is not an acceptable expression of pluralism. Sometimes, it is necessary to make a correction by a public statement, perhaps not so much with respect to an individual person but perhaps for a whole complex of questions that arises. And we sense this. On the one hand, you find that there may be a whole area of teaching that somehow is slipping away because of questions people are asking, comments priests are making. On the other hand, there are areas that you would think are comfortable.

In Mobile some years back, we had a famous case of a lynching. Something like that hadn't taken place, I guess, in twenty, thirty years. But a black man was lynched. And a member of the Ku Klux Klan was apprehended and his family was involved.

The family was Catholic. They went to trial and the man's father said, not on the stand in the court room, but later in the corridor, yes, he was a Roman Catholic and there was nothing in his Catholicism that in any way stood as a contradiction to his membership in the Ku Klux Klan.

Our switchboard "lit up"—we don't have a switchboard, we just have three lines—but they were all busy. And our black parishes wanted to know, "Is this true?" Of course, we know it was not true. But I hunted for the statement whereby the Catholic Church specifically repudiated membership in the Ku Klux Klan. I couldn't find it. Because the question had never arisen.

You know, Catholics were never invited to join the KKK in the old days. They used to chase us, too. But not finding anything, I very quickly proposed a response that contained the censure that not only is it not possible but any Catholic would be refused the sacraments if they were known members of the Ku Klux Klan.

It caused the mother of the man indicted, the wife of the person on the stand, to leave the Roman Catholic Church. And she died shortly thereafter and was buried from a Protestant church. That's the kind of stand sometimes it is necessary to take, the kind of stand that is unmistakable.

As another example, a similar public statement through a weekly column that I write when the recent question of reexamining the *Roe vs. Wade* decision came up. There had been, I had felt for some time, a kind of a growing sense that maybe there is a free choice position with respect to abortion because so many people were saying, "Catholics can do this." Such misrepresentation was getting national advertising. I wrote the column and called it, "Not Since Dred Scott." I thought that was an interesting way to get their attention. I spoke about the moral teaching of the Church on abortion and the recent document from the Vatican concerning human life from the moment of conception, to be able to strengthen the teaching.

A diocesan Bishop can accomplish a number of things when he writes, officially, as the teacher. If people are teaching otherwise in the diocese, at once and instinctively, individuals have a test: this is what the Church is teaching because this is what the Bishop has said clearly, for everyone, priests and people alike, to see. And that test is something you can measure other teaching against. One then questions the sources for unacceptable teaching.

Difficulties should be addressed promptly and honestly. Reach out to the priests, the people, the college, the teaching institutes, and try to find out just what has been said. Then examine what has been said to see whether or not there is a misunderstanding. Clarify the terms. Perhaps it is that the teaching has been misunderstood. Then the person who has taught has an obligation to refer to the perennial teaching and place in high relief the authentic teaching of the Church. But perhaps the controversial point has been exactly what he said, or she said. Then you must test it against the accepted teaching of the Magisterium and here the Bishop is important and the Bishop must have a care to know what that teaching is with its nuances, with its old theological notes.

How much of it is, not so much irreformable or infallible, but how much of it is binding, a much broader term. And I think this should be clearly stated in such a way that the issues are easily available, not only to the technicians, to the professionals, but to the people in the pews. At the level of the diocese, we are not dealing with seminary personnel; we are dealing with a pastoral situation in which the lowest possible common denominator has a right to the teaching of the Church in language that can be easily understood. And questions should be formed that can be answered so that people are not confused but led along paths that they would not otherwise choose.

Once this consonance with the teachings of the Church has been determined, then there is the practical outcome. Do you censure the teaching as false and erroneous teaching? Do you tell the individual I'm sorry, you can no longer teach? Those are extremes. Certainly, if damage has been done, it seems to me the diocesan Bishop has an obligation to repair the damage. Possibly, the most effective cases for such action are in workshops for the clergy. This is a remarkable avenue. But it has its own pitfalls. I know we all invite speakers of expertise, notoriety, if you wish—something that brings a person into the diocese with a hoped for sense of vision, enthusiasm. Sometimes the vision and enthusiasm cannot be exactly where Holy Church is willing to go. If that happens, then I think the Bishop must challenge, publicly if necessary, at the cost of great embarrassment, perhaps. You can do it as nicely as possible. But stand on that occasion and take issue. I have done that on one or two occasions and it has not earned me many friends, but it has at least earned me a certain respect.

If I go to meetings and something comes up so that the teaching of the Church is challenged, I would not let it go by since my silence confirms it. This places a great burden on the diocesan Bishop. It sometimes may lead to invitations not being extended too readily but, if they are our own workshops with our own priests, we should and could be a part of them and a participating part.

Finally, let me just say that we need to build up and represent a Magisterium that is admittedly countercultural. That term has been used a couple of times here in Dallas and it's very right. I think that a Bishop, in trying to be faithful to the Magisterium, in our day and age, is going to have to be countercultural.

All around us there are areas of taking short cuts in questions of morality. They have become part of our way of life. We are not hunting for hard things but neither can we accept "short cuts" in the process of becoming Christians worthy of the name and Catholics true to the gifts that have been our tradition.

We must insert moral theology into the wider context of the gifts of any Catholic tradition. Remember, no one reaches out and adheres to moral theology in a vacuum. It is impossible without the other dimensions of our Catholic teaching and the Presence of Christ that enable us to live as Christ would have us live. Bishop Murphy put it this way, "Moral theology cannot be separated from dogmatic and spiritual theology as people experience Christian growth in a spirit of genuine love." And later, he said, "It is really an issue of discipleship and the costs involved in being a follower of Christ."

My brother Bishops, my friends, theology is a matter of faith and so is moral theology. We have somehow, because of the advances in all the sciences that assist moral theology, and the historical/critical methods that have been so fruitful, come to a methodology whereby scholarship has almost taken the upper hand in giving us moral truth. This cannot be so. Because always, in a dimension of faith, our answers are not those that are so evidently certain that God's challenge to do the loving thing is precluded. This is true in the act of faith wherever you find it. It is no less true in moral theology.

Earlier last month, I had a conversation with a moral theologian of great note. And we differed on some matters. And he kept saying, "It is the force of the argument that is persuasive." I said, "No. It is the force of the argument that is important but it is the gift of faith that is persuasive."

That gift of faith is the heart and kernel of the Magisterium in challenging us to something we might not be able to see so clearly but that we can accept because of God's love for us. It is, perhaps, the Ninth Beatitude of which Father Groeschel spoke so powerfully.

Thank you very much.

II. Archbishop Murphy

In the Handbook for this 1989 Bishops' Workshop, there is an overview offered regarding the theme of the Workshop in which we have taken part these past few days—CRITICAL ISSUES IN CONTEMPORARY HEALTH CARE. We have discussed many issues—artificial provision of nutrition and hydration, institutional ethics, fetal and newborn tissue donation, and issues facing the health and psychosexual development of priests. We come to this final session which is described as "THE GRAND FINALE."

The use of the term, "the grand finale," cannot help but recall the Broadway production of some years ago called, "Pippin." It is the story of Charlemagne's son who is looking for meaning in his life. He becomes convinced that such meaning will only come by taking part in a grand finale which results in his own self-destruction by being consumed in a ball of fire. We are not sure if the reference to the "grand finale" listed in the program has any reference to Pippin, but Pippin comes to the end of the play, only to decide he will continue life in an ordinary way. Yet, he comes to the end of the play and asks if there is any real meaning to life, and concludes with the simple statement, "Maybe!"

In many ways, the "maybe syndrome" is the reality we face as we look for ways to seek consistent pastoral application of the moral doctrine of the Church in a milieu of great theological diversity. How do we insure fidelity to Catholic teaching and the Magisterium in the preparation of candidates for priesthood and in the ministry offered by priests and deacons in service to the people of God?

At the heart of this response is the need to realize that the priest is a public person whose ministry must be seen and understood in the context of the Church. As a public person, the priest has the obligation to speak on behalf of the Church, to share its teaching and to call people to be faithful to the moral imperatives which are part of our tradition as a community of faith.

There have been many benefits to the Church and to the seminary community as a result of the Visitations that have taken place to each seminary program at the college and theologate level in the United States over the past few years. As a Church and especially in our ministry as Bishops, we have been reminded of the importance of seminary formation and education, and we have become familiar once again with the many documents related to the preparation of candidates for priesthood. To achieve a consistent pastoral application of the moral doctrine of the Church, it is essential that the way in which this can become a reality must begin in the formation and education process of candidates for priesthood.

In the Basic Plan for Priestly Formation, issued by the Sacred Congregation for Catholic Education in 1970, there are clear statements regarding theological education, and the expectations of the place of Moral Theology in the theological enterprise. It states, "The whole of four years at least must be devoted to theological studies. Their purpose is to enable students to make as profound a study as possible of the Divine Revelation in the light of faith and under the guidance of the authoritative magisterium, nourish their own spiritual lives with what they have learned, guard it in their priestly ministry, and proclaim and expound it for the spiritual good of the faithful."[1]

In speaking of moral theology, the Basic Plan for Priestly Formation insists that moral theology should be animated by the teaching of Sacred Scripture. It goes on to say that moral theology "has to demonstrate how the Christian's vocation is founded on charity and give a scientific explanation of the obligations incumbent on the faithful. It should endeavor to discover the solution to human problems in the light of Revelation and make eternal truths relevant in a changing world. It should seek the assistance of reliable and modern anthropology in its efforts to restore a sense of virtue and of sin to peoples' conscience. The teaching of morals finds its completion in the study of **Spiritual Theology** which, in addition to other matters, should include a study of the theology and spirituality of the priesthood and of a life consecrated to God by the following of the evangelical counsels, in order that spiritual direction can be given according to one's state of life."[2]

The Program of Priestly Formation from the NCCB recognizes the wisdom found in "The Basic Plan for Priestly Formation," and maintains that moral theology must be presented in the context of an intimate relationship between belief and life. Moral Theology cannot be separated from dogmatic and spiritual theology as people experience Christian growth in a spirit of genuine love.[3]

If we are to hope for a consistent pastoral application of the moral doctrine of the Church in pastoral situations in the midst of great theological diversity, it must begin in the programs of formation and education of candidates for priesthood. We must convey to candidates for priesthood and priests themselves that they will be or are public persons in holy orders who have an obligation to contribute to the order of the Christian community. This is incumbent not only on candidates for priesthood and priests themselves, but on those responsible for seminary education and ongoing education of clergy.

However, as we try to achieve this goal, we must be faithful to what the "The Basic Plan for Priestly Formation" describes. Our presentation of moral theology must be rooted in charity and must be accompanied by scientific explanations. We must recognize the ongoing journey we take in trying to discover the solution to human problems in the light of revelation. We are reminded that the solutions must be "relevant in a changing world." Most of all, there is the absolute need to "seek the assistance of reliable and modern anthropology" in recapturing an appreciation for virtue and the reality of sin in helping people form their conscience.

However, at the heart of developing a truly Catholic appreciation of moral theology and a consistent pastoral application of the moral doctrine of the Church is the need to incorporate a spirituality of priesthood and an appreciation of the spiritual life rooted in the evangelical counsels for living out priesthood and calling others to a growth in Christ. It is really an issue of discipleship and the costs involved in being a follower of Christ. The cost of discipleship calls for a spirit of self-sacrifice which is a genuine asceticism. Fidelity to Gospel ministry in 20th century society, especially in being faithful to Christian morality, might indeed be countercultural. The Good News was countercultural in Jesus' time and remains so today.

Modern men and women can identify with Pippin as they look for the meaning of life. They could well come to a conclusion of "Maybe" as Pippin did. But if the ideals of our tradition in Catholic moral teaching are to have an impact on peoples' lives, as well as the world and culture in which we live, then we must share that tradition and teaching with faith and courage with those preparing for priesthood as well as in ongoing continuing education programs of priests in ministry today.

How we do this leads me to introduce the next part of the Grand Finale, Bishop DiLorenzo.

Notes

(1) The Basic Plan for Priestly Formation. Sacred Congregation for Catholic Education, 1970, para. 76

(2) ibid, para. 79

(3) The Program of Priestly Formation, NCCB, 1981, para. 158

III. Bishop DiLorenzo

Our task as panelists is to share some strategies as to how a diocesan bishop can assure a consistent Moral Theology in his diocese given the pluralistic background of his clergy. In this panelist's opinion, the essential word is *consistent*. Of the many ideas associated with this word in this context, the following presents itself. *Consistent* could signify an authentic and religious moral discernment process that will put one in touch with God's loving will and is faithful to the Magisterium.

Certainly a diocesan bishop would want to assure this, but the perception can and does exist that parishes, seminaries, colleges and universities all have a plurality of viewpoints concerning just what is a consistent Moral Theology.

Some indications, which would support these concerns, are found in some of the trends over the last 30 years. Many researchers believe that the parish context from which this generation of Catholics has sprung is substantially different from the parish life of the late nineteenth and early twentieth centuries. This appears to be the conclusion of Jay Dolan and David Leege, authors of the second report of the *Notre Dame Study of Catholic Parish Life* (1985). They state,

> "Given this composit demographic profile of Adult Catholics in the United States in the 1980's, it is hardly surprising that Catholics increasingly populate the boardrooms of large corporations and policy-making councils of the White House and Capitol Hill. Catholics, with the exceptions of the newer ethnic groups—Hispanics, Asians—are in the mainstream of American life."[1]

The report continues and informs us that Catholics are not too distinguishable from Protestant Americans with all their strengths and weaknesses. The Catholic Church in America will face the struggle for the minds and hearts of the people that Protestant Churches face—whether it be in uplifting liturgies, effective socialization, or transforming social ethics.

The experience of many priests and bishops seems consistent with the above mentioned trends. At the very least, Catholics in America are becoming very comfortable about more liberalized viewpoints concerning Church authority and who exercises it, contraception, divorce and subsequent invalid second or third marriage, married priests, and intercommunion in an ecumenical setting, to mention a few.[2]

There is another indicator which would support the concerns of bishops who are seeking a consistent Moral Theology. This is found in the field of Moral Theology itself. With the call of the Second Vatican Council to renew Moral Theology, many attempts have been made to do just that. Some of these attempts have been helpful and others have been bitter disappointments. The attempts included Consequentialism, Proportionalism, the Theology of Compromise, Theology of Overriding Right, and the Creative Integration Model.[3]

While these models were being proposed, many seminarians were interiorizing such during their seminary years. Obviously this has had a profound impact on their personal religious formation and their attempts to minister to their parishes and/or students.

At this time it should be mentioned that many religious studies programs had been springing up throughout this country. The students who populated these were layfolk, men and women religious, and diocesan clergy. Hence these newer trends in Moral Theology were learned and, in turn, passed on to students in the high schools, colleges, and universities. No doubt these newer, untested moral theories were being well received by a Catholic population whose viewpoints on religion and morality were becoming more liberalized.

The final indication which supports the concerns of many bishops can be found in Cardinal Baum's letter on September 14, 1986, regarding the state of theologates here in the United States. After much self-study, visitations and exit reporting, the results came back to the U.S. bishops. When addressing the state of Moral Theology in American theologates, the letter raised the following issues:

There seemed to be concerns in a few instances of dissent from the Magisterium in the teaching of Moral Theology. In a few cases, Cardinal Baum's Congregation "recommended that seminary authorities act to resecure the Magisterial integrity of the teaching of Moral Theology."[4] When discussing the issue of dissent in seminaries, the letter pointed out this concern. At the end of their courses in Moral Theology, seminarians were not sure of what the Church taught in a particular matter, or there were some seminarians who thought that the Church's teaching is only one theological opinion among a number of other equally valid theological opinions. The letter stated that this issue needed emphatic clarification and redress.[5] Finally the letter raised concerns that there was an impression and/or perception in some seminaries that an authentic non-infallible statement is not binding. The letter stated that to propose this was a great disservice not only to the seminarian but also the persons he will minister to later on.[6]

346

In reviewing the above mentioned data, it is the opinion of this panelist that there exists a solid basis for concern. Most fair-minded persons, in reviewing the existing data that underlies these indicators, will see the basis for concern. Priests and parishioners are living in a changing environment where traditional religious and moral values are being questioned. This change process no doubt has an impact on both priests and parishioners as has been indicated. From this context, potential future priests come to seminaries. The teaching of Moral Theology in some of these seminaries has raised some concerns. Hence, what is a bishop to do in the midst of this situation?

Earlier in this presentation, the significance of *consistent* Moral Theology was defined as an authentic and religious moral discernment process that will put one in touch with God's loving will and is faithful to the Church's Magisterium. One can approximate assuring a consistent Moral Theology in the following ways:

A. *Explore the Essential Elements of a Consistent Moral Theology.* Any religious discernment process assumes that the person has a deepening faith, hope, and love in and for Christ and His Body, the Church. Persons with this religious moral orientation have arrived at the conviction that there are certain moral insights that lay claim on them as persons in the context of an ecclesial community. The significance, importance, and depth of these moral insights are seen as objective, eternal, and universal. They are seen as unchanging and unchangeable; timeless, rather than timely.

Persons with a religious moral orientation have developed a nuanced sense from where these values spring. They look to the life and words of Christ—the moral messages found in Sacred Scripture, and the moral heritage coming from the living voice of the Spirit filled Church of Jesus Christ known as the Magisterium.

A religious moral person should be conscious of the unity that must exist in Christ's Church. This unity, willed by Christ, takes the following form. One professes a creed in unity with one's brothers and sisters in the Lord. One unites oneself with those who have the authentic and authoritative ministry of teaching, governing, and sanctifying the Church. And finally one is united to one's brothers and sisters by virtue of their own common Baptism, participation in the Eucharistic Liturgy, and the other sacraments.

Persons with a religious moral orientation develop a nuanced sense of their responses to infallible and authentic non-infallible Church statements.

Finally, persons with a religious moral orientation develop an understanding for natural law insights.

There are other significant and essential elements that are to be found in a consistent Moral Theology. Some of these would be the relationship of the social sciences with moral theology, the theology of conscience formation, the reality and experience of human freedom, circumstances in which the moral persons find themselves and, finally, the meaning of sin and grace for the person.

B. *Explore How Significant Teaching Centers Within a Diocese Actually Model Religious Moral Discernment and Their Evaluation of the Church's Magisterium.* Obviously some of these centers can be identified as college seminaries and theologates, colleges and universities and, finally, religious education institutes who prepare teachers and catechists for primary and secondary grade levels.

Since the discussion of the rough draft, *Doctrinal Responsibilities; Approaches to Promoting Cooperation and Resolving Misunderstandings Between Bishops and Theologians,* we have initiated a dialogue in the Diocese of Scranton with several clearly identifiable theological communities. These various theological communities expressed a willingness to come together with their colleagues and the two bishops of the diocese. In these discussions we hope to explore their reflections on certain designated theological topics, including Moral Theology.

As bishops, we hope to listen carefully and respectfully to what is being said. We will not shrink from exploring biases that may well be built into their moral methodology. At the same time, we welcome their observations and responses, centering on their legitimate research and findings as Catholic Theologians. To be sure, a clear picture will definitely emerge from the different Theological Communities. This leads one to the next part of this strategem.

C. *Synthesize the Findings to Determine the Actual Situation in One's Diocese.* It will not be difficult for a perceptive and well educated bishop to determine just what is the situation in his diocese.

If a portrait emerges that suggests there are actual problems, then problem resolution is essential. Avoiding a confrontation is counterproductive, as most bishops know. To be avoided also is a war of wits that generates more heat than life. The best approach, in this panelist's opinion, is to address each problem on an issue-by-issue basis in a theological forum. It is wise to have some theological advisors who are properly credentialed and can articulate well what is the Church's position in a given area. By doing this, one adequately assures oneself that one has dignified the situation with a proper preparation and the discussion can flow well.

SUMMARY

The original task of this short exposition was to outline how diocesan bishops can assure a consistent Moral Theology in their dioceses, given the pluralistic background of their clergy. The following was suggested as a strategy:

1. Explore the essential elements of a consistent Moral Theology.
2. Explore how significant teaching centers within a diocese actually model religious moral discernment.
3. Synthesize the findings to determine the actual situation in one's diocese.

If there are problems, deal with them forthrightly. If there are no problems, blessed are you!

NOTES

1. Jay Dolan and David Leege "A Profile of American Catholic Parishes and Parishioners: 1820's to 1980's" in *Notre Dame Study of Catholic Parish Life* (Notre Dame, IN.: U. of Notre Dame, 1985) p. 8.

2. David Leege and Joseph Gemillion "The People, Their Pastors, and the Church: Viewpoints on Church Policies and Positions" in *Notre Dame Study of Catholic Parish Life* (Notre Dame, IN.: U. of Notre Dame, 1986) pp. 3 ff.

3. A source of these attempts at renewal can be found in the works of the following: Richard Gula "Shifts in Catholic Moral Theology: A Primer for the Perplexed Personalist" *The Living Light,* (Winter, 1981) pp. 296 ff.

Kevin McDonald, "Moral Theology: Retrospect and Prospect" *The Clergy Review* (February, 1982) pp. 41–48.

Norbert Rigali, S.J. "After the Moral Catechism" *Chicago Studies* (1981) pp. 151–162

John Connery, S.J. "Catholic Ethics: Has the Norm for Rule Making Changed?" *Theological Studies* (June, 1981) pp. 232 ff.

Richard McCormick, S.J. "Notes on Moral Theology: 1981" *Theological Studies* (March, 1982)

Philip Keane, S.S. "The Objective Moral Order: Reflection on Recent Research" *Theological Studies* (June, 1982) pp. 260 ff.

Karl Peschke *Christian Ethics: Moral Theology in Light of Vatican II* (Alcester and Dublin: C. Goodliffe Neale, 1986) pp. 1–12.

Francis X. Meehan, S.T.D. "Spirituality and Discernment in Moral Theology" in *The Catholic Theological Society of America: Proceeding of the Forty-Third Annual Convention* (Louisville, KY.: Bellarmine College, 1988) pp. 145 ff.

4. William Cardinal Baum *Sacra Congregatio Pro Institutione Catholica* Prot. N. 982/80 Page 15

5. Op. Cit. p. 16.

6. Op. Cit. p. 16.

Index

351